NUTRITIONAL SUPPORT IN NURSING

JO ANN GRANT, RN, BSN

Research Service, San Diego Veterans Administration Medical Center
Department of Psychiatry, School of Medicine
University of California at San Diego

CHRISTINE KENNEDY-CALDWELL, RNC, MSN, CNSN

Doctoral Student, Brown University,
Provident, Rhode Island

GRUNE & STRATTON   1988
An Imprint of the W. B. Saunders Company

Harcourt Brace Jovanovich, Publishers

Philadelphia   London   Toronto   Montreal   Sydney   Tokyo

Library of Congress Cataloging-in-Publication Data

Nutritional support in nursing.

Includes index.
1. Artificial feeding.   2. Artificial feeding—Moral
and ethical aspects.   3. Nursing.   I. Grant, Jo Ann.
II. Kennedy-Caldwell, C. (Christine) [DNLM: 1. Enteral
Feeding—nursing. 2. Parenteral Feeding—nursing.
WB 410 N976]
RM222.5.N88 1988   615.8′54   87-24773
ISBN 0-8089-1889-3

Grune & Stratton
Philadelphia, PA   19105

Library of Congress Catalog Number 87-24773
International Standard Book Number 0-8089-1889-3
Printed in the United States of America
88 89 90   10 9 8 7 6 5 4 3 2 1

To George and Ann Nallinger with loving memory
and
To Igor with love

JAG

To Eugene and Marjorie Kennedy whose encouragement sustained me.

To all those in my family who listened to "I can't do that. I'm working
on the book"—Ann, Bridget, Camper, Colleen, Erin, and Michael.

And to my husband, Michael, for everything else!

CKC

Contributors

Nancy Bergstrom, RN, PhD
Associate Professor and Interim Dean
Nursing Research Center—College of Nursing
University of Nebraska Medical Center
Omaha Nebraska
Basic Principles of Nutrition

Carla S. Bour, RN, MSN
Abbott Laboratories
Abbott Park, Illinois
Psychological and Social Responses to Nutritional Support

Linda Carrick Torosian, RN, MSN
Clinical Director, Surgical Nursing
Hospital of The University of Pennsylvania
Philadelphia, Pennsylvania
Nutrition Support Nursing in a Changing Health Care Environment: Administrative Issues

Mary Williams Cazalas, RN, JD
New Orleans, Louisiana
Nutritional Support Nursing: Medico-Legal Concerns

Kathleen S. Crocker, RN, MSN, CNSN
Director of Nursing
New England Critical Care, Inc.
Marlborough, Massachusetts
Metabolic Monitoring During Nutritional Support Therapy

Margaret Cunliffe, RN, MSN
Formerly, Nutritional Support Nursing Coordinator
Hospital of The University of Pennsylvania
Philadelphia, Pennsylvania
*Nutrition Support Nursing in a Changing Health Care Environment:
Administrative Issues*

Leah Curtin, RN, MA, MS, FAAN
Nursing Management
Cincinnati, Ohio
Ethical Issues in Nutritional Support: Should We Feed Baby Doe?

DeAnn M. Englert, RN, MSN
Houston, Texas
Ambulatory Home Nutritional Support

Loretta Forlaw, RN, MSN, CNSN, LTC, ANC
Nutritional Support Clinical Nurse Specialist
Department of Nursing
Walter Reed Army Hospital
Washington, D.C.
Nutritional Assessment

Jo Ann Grant, RN, BSN
Research Service
San Diego Veterans Administration Medical Center
Department of Psychiatry
School of Medicine
University of California at San Diego
Historical Perspectives in Nutritional Support

Barbara A. Griggs, RN, MA
Associate Director
Nutritional Support Department
University of Cincinnati Medical Center
Cincinnati, Ohio
Indications for Nutritional Support in the Adult Patient

Barbara C. Hansen, RN, PhD
Vice Chancellor for Graduate Studies and Research
University of Maryland Graduate School
Baltimore, Maryland
Research Opportunities: Dimensions in Nutritional Support Nursing

Mary C. Hoppe, RN, MSN
Abbott Laboratories
Abbott Park, Illinois
Psychological and Social Responses to Nutritional Support

Christine Kennedy-Caldwell, RN, MSN, CNSN
Doctoral Student, Brown University
Providence, Rhode Island
Pediatric Nutritional Support

Millie Lawson, RNC, MS, CRNI
Clinician IV, Infusion Therapy Teams
Division of Nursing
M. D. Anderson Hospital and Tumor Institute
Houston, Texas
Ambulatory Home Nutritional Support

Bonnie L. Metzger, RN, PhD
Associate Professor, School of Nursing
University of Michigan
Ann Arbor, Michigan
Research Opportunities: Dimensions in Nutritional Support Nursing

Marsha Evans Orr, RN, MS, CNSN
Associate Director, Home Care
St. Joseph's Hospital Health Center
Syracuse, New York
Future Directions

Rhonda S. Patterson, RN, BSN
Director of Nursing
Intravenous Home Care, Inc.
The Woodlands, Texas
Enteral Nutrition Delivery Systems

Marcia A. Ryder, RN, CNSN
Nutritional Support Nurse Specialist
Santa Clara Valley Medical Center
San Jose, California
Parenteral Nutrition Delivery Systems

Jack L. Smith, PhD
Jack L. Smith & Associates, Inc.
Medford, New Jersey
Basic Principles of Nutrition

Foreword

The genesis of the field of nutritional support nursing occurred in 1967 when Jo Ann Grant was first recruited by Dr. Stanley Dudrick to become a Research Nurse at The Hospital of the University of Pennsylvania. During the next several decades, a nucleus of dedicated professional nurses has remained committed to the premise that optimal nutritional and metabolic support of patients with varying degrees of gastrointestinal dysfunction will have a crucial impact upon their clinical outcome and prognosis of their primary disease process. These determined nurses have collaborated with other members of the multidisciplinary health team to make a number of important contributions in the care of countless numbers of patients with metabolic and nutritional disturbances.

Indeed, it has been the expertise, ingenuity, energy, and leadership of our nursing peers who are responsible for these prospective accomplishments and future developments in this exciting area of medicine. Organizations such as The American Society for Parenteral and Enteral Nutrition have provided opportunities for comradery during Annual Congresses and other symposiums and meetings as we share modifications, improvements, and empirical findings in our nutritional support experience. As our nursing specialty has proliferated and become increasingly sophisticated, Nutrition Support Nurses now have a certification process to acknowledge their clinical and scientific expertise and experience among other nursing colleagues. There is no doubt in my mind that this noteworthy book, which Jo Ann Grant and Christine Kennedy-Caldwell have co-edited with contributions from major nursing leaders in the field, will generate a great deal of excitement and enthusiasm among involved and interested nurse clinicians, teachers, and researchers and will serve as a basis for an evolving new science in nursing.

DeAnn M. Englert, RN, MSN, CNSN

Preface

Although the nursing specialty of nutritional support has existed for less than 20 years, nurses have been providing care for patients with nutrition problems for decades. While the professional health literature is replete with articles and books about nutrition, they either are about normal and therapeutic dietetics or are written for the practicing physician. It is our belief that professional nurses of every health care team must have a working knowledge of both the identification and the management of nutritional problems which already exist or may develop in the patients under their care. Thus the purpose of this book is to improve the *nursing* care given to patients who require specialized nutritional intervention and their families and to promote excellence in the specialty of nutritional support nursing.

As the first nurse-authored text in the field, this book is primarily intended to assist the staff nurse and clinical nurse specialist involved in "high tech" nutrition support and intravenous therapy. It can serve as a reference for nurses who are working in a variety of settings—not only the acute care hospital but the community and the private health care sectors. Because it is comprehensive in its review of both the "art and science" of nutrition and nursing, faculty will find it a useful resource during the development and teaching of both undergraduate and graduate nursing curricula.

The first section of the book presents a historical review of nutritional support, the principles of basic nutrition, indications for nutritional support, assessment of nutritional needs, and all aspects of clinical management of both adult and pediatric patients. The second section deals with a variety of issues of concern to the Nutrition Support Nurse. Ethical, medico-legal, and administrative aspects of nutrition support nursing are covered as well as research opportunities and a look to the future of nutrition support nursing.

The book is authored by several leading nurse experts in this field. We gratefully acknowledge the support given the authors by the institutions in which they work. Throughout the lengthy process, the authors maintained their commitment to excellence, their patience, their persistence, and best of all their sense of humor! We would both like to acknowledge the constant interest, support, and encouragement of professional colleagues associated with the American Society of Parenteral and Enteral Nutrition. Noted among these were members of the Nurses Committee and also Dr. Stan Dudrick and DeAnn Englert, RN, MSN, CNSN. In addition many thanks to Barbara Davis and to the staff of Grune and Stratton, especially Tom Eoyang, without whom this book would be just another great idea. Finally, a special word of thanks must go to our husbands, Igor Grant, MD and Michael Caldwell, MD, PhD. Not only did they assist us by providing scientific input but they also were unrelenting in their enthusiasm and encouragement of this project.

Jo Ann Grant
Christine Kennedy-Caldwell

Introduction

When I first met Jo Ann Nallinger Grant on the medical service of the Hospital of The University of Pennsylvania in 1961, she was a second-year student nurse, and I was a rotating intern. We shared the management of many of the 40 patients on that traditional Florence Nightingale ward, and it was there that I gained great respect and admiration for this outstanding young woman. Most of our patients were elderly, debilitated, and indigent human beings with multiple and interesting medical problems that were frequently complicated by some degree of malnutrition or starvation. Standard intravenous therapy at that time consisted of 5 percent dextrose in water, or in quarter strength to full strength 0.9 percent sodium chloride solution, infused by gravity through a metallic needle inserted into one of the small peripheral veins of the extremities. In some of the bottles of solution, 20 to 40 mEq of potassium chloride and 1 to 2 ml of water-soluble (B-complex and C) vitamins were added to the usual 2 to 2½ liters of fluid daily. Rarely, calcium, magnesium, or iron-dextran were added to the regimen in patients with specific deficiencies; more often these were given as a bolus than as an additive to the reservoir bottle. In some critically ill patients, blood, plasma, and albumin were sometimes infused for nutritional purposes. Protein hydrolyates of fibrin or casein were only rarely given together with 5 percent dextrose to provide amino acids and short-chain peptides to the most critically protein-depleted patients. Intravenous fat in the form of a soybean oil emulsion (Lipomul) was available in limited quantities for experimental use for a few years but was eventually taken off the market because of the unacceptable incidence of adverse reactions. Infusion pumps, in-line filters, and central venous feeding catheters were not in clinical use. Feedings of blenderized foods via nasogastric or gastrostomy tubes were administered by gravity or syringe bolus to patients with functioning alimentary tracts; jejunostomy or other enteral feedings were accompanied by a high incidence of complications and were used less frequently, and there were virtually no commercially produced special nutrient formulations available for either of these feeding techniques.

We were often frustrated in those days by our inability to provide enteral or parenteral nutritional support to meet either the ordinary or the extraordinary nutritional requirements of our patients. It was obvious that nutritional support technology lagged far behind the rapidly advancing pharmacologic and technical medical and surgical armamentarium. Nonetheless, we coped with the problems as best we could with available resources and improvisations and searched for better ways to provide our patients' nutritional needs in the future.

Five years later, Jo Ann Nallinger Grant was working in the Emergency Department of the Hospital of The University of Pennsylvania, while I was beginning my final year training as Chief Resident in Surgery. By that time, total parenteral nutrition, or intravenous hyperalimentation, had been clearly demonstrated to be possible and also practical by supporting the normal growth and development of beagle puppies for more than 250 days. I was able to accomplish this with the confidence and support of my co-workers, Dr. Jonathan E. Rhoads and Dr. Harry M. Vars. Application of this laboratory technique to the clinical situation represented a revolution in patient care and could not possibly have succeeded without the invaluable contributions and dedication of nurses, who are so essential to the optimal minute by minute care of patients. We recognized prospectively that this was the case, and, accordingly, Dr. Rhoads, my mentor and Chairman of the Department of Surgery, authorized me to recruit a research hyperalimentation nurse to the Harrison Department of Surgical Research. Because Mrs. Grant and I had discussed on several occasions the possibility that we might work together someday, and because of the high regard in which she was held personally and professionally in the hospital, I avidly recruited her to our team and was successful in my efforts. With the acquisition of a top-flight nurse, the nucleus of our physician-basic scientist-pharmacist-technician-nurse hyperalimentation team was complete.

Florence Nightingale is widely recognized not only as the founder of nursing but also as the founder of dietetics. Thus, attention to the nutritional needs of patients was originally established as a foremost priority of nurses. As the prototype hyperalimentation nurse, Jo Ann Nallinger Grant also became a pioneer nutritional support nurse. Because her initial role and responsibilities were only partially defined, she used her skill, dedication, and ingenuity to establish not only the principles and standards for clinical nutritional support nursing, but also the nurse's role in clinical nutrition research.

Throughout the years, nursing heritage and education have been such that nurses have made, are making, and will continue to make significant contributions to clinical nutrition and nutritional investigation. The initial history, physical examination, and nutritional assessment are made by the admitting nurse. The final common path of the physician's prescription, the pharmacist's formulation, and the dietician's nutrient regimen for the patient is through the nurse, who administers, supervises, and documents the patient's infusion or intake of nutritional regimens. Nurses make critically important evaluations of the acceptance, utilization, and efficacy of dietary rations and can offer useful recommendations for improving nutritional intake and status. The many conscientious recordings of observations and data by nurses are invaluable to the success of research protocols. Finally, the contributions of nurses in the important area of nutrition support are limited only by their ingenuity and ambition.

In this day of increasing specialization, nurses have eagerly seized the opportunities to excel in areas such as nutritional support, nutritional support research, home nutritional support, and industrial or corporate nutritional support. Even more highly specialized areas of nutritional endeavors for nursing have developed, including critical care, cardiovascular, pulmonary, renal, hepatic, infectious disease, trauma, oncologic, pediatric, geriatric, and psychiatric nutritional support nursing. I am sure that this list is already incomplete and will certainly continue to grow.

The importance of the nurse as a patient advocate, communicator, and teacher cannot be overemphasized in any aspect of patient care, but it is especially obvious in the management of nutritional problems. It is often the nurse who provides the first insight, information, or data regarding the patient's nutritional status or response to therapeutic nutrition endeavors. It is often the nurse who is the most effective communicator with the patient and family regarding inpatient and outpatient management after physicians and other health care personnel have delineated their instructions. It is often the nurse who must teach the patients and their families or friends the many theoretical and practical essentials to the success of their prescribed management. It is often the nurse who first calls attention to the moral, ethical, psychological, physical, social, political, economic, and religious aspects of the patient's care, including the optimal provision of their nutritional requirements. Clearly, the nurse is an invaluable, and perhaps the most important, member of the nutritional support team.

Just as it is incredible now to realize that 25 years ago medicine and nursing were practiced without the highly beneficial and potentially life-saving tools of total parenteral nutrition and many other specialized forms of nutritional support, it would have been incredible then to imagine what is currently available to us and to our patients in these areas today. Although it is impossible to predict what new developments will be made in the next decade and further into the future, it is inevitable that significant advances and changes will occur. With the increasing sophistication of nutritional support technology, the practice of nutritional support will become the practice of clinical biochemistry, in which the precise nutritional requirements for all physiologic and pathophysiologic conditions will be understood, acknowledged, and provided, so that truly optimal nutrition can be provided to all patients, under all conditions, and at all times. We owe Jo Ann Nallinger Grant and Christine Kennedy-Caldwell and the outstanding group of nurse-authors they have assembled in producing this outstanding volume our admiration and gratitude for their signal contributions to this lofty goal.

Stanley J. Dudrick, M.D.
The University of Texas Medical
School at Houston

Contents

Part I

Aspects of Clinical Management

Jo Ann Grant

1

Historical Perspectives in Nutritional Support

T he offering of conscientious nursing care is a significant element in our social history. Predating the practice of medicine, nursing emerged from humanity's basic need for comfort and care and has evolved through social and political changes as well as progress in science and medicine to its present form as an adjunct to the establishment of sound medical practice. Throughout this history, the nutritional support for the ill and injured has been an integral part of medical theory and practice and of the practice of nursing.

PREHISTORIC ERA

From the dawn of humanity, the acquisition of food has been a primary concern to all peoples. During early human history, geographic location, climate, proximity to water, and the variety of vegetation determined what would be eaten. It was during the Neolithic Age (7000 BC–3000 BC) that people began to grow their own food rather than merely gather it. As a result, nomadic life began to decrease, farming villages appeared, and animals were domesticated.

Nursing of the ill and injured in these prehistoric times most likely developed from the concern and care felt by family members, with the actual caregiver being the wife/mother. Such caregiving was an intuitive behavior resulting from the need to keep people healthy and the desire to provide care and comfort to the sick, thus fulfilling a fundamental family need.[1] Women who displayed more nurturing behaviors and who proved to be more skillful and successful than others were then called on by friends and the community to nurse their sick.

NUTRITIONAL SUPPORT IN NURSING
ISBN 0-8089-1889-3

Because medical knowledge was nonexistent, the care given by these early practitioners was limited to listening, comforting, cleansing, and feeding their charges. In time, however, they became knowledgeable about the medical properties of the roots, nuts, berries, herbs, and foods available to them. They learned which foods were better for specific complaints. Food was recognized as being not only essential to life, but also as having curative powers.

EARLY ANCIENTS

The Egyptians, highly civilized among early societies, introduced medical specialization and outpatient medicine as well as public health principles, evidenced by their irrigation of crops and sanitary methods of food storage. Papyrus documents indicate that special diets were prescribed for some patients under the direction of a nurse.[2] Egyptian arts of mummification, wall murals, and paintings have provided us with a record of the diseases of the times. According to these sources, much of the nursing care was the task of servants or slaves.

The Mosaic Health Code of the ancient Hebrews included principles of personal hygiene, food inspection, reporting of disease, isolation and quarantine of communicable diseases, and disposal of excreta. The high priest served as health inspector and physician. Certain Hebrew women served as nurses, visiting and caring for the sick in their homes, promoting public health practices, and stressing health education.

GREEK MEDICINE

As the influence of Greek civilization grew, so, too, did the emphasis on good health maintenance as a necessity for a high quality of life. Three gods of Greek mythology personified this concern: Asklepios, god of medicine and son of Apollo, and his daughters, Hygeiea, goddess of health maintenance (nursing), and Panacea, goddess of medication (pharmacy). Within the walls of the temples created to honor these figures, patients were treated by the temple priests in the name of the gods.

It was during this era of mythical influence that Hippocrates (460 BC) was born. He became a free thinker whose influence would prove to be far more lasting than that of the gods. His contributions to both medicine and nursing were abundant.

Hippocrates paid strict attention to his patients' diets. Because he thought that certain foods caused certain diseases, he instituted the first form of diet therapy, giving specific instructions to the medical student nurses as to each patient's food intake. He held the view that the innate heat of the body was generated by air and, most importantly, food.

Various texts in the Hippocratic corpus and the Cnidus works indicate that early Greek medicine conceived of disease as a process that ran a predictable course and for which diet was emphasized as a major therapy.[4] These ideas were quite distinctly Greek. As a result, dietetics has been described as the "greatest dynamic element within Greek medicine."[4]

Food and diet were closely associated with the theory that the elemental components of man were fire (hot and dry) and water (cool and wet). Diets of specific foodstuffs were prescribed for specific diseases to heat, dry, cool, or moisten the body in order to maintain or regain a healthful equilibrium. The healthy diet was modified and presented to the patient in three different forms with varying consistencies: solid food (SITION), slops or gruel (RUPHEMA), and drink (POTION).[4]

Philosophers of the fifth century BC thought of health as a "balance of forces," and nutrition as an "attraction of like to like"; that is, each part of the body attracted the specific substance needed for growth from the absorbed food. By the end of the 4th century BC, Greek philosophers had proclaimed that:

- After being eaten, food was dissolved and transported to the tissues where it was assimilated
- Food supplied both energy and building material
- Each person had both individual energy and building needs[5]

Aristotle further advanced the theory of innate body heat by proposing that it explained the functions of nutrition, sensation, movement, and thought in humans. He also proposed that the heart, as the origin of the blood and all its containing vessels, collected the fluid made elsewhere in the body from ingested food and turned it into blood by the action of the vital innate body heat that was centered in the heart.

The seething of the blood in the heart from the vivifying heat was manifested in the patient's pulse rate. Because Aristotle thought of blood vessels as sensory paths that connected all organs with the heart, he believed that the heart was the lifelong seat of both nutrition and the sensory soul.

The nurse played an important role in upper class Greek society. Assigned to give exclusive care to an infant, she then continued to nurture that person throughout childhood and adult life. Most nursing was the responsibility of household slaves, although some especially skilled nurses were paid. Virtually all nursing was carried on in the home. Nursing of the lower classes was carried out by family members while slaves nursed each other.

ROMAN ERA

Despite the decline of Greek influence and Greece's defeat at the hands of the Romans, Greek culture and knowledge remained influential. As the Romans rose to power, they retained and practiced Greek methods of medicine.

Galen (130–201 AD) was the most reknowned Greek physician of his time and served as physician to Emperor Severus. He was convinced that all parts of the body had been created by God for a specific purpose. He sought to explain the structure of each body organ in terms of what he thought its function to be. Because the body was constantly ridding itself of waste material, Galen believed that the ultimate purpose of food or nourishment was the replacement of losses—a metabolic process of replenishing by assimilation in the tissues. The preparation of food for this assimilation took place in the mouth and stomach where the foodstuffs were not merely broken down, but changed into very different substances. These new compounds were then absorbed by the veins and transported to the liver where they were converted into blood. Although Galen held the erroneous belief that the liver was the central source of the blood, he seems to be the first to describe the fact that both the veins and arteries carry blood and that blood itself carries vital nutrients.

EARLY CHRISTIAN INFLUENCE

There did not seem to be organized groups of nurses before the Christian period. With the teachings of Christ came a new awareness of the plight of humanity. Despite the wealth and glory of Rome, most of the citizenry lived in disease-ridden slums, poor and neglected. By personal example, Christ taught kindness, charity, love, and the dignity of individual human worth. He was particularly compassionate toward the sick and chronically ill. He preached that women could be equal partners with men in life's endeavors and that they should be treated with respect and consideration, not as possessions to be shut up at home. Single women were given the opportunity to pursue humanitarian endeavors and social service. Many chose to enter nursing.

The first nurses to organize for the visiting of the sick were the order of Deaconesses in approximately 58 AD. Their code of practice, The Corporal Works of Mercy, included the responsibility to "feed the hungry" and "to give water to the thirsty."[1] They gave of themselves to help heal the sick and recognized the need to feed the malnourished both physically and spiritually. Kindness, empathy, and service to others through charitable works were the foundation and purpose of their nursing. The order consisted of men as well as women who made the care of the sick their life's work. As people sought to atone for their sins and follow Christ's teachings, the work of the deacons and deaconesses spread throughout Europe—west to Ireland and east to the Middle Eastern parishes.

The position of women in upper class Roman society was much above that of previous times. In this society there emerged a group of Roman matrons, converts to Christianity, whose wealth, intelligence, and social leadership enabled them to help ease the suffering of the sick and poor. St. Helena, Empress Facilla, St. Marcella, St. Fabiola, and St. Paula were but a few who established hospitals and shelters where they visited daily to prepare food, feed the sick, and wash and tend the patients.

These women, and others of high social standing, gave up their wealth to devote their lives to others in need. Their high intellectual ability and excellent education set an appropriate standard for the nursing profession. Their attention to detail, their skills in assessment, observation, administration, and teaching, and their effect on social welfare had a lasting impact on history in general, and on nursing in particular.

THE EARLY MIDDLE AGES

The Dark Ages following the fall of Rome was a period of decline and deterioration. Toward the end of the first millennium AD, the medieval period ushered in feudalism and monasticism. Only through the founding and organization of the monasteries could Christian men and women pursue a life of service. Beyond serving as repositories of ancient learning and culture, the monasteries provided the poor and suffering with medical care, nursing, medicines, and compassionate attention.

THE LATE MIDDLE AGES

The ensuing centuries brought many changes. As the shift of population from the rural areas to the cities concentrated the poor in crowded and unsanitary conditions, more hospitals were built. The ravages of leprosy, syphilis, infectious diseases, and the Great Bubonic Plague of the 14th century brought devastation, fear, and misery. Many people turned to religion for comfort and nursing care.

Meanwhile, medicine continued to remain fettered by its steadfast belief in the Greek theory of the four bodily humors that fire, water, earth, and air contributed to an equilibrium of internal forces. Illness was considered the manifestation of an imbalance in these forces. Treatments still consisted of attempts to restore the balance of humors and extract offending ones from the body by bleeding, purging, cupping, and leeching. This was the accepted method of treatment, and practitioners were content to continue them without question.

THE RENAISSANCE AND THE REFORMATION

Complacency with Greek theory was soon to change. The 1500s saw a rekindling of curiosity and individual thinking in Western civilization. The Renaissance spawned expansion of trade, exchange of ideas, receptiveness to invention, and growth in printing, art, and literature. Medicine and nursing benefited greatly from this interest in exploration in the fields of science and the mechanisms of the human body.

Another movement of this time, however, had a devastating effect on nursing. The Reformation, a church reform movement, closed and/or destroyed the Catholic monasteries and hospitals in northern Europe without providing adequate alternative care for the poor and sick. Inexperienced lay people were appointed to run the existing hospitals. The wealth of the monasteries was turned over to secular institutions. This was particularly unfortunate for women because without the monasteries, education for women and girls became unavailable. As a result, few educated nurses were availabe to assist physicians.

Since nursing was no longer attached to the church, nurses suffered a loss of education and of social standing; consequently, nurses increasingly has to be recruited from the illiterate classes. Careers for upper class women were unthinkable—a woman's place was in the home. Nursing came to be considered a type of domestic service. This attitude, along with low pay, long hours, poor food, and cheerless, monotonous work, drove many of the lower class nurses to seek solace in drink, often neglecting their patients.

DIETS OF PATIENTS DURING THE MIDDLE AGES AND THE RENAISSANCE

There were detailed descriptions of daily life in the average medieval monastic hospital.[2,6] Most hospitals served two meals daily, consisting for the most part of bread and salted meat. Fresh meat and fish were served when available. Fresh fruit and vegetables were included in most meals as were eggs or cheese, all of which were produced on the monastery's lands. Beer was often included in the daily menu.

By the mid 1600s there had been some changes in hospital diets.[7] Most notable was the absence of fresh fruit and vegetables, which caused major vitamin C deficiencies in the patients. The diet supplied approximately 2350 calories and 70 g of protein and 80 g of fat. It included $1\frac{1}{2}$ ounces of cheese, 1 pint of milk pottage, 4 ounces of beef or mutton, 1 pint of broth, 1 ounce of butter, 10 ounces of bread, and 3 pints of beer (given to children as well as adults).

The 1800s introduced tea and milk into the hospital diet. As an economic and, possibly, therapeutic move, less expensive foods in smaller portions were used.[7] Half rations were given to the seriously ill, and pap and cereals boiled in water were introduced. Pap consisted of bread or flour cooked in water or occasionally ale and spoon-fed to the patients. Panada, a variation of pap, combined flour, bread, or cereal with either milk or broth and sometimes butter.[8]

As more attention was paid to the patient's diet, specific diets for specific diseases were more routinely recommended. For example, diets for fevers included cereal broths mixed with wine, lemon or orange juice, and currant or fruit jellies, but excluded meat broths.[7] As many patients relied on food gifts from outside the hospital or purchases from food vendors who made rounds on the wards, the enforcement of special diets presented problems.

EARLY EXPERIENCE WITH INTRAVENOUS TECHNIQUE

In the spirit of the Renaissance, man began to look more intently at his relationship to the world about him, using observation and experimentation. As a result of the revival of the scholarship of the classical era in the universities, there was a renewed interest in blood as the source of life. In 1489 an Italian philosopher suggested giving the blood from the veins of healthy youths to the aged by means of suction.[9] Pope Innocent VIII was reputed to be the first recipient of a blood transfusion in Rome in 1490.[9] Blood from three young boys was used, but records are unclear as to whether the blood was given as a draught or an intravenous injection, or if, in fact, this actually occurred.

German physicians of the early 1600s reported on their experiments with the intravenous transfusion of blood in humans.[9] But it was in 1616 that the English physician, William Harvey, made a discovery that would change the course of medicine: he described the circulation of the blood. Although not published until 1628, this breakthrough provided the answer to the question of how water, oxygen, and nutrients reached the cells and how metabolic waste products were eliminated. It made blood transfusion feasible and opened the door for scientific studies on the infusion of various substances in the blood. Capillary circulation was discovered with the aid of the newly invented microscope, thus completing Harvey's theory.[10]

The first detailed description of an intravenous infusion has been credited to Sir Christopher Wren, the famous London architect.[11] Proposing that it would be easy to inject any liquid into the blood stream, this self-styled scientist injected wine and ale into a vein of a living dog in 1658 using the hollow quill of a bird's feather attached to a pig's bladder. Boyle (1659), Scotus (1664), and Lower (1665) reported additional experimental intravenous injections in dogs.[10,12]

Learning of his English colleagues' work, Jean Denis, physician to Louis XIV of France, published an account of his 1667 transfusion of lamb's blood into the veins of a youth.[13] The boy made an excellent recovery from his obscure fever, but the procedure caused such controversy that the practice was later prohibited in France.

Due in part to unsuccessful experiments and in part to religious objections, the use of blood transfusions declined in England and France until interest was revived by the animal experiments of Harwood in 1785.[13] Blundell, a London obstetrician, successfully transfused blood from one human to another in 1818 to replace blood lost through puerperal hemorrhage.[14] By 1830 it was clear that blood from animals should not be infused into humans.

BEGINNINGS OF INTRAVENOUS FEEDING

Although much was learned about intravenous techniques from early blood transfusions, it was not until progress was made in understanding the energy and fluid needs of the body and the chemical composition of foods that infusions of other fluids became practical. The numerous experiments and discoveries that have immeasurably increased understanding of the physiology of nutrition have been well-chronicled.[11,12,15]

The first to give a nutrient substance intravenously was the noted French physiologist, Claude Bernard. His 1843 experiments, although not conducted for nutritional reasons, included the injecting of cane sugar solutions into animals and monitoring the amounts of sugar excreted in the urine.[16] By then injecting a similar cane sugar solution previously treated with gastric juices and showing that the sugar did not appear in the urine, he demonstrated that the gastric juices converted the sugar into glucose for assimilation in the blood. In 1856 he described the liver's function in the formation and storage of glycogen.

Milk, rather than blood, was used as fluid replacement in cholera patients by Hodder in 1873. He successfully treated two out of three patients by injecting warm milk into an open arm vein with a syringe.[17] In an attempt to prevent a patient's suicide by starvation, Krueg (1875) administered subcutaneous injections of oil followed by beaten egg. Hypodermic injections of milk alternating with beef extract and cod liver oil were used by Whittaker (1876) to help nourish an extremely emaciated patient with epigastric pain. Eichhorn reported (1881) that he maintained the weight of rabbits for 30 days using subcutaneous injections of milk, olive oil, egg albumin, and peptides.

The work of two investigators outside the field of nutrition research has had a profound effect on the success of intravenous nutritional support, as well as on medicine in general. In 1857 Pasteur proved that living organisms could be found in liquids following fermentation, and he hypothesized that they were germs that came from the air. He felt that these organisms, bacteria, spread disease but that they could be controlled and killed. Utilizing this theory, Lister proposed that the formation of pus was due to bacteria and that these germs were carried by people, resulting in cross-contamination. Therefore, he introduced the use of antiseptics for hands, bandages, and instruments.

REVIVAL OF PROFESSIONAL NURSING IN THE VICTORIAN ERA

Skilled nursing of the early 19th century was practiced for the most part by the various Catholic and Protestant religious orders. The terrible conditions and poor quality of care in lay hospitals prompted compassionate inquiry and an awakening of social conscience. The concerned public began to look toward helping their fellow citizens, and attempts were made to relieve the suffering.

As the need for skilled nursing and the desire for acts of charity grew, the ancient order of Deaconesses was revived. Pastor Fliedner and his wife opened the Kaiserwerth Institute for the Training of Deaconesses in 1836. There they not only trained healthy, moral, and energetic women over 25 years old to be teachers, but also established a hospital and a school for nurses. Many nurses who trained at Kaiserwerth went out to establish chapters and hospitals worldwide. Anglican deaconesses under Dr. William Muhlenburg founded the St. Lukes Hospital in New York City in 1858.

Of note are Muhlenburg's progressive ideas on nursing. He advocated skill training for nurses and medication administration by nurses utilizing a time schedule, and he emphasized the importance of diet in each patient's plan of treatment. He maintained that only the best prepared and most capable nurses assumed this latter responsibility.

FLORENCE NIGHTINGALE

The year 1820 saw the birth of a most remarkable woman—one who would advance the position of women and set the course of modern nursing— Florence Nightingale. Born of a well-to-do English family, she possessed both an intelligent, inquiring mind and a father who, despite Victorian convention, encouraged the formal and liberal education of his daughter. Florence desired to serve humanity, and to this end she applied all her charm, brilliance, enthusiasm, cleverness, and courage. She spoke of a woman's obligation to improve society and lamented woman's traditional lack of political power.

Despite the objections of her family, Nightingale studied and observed the art of caring for the ill and downtrodden in various hospitals in England and on the continent. She spent three months in nurse's training at Kaiserwerth and studied in Paris with the Sisters of Charity. She spent brief periods as superintendent of nurses at two hospitals.

In 1854 world events focused attention on the field of nursing. Following England's entry in the Crimean War, appalling accounts of poor medical care and dreadful conditions for the British soldiers caused much indignation and public outcry in London. Nightingale was called on to supervise the British military hospitals in Turkey and to organize a group of skilled nurses to accompany her to tend the wounded.

Her many achievements at Scutari are well documented. Of special interest is her work concerning the nutrition of the hospitalized soldiers. On arrival she found existing conditions grossly inadequate. Because there was only one kitchen located at the extreme end of the barracks hospital and 3–4 miles of sick and wounded in the long wards and corridors, it took 3–4 hours to serve the two meals a day to all the men. All cooking was done in only eight huge copper pots, and all meals consisted of boiled beef and the occasional vegetable with no variety or light meals available.[18]

Nightingale set her hand to remedying this situation despite lack of cooperation from the medical staff. A diet kitchen was immediately set up to prepare such light foods as gruel, beef tea, arrowroot, lemonade, and rice pudding using stoves the nurses had brought from England. Within a week smaller boilers and other equipment had been obtained to begin operating two additional diet kitchens and a third for the making of liquid diets. All of these activities were under the direction of the nursing staff.

Nightingale's knowledge of chemistry and nutrition and her experiences in the Crimea shaped her ideas on the importance of proper nutritional support for the ill and injured. She believed that the physician should prescribe the diet but that the science and art of feeding patients was an essential part of nursing. She emphasized the importance of proper food selection, preparation, and service. In her "Notes on Matters Affecting the Health, Efficiency, and Hospital Administration of the British Army," written for a Royal Way Department Commission, she devoted two of the eighteen chapters to diet.

Her best-known book, *Notes on Nursing—What It is and What It Is Not* (1859), contains two chapters on the patient's diet.[19] In Chapter IV, "Taking Food," she observes that "in chronic cases, lasting over months or years . . . the fatal issue is often determined at last by mere protracted starvation." In stating that "every careful observer of the sick will agree in this that thousands of patients are annually starved in the midst of plenty," she goes on to emphasize that:

1. large meals should not be served early in the morning;
2. ingenuity is needed in the timing and amount of food served;
3. punctual service of food is important;
4. "let food come at the right time and be taken away, eaten or uneaten, at the right time; but never let a patient have something always standing by him";
5. the patient must not see or smell the food of others;
6. there must be no ward activity during meals;
7. all food presented must be food of high quality—fresh and not spoiled;
8. there must be accurate observations of the patient's daily food intake.

Chapter VII, "What Food?", discusses various components of sick diets such as beef tea, meat, vegetables, dairy products, arrowroot, sweets, jelly, tea, coffee, and bread. The need for conscientious observation of the benefits of the diets is stressed:

> I should therefore say that incomparably the most important office of the nurse, after she has taken care of the patient's air, is to take care to observe the effect of his food, and report it to the medical attendant. It is quite incalculable the good that would certainly come from such sound and close observation in this almost neglected branch of nursing, or the help it would give to the medical man.

Through her example and her teachings, Florence Nightingale demonstrated how well-educated women could benefit society. They must possess the ability to analyze situations accurately; formulate a plan of action; document, present, and publish facts; and direct others efficiently. Those traits, when embodied in nursing in general and nutritional support nursing in particular are the foundation of intelligent nursing care. Nursing had become a viable career for intelligent, clearheaded women.

Donations by government and private sources enabled Nightingale to establish the Nightingale Training School for Nurses (1860) in affiliation with St. Thomas' Hospital in London. This first school specifically organized for the education and preparation of skilled nurses was to serve as the model for subsequent nursing schools the world over, especially in the United States.

NURSING EDUCATION IN THE UNITED STATES

Nursing in the late 19th century was recognized as an acceptable vocation for women. In addition, it became clear that a skilled and efficient nurse was a well-educated nurse. The continually increasing number of hospitals demanded more trained nurses to staff them. By 1873 four training schools for nurses operated in the northeastern United States. By 1900 that number had increased to 400. Because some hospitals had no cooks, cooking became an essential part of the nursing school curriculum.

THE NURSE AND THE DIETITIAN

During this time there was an increasing awareness of the role of good nutrition in health care and recovery from illness. Florence Nightingale's *Notes on Nursing* was the first clear indication of the nurse's responsibility in this area. Noted cooks were also becoming aware of the need for special foods for the ill. Catherine Beecher's cookbook, *Miss Beecher's Recipe Book*, written in 1842, contained a chapter entitled, "Recipes for Food and Drink for the Sick." Physicians began to regard good nutrition as a vital part of good health. For example, Dr. Pavy of the Royal College of Physicians wrote a paper on food and dietetics in which he stated that "ill management of food kills off the weak and ruins the middling." Dr. Fothergill, superintendent of London's Guy's Hospital, gave lectures on foods and nutrition to his students.[6]

In 1873 the physicians at the Dewitt Dispensary in New York City sought the help of some prominent women in obtaining nourishing food for the poor, and the Diet Kitchen Association of that city was born. The next year the South End Diet Kitchen began to supply nourishing food for specific patients at the Boston Dispensary, and in 1882 the General Hospital of Rochester opened a diet kitchen where student nurses worked for one month on a rotating basis.

Interest in nutrition and food preparation as well as desire to improve home cookery were motivating forces behind the development of cooking schools.

Some classes included nursing students, and a number of graduates of these cooking schools gave instruction to nurses in the preparation of food for the sick—then called *invalid cookery*.

Cooking schools established in New York City (1876), Philadelphia (1878 and 1882), and Boston (1879) were pioneers in this effort. Martha Byerly, as the first graduate of the Philadelphia Cooking School, taught nursing school seniors at Pennsylvania Hospital and served as "Superintendent of the Diet" at the Presbyterian Hospital. As "Instructor of Cooking" at Johns Hopkins Hospital Training School for Nurses, Mary Boland prepared a *Handbook of Invalid Cookery* for the use of "nurses in training schools, nurses in private practice, and others who care for the sick."[20]

These and other newly formed cookery schools graduated women now educated in all forms of cookery. Many graduates of these schools sought jobs in the diet departments of hospitals run by nurses. A trend was building to have a person specifically educated and trained in foods and food preparation in charge of the diet kitchen rather than the nurse. Hospitals themselves began to initiate courses to train dietitians with the aim of filling the increasing need for knowledgeable personnel to organize special diets for a variety of disease states. The Department of Public Charities of New York City (1903), the Jefferson (1911) and Pennsylvania (1916) Hospitals of Philadelphia, and the Massachusetts General Hospital gave the first in-hospital training courses for dietitians.

As the number of specifically trained "dietitians" who sought employment in hospitals grew, the traditional role of the nurse as head of the kitchen and food service began to diminish until the nurse relinquished all such duties to this new professional food expert. The American Dietetic Association was founded in 1917. Concurrently, the knowledge and responsibilities of the nurse were rapidly expanding, and her time and interest were being pulled in a variety of other directions. Therefore, until the development of parenteral alimentation, the nurse took a more passive role in the nutritional care of her patients.

NUTRITION IN NURSING EDUCATION

Despite the emergence of the dietitian role, the nurse still required a thorough background in nutrition and diet and their relationship to health. By 1910 most of the nurses' training schools has courses in food for the sick and the basics of food preparation. Hospital schools of nursing planned their nutrition courses to teach students how to prepare and serve meals, set up trays, and physically feed the patients. The first planned diet kitchen program gave students actual food preparation experience.[21] For the most part, the length of time spent in lectures and the cooking experience varied among schools.

After 1920 the educational emphasis on invalid cookery and complete food preparation shifted to the teaching of diet therapy and the basic principles of the newly expanding science of nutrition.[22] The length of the diet kitchen experience decreased in the mid 1930s and the use of the food laboratory was initiated. In order to make nutrition a more meaningful experience for nursing students, the case study/conference system was adopted. As early as 1917 nursing curricula in some schools included a 40-hour course in nutrition and cookery and a 10-hour course in the diet in relation to disease.[23] This was the beginning of the integration of the nutrition and diet experience with the medical curriculum. As the apprenticeship form of nurses' training was slowly being replaced by the more organized system of theoretical and practical education of the 1920s and 1930s, the need for these and other modern teaching methods became evident. Emphasis was placed on the direct application of theory to practice. Student nurses were given the opportunity to directly relate classroom knowledge of nutrition to the clinical situation.

THE EVOLUTION OF MODERN PARENTERAL ALIMENTATION

As nursing practice and nursing education underwent the changes and improvements that would provide nurses with the theoretical and practical skills to play a vital role in nutritional support, the early 20th century also brought many advances linking medicine and nutrition, giving physicians more insight into the complexities of the nutritional state of their patients.

Until this time, the relationship of food to health was not well understood in specific terms. It was clear that food contained dietary constituents necessary for growth and health and that the lack of some substances in foods was the cause of specific diseases. Two unknown but essential factors were identified by McCollum and Davis in 1913 and Osborne and Mendelin in 1915: vitamin A and vitamin B, respectively. Vitamin C was discovered in 1917, followed by vitamins D and E in 1922. It took until 1947 to identify all the components of the B vitamin complex.

In 1899 Lilienfield showed that glucose could be given safely by intravenous means, but that similarly administered hydrolyzed protein produced toxicity. In 1887 Landerer administered 300 cc of 3% glucose intravenously to a patient with severe postoperative hemorrhage to help combat shock. In addition, he described glucose as a source of parenterally administered food and conducted further studies on his "artificial nutrition."[24]

The use of parenteral solutions gained acceptance. P. L. Friedrich, Professor of Surgery at the University of Leipzig, issued a report in 1905 entitled "Artificial Subcutaneous Nourishment in Practical Surgery." He described experiments in which solutions of water, salt, carbohydrates, fats, and peptones were injected subcutaneously into a patient whose condition prohibited oral intake. A. E. Barker reported on his use of subcutaneous injections of saline and glucose in 1905 and predicted that humans would "devise some solution which, when injected subcutaneously, would bring to the system other more complex foods."[24]

Solutions of glucose were by far the most common form of parenterally administered nutrients. Kausch (1911) believed that patients who were unable to take food by mouth necessitated artificial feeding. He administered three liters of a 10% glucose solution intravenously daily for 6 days with no sugar spill in the urine. Woodyatt demonstrated that glucose could be given intravenously at a rate of 0.9 g/kg body weight/hour without glycosuria (1915). He called this "intravenous nutrition."[25]

With the identification of the amino acids (1906, 1916, 1938) came the realization that they are not synthesized in the body and, therefore, had to be supplied by the diet. Although the key role played by protein in the body's nitrogen balance had been demonstrated as early as 1852, it was not until after the turn of the century that the medical community became interested in the use of nondietary protein for nutritionally needy patients. Protein casein was treated with mild alkali hydrolysis and successfully administered to animals without toxicity—but also without positive nitrogen balance.[26] Other experiments used intravenous solutions of enzymatically digested protein.[12,26]

Studies of amino acid metabolism and requirements in the human body suggested the strong possibility that the intravenous use of amino acids delivered with sufficient calories would fulfill the needs of nutritionally depleted patients.[27] Then, in 1937, significant experiments with a parenterally administered solution of amino acids and glucose demonstrated positive nitrogen balance in postoperative patients.[28] This solution used by Elamn was prepared by the acid hydrolysis of casein with the addition of tryptophan and cystine. The field of parenteral nutrition was further advanced by the development of inexpensively produced crystalline L-amino acids by Japanese researchers. During the 1930s and 1940s much work was done to show the importance of positive nutritional balance and the grave consequences of hypoproteinemia in surgical and trauma patients.[29–32]

Although use of this amino acid solution met with success, researchers still looked for a way to add more calories to the regimen. Glucose, with its delivery of 4 kcal/g, had long been used as the major intravenous calorie source. In a quest for a method of greater intravenous calorie intake, researchers turned their interest to other substances. Oral ethyl alcohol (7 kcal/g) as a calorie source was explored in 1891.[33] The first parenteral use of ethyl alcohol for nutritional repletion, however, was not reported until 1952. The study stated that if the alcohol was infused slowly (700 cal/day) along with invert sugar, protein hydrolysates, electrolytes, and vitamins, patients could maintain a positive nutritional balance without reaching intoxicating blood levels.[34] Commercially prepared intravenous alcohol as an inexpensive calorie source enjoyed wide use until its hepatotoxic and adverse metabolic effects were demonstrated by further research.[35]

Another intravenous calorie source explored was the use of parenteral fat solutions that could not only deliver 9 kcal/g but also supply essential fatty acids. Early experiments with natural fats were unsuccessful.[36] Japanese researchers began experiments with artificial fat emulsions in the 1920s.[36] Investigation began in the United States in 1935 with the administration of intravenous homogenized fat emulsions to pediatric patients.[37,38] Other studies demonstrated the ability of a water-oil-lecithin emulsion to prolong the life of starving laboratory dogs and to reduce their eventual weight loss.[39] Soya bean phosphotide emulsions were introduced in 1943 and met with varying success. Numerous successful clinical and research experiments using a cottonseed oil emulsion, Lipomel (Upjohn Company, Kalamazoo, MI), were reported at 1957 symposia on the use of intravenous fats.[40] Shortly thereafter the long-term effects of intravenous fats—fat overloading syndrome—were demonstrated.[40,41] This plus the reports of other complications of fat infusions resulted in a marked decrease in use and an eventual ban by the United States Food and Drug Administration. A well-tolerated 10% soya bean and egg yolk phospholipid emulsion, Intralipid (KabiVitrum, Inc., Alameda, CA), was developed in Sweden, marketed in Europe in 1962, and became available in America in the mid 1970s.

THE BREAKTHROUGH

For several decades nursing school nutrition courses provided limited integrated knowledge about the complex nutritional aspects of health and nursing care. The study of vitamins and their related deficiency diseases, disease-specific diet calculation, and procedures for enteral tube feedings constituted much of the material presented. As medicine was demonstrating experimentally the importance of nutritional status in a patient's overall care, nursing education was beginning to upgrade and expand the nurse's understanding of and participation in nutritional support. Recognizing areas of deficiencies, many schools of nursing reorganized their nutrition courses based on reevaluation, conferencing, and current research findings.[42-46] Unknowingly, nursing was preparing to step forward into an expanded and rewarding role in the nutritional support of the patient. Medicine would soon provide the practical means to achieve that transition.

Intravenous feeding studies began at the University of Pennsylvania School of Medicine in the 1940s. In one study, healthy subjects received peripheral solutions of 10% glucose with 5% hydrolyzed protein in high volume (5–6 liters/day) in experiments designed to ensure a high protein-calorie intake.[47] Although the disposal of excess fluids was facilitated by the use of diuretics, the potential dangers of fluid overload and electrolyte imbalance precluded the use of this method as a routine treatment.

It was clear that two major stumbling blocks had to be overcome before the full scope of these ideas could be explored. Availability, inexpensiveness, and relative safety made glucose the calorie source of choice, but to alleviate the problem of fluid overload, a more highly concentrated solution was indicated. Concurrently, a safe and efficient intravenous route of administration was necessary to enable the delivery of this hypertonic nutritional solution.

Previous scientific and medical knowledge and the beginning of effective intravenous nutrition were brought together in a series of experiments conducted at the Harrison Department of Surgical Research at the University of Pennsylvania. Experiments were begun by Dr. Stanley J. Dudrick in 1964 using beagle puppies to determine whether positive nitrogen balance, growth, and development could be achieved by intravenous means alone.

A basic hypertonic dextrose, protein hydrolysate, and electrolyte solution was formulated in the hospital pharmacy based on diet requirements for growing puppies as recommended by the Food and Nutrition Board of the National Research Council. An infraclavicular subclavian vein catheterization technique was used to deliver the solution. Twelve-week-old litter mates were paired; one puppy received an oral diet and the other received an identical intravenous diet. A total of 6 sets of puppies were studied in a series of experiments lasting 70–256 days. The results indicated that the paired sets paralleled each other in growth and development. For the first time in medical history it was shown experimentally that long-term total intravenous feeding could sustain and nourish growing animals.[48]

The next step was to apply these techniques to the care of humans. Selected patients in dire medical condition and suffering profound depletion of nutrients were started on a regimen of "parenteral hyperalimentation," a phrase coined by Drs. Dudrick and Rhoads. To a 10% glucose and 5% amino acid solution formulated in the hospital pharmacy, electrolytes, vitamins, and minerals were added according to each patient's individual metabolic needs. A percutaneous infraclavicular subclavian vein catheterization placed the tip of the catheter in the superior vena cava thus ensuring the immediate dilution of the hypertonic nutritional solution.[49] This solution was delivered through a microdrip chamber administration apparatus. Alterations in the patient's carefully monitored serum chemistry values were quickly corrected by appropriate changes in the intravenous admixture. Each patient was closely observed for any sign of metabolic, systemic, or equipment-related complications.[50]

THE NURSING ROLE BEGINS

As clinical responsibilities involving parenteral hyperalimentation increased and varied, Dr. Dudrick recognized that a nurse would be essential to the success and continuance of this new form of therapy. Anticipating the scope and potential of this therapy for patients who were unable to take oral nourishment due to trauma, surgery, or disease process, he saw that nursing could play an invaluable role in assuring optimum nutritional support in the care of their patients.

Two decades earlier, two nurses had been hired by the University of Pennsylvania to work with physicians in their nutrition-oriented clinical research.* In the 1940s Marie Barnes assisted in clinical trials on selected patients using a 15% cottonseed oil emulsion or a 10% sesame oil emulsion.[51] Eina Goulding assisted in an experiment that force-fed preoperative patients in order to offset postoperative negative nitrogen balance.[52] With these precedents, the Chairman of the Department of Surgery, Dr. Jonathan Rhoads, authorized the hiring of a nurse in 1967 to work with the parenteral hyperalimentation team.

Dudrick identified the need for an extremely competent nurse in order to help show the therapy to its best advantage as well as one who could elicit the respect and cooperation of the nursing staff. When approached, the hospital nursing service was unwilling to relinquish one of its nurses to what it considered a non-hospital oriented, non-nursing position in research.† Therefore, the Harrison Department of Surgical Research employed me, an emergency room nurse, to be the first nurse hired exclusively for work in this new form of nutritional support.

DEVELOPMENT OF NURSING RESPONSIBILITIES

Until this time the parenteral hyperalimentation team consisted of Dudrick, a surgical resident, and a laboratory technician. I joined the team to oversee the nursing care of the patients receiving this new nutritional support therapy. Although in this initial period the nurse's duties varied widely, the basic responsibilities of a nutritional support nurse became more clearly defined as I worked with the first patients receiving this nutritional support.

My first and foremost responsibility was the care and maintenance of the intravenous delivery system of the nutritional solutions. Present at all subclavian vein catheter insertions, I prepared the patient and assisted the physician with the procedure. The catheter dressing became my prime responsibility. These dressings were inspected twice daily, and the site was completely redressed at least three times a week or as needed to ensure the asepsis of the catheter and the delivery line. All aspects of catheter dressing care, now routine, were tested, improved, and standardized during this early period. Methods of protecting the dressing also evolved, specifically, the use of plastic adhesive operating room drapes to provide waterproof protection for the dressings of patients with head and/or neck wounds or tracheostomies. Catheter removal was performed by the nurse, and each catheter tip was cultured in conjunction with the research protocols.

---

* J. E. Rhoads: Personal communication, February, 1985.
† S. J. Dudrick, M.D.: Personal communication, February, 1985.

Another identified duty of the nutritional support nurse as I practiced it was the observation and assessment of the patients and their response to therapy. The present-day parameters of detailed nutritional assessment were not in use in the late 1960s; nevertheless, the importance of an accurate evaluation of the patient's reactions to the intravenous nutritional regimen was recognized and carried out. The nurse, as well as the physician, was also alert to the signs of sepsis, catheter displacement, electrolyte imbalances, mechanical problems with the delivery system or equipment, and allergic reactions to the nutritional solution, adhesive tape, antiseptics used in the catheter site redressing, and so on.

Another aspect of this new nursing role was in the area of education and consultation. In addition to the nutritional support team physicians who were continually educating their peers, the team nurse was also responsible for physician education. The medical house staff's in-depth understanding of the procedures and ramifications of this advanced form of nutritional therapy was essential to present and future successful applications. In an effort to familiarize the medical staff with acceptable dressing change technique, I addressed the Hospital of the University of Pennsylvania's Surgical Grand Rounds to explain the procedure. Daily discussions with the house staff also served to reinforce the principles of the nutritional therapy.

It became increasingly evident to the team that without the interest, cooperation, and diligence of the nursing staff the therapy would founder. Some members of the nursing staff resisted the changes and additions to routine patient care that this new regimen demanded. The metabolic implications of deviation in the intravenous fluid's mandatory continuous-flow rate and the systemic consequences of contamination of the dressing or solution had to be reiterated and emphasized. But as staff nurses became acquainted with and interested in nutritional support, they began to help educate their colleagues and improve the quality of patient care.

The lack of involvement of the Department of Nursing in the nursing role on the nutritional support team precluded any formal teaching or inservice for the nursing staff by the team nurse. However, I initiated one-to-one or small group teaching in the clinical setting and attended ward nursing case conferences on patients receiving intravenous nutritional therapy. I met with the staff informally to explain rationales and procedures and, most importantly, to work with these nurses to solve the everyday practical nursing care problems that arose.

As the parenteral hyperalimentation nurse, I was also responsible for coordinating and promoting good patient care. My duties included integration of the unique requirements of the parenteral hyperalimentation therapy with standard nursing care. I acted as a liaison with the hospital pharmacy regarding the patient's individualized solution requirements and the addition of solution additives on the nursing unit. A laminar air flow hood was obtained for one of the nursing units, and the nursing staff was instructed in the acceptable method of introducing additional additives to the nutritional solutions. I made certain that the patient's fluid intake and output and daily weights were measured and accurately recorded, that the ordered laboratory tests were completed and reported, that fractional urine tests were performed and recorded and that appropriate occupational and physical therapy programs were instituted and maintained for those patients receiving parenteral hyperalimentation.

As this new form of nutritional therapy was being developed, the team nurse took on the additional role of researcher. In the initial clinical applications of parenteral hyperalimentation, each patient was monitored according to research protocols. Detailed records were kept of the patient's intake, output, and daily weight. In addition, all patient output—urine, feces, drainages—were collected daily for later analysis by the team laboratory technician. All relevant laboratory data were recorded. The compilation of the collected data, the preliminary graphing of the data for the medical artist, and numerous library searches contributed to several early publications in this new field. I also was active in the experimental research laboratory, giving assistance with operative procedures, vein cannulations, and the mixing of nutritional solutions for the animals.

A final, but no less important, major aspect of this role was the nurse's responsibility for the psychological and supportive care of the patient receiving parenteral hyperalimentation. Because this was a complicated technique used mostly for very ill patients, the team nurse had frequent, daily contact with the patients. In the continually changing world of a hospital staff (because of days off, vacations, shift changes, and reassignments) the team nurse provided a continuing and familiar presence in the hospital lives of these patients. By virtue of training and accessibility, the parenteral hyperalimentation nurse was afforded an opportunity to educate and support the patients and their families throughout the therapy.

GROWTH IN THE FIELD

As the benefits and techniques of this nutritional therapy were reported and its potential for future applications became evident, physicians and reserachers in other medical centers began extensive investigation into the theory and application of nutrition for the hospitalized patient, and parenteral hyperalimentation teams were begun. Several interested physicians (along with one nurse) visited the Hospital of the University of Pennsylvania to gain first-hand knowledge of this therapy and to observe the daily activities of the first nutritional support team.

Nurses also played an important role in the development of nutritional support teams throughout the country. Rita Colley, a respiratory intensive care nurse, worked with the team at Massachusetts General Hospital (1970) and was joined by Karen Phillips one year later. Dorothy Godfrey, head nurse of the Intravenous Team at Johns Hopkins Hospital, became the first parenteral hyperalimentation nurse at that institution in the early 1970s. DeAnn Englert joined Dudrick's team at his new location at Hermann Hospital at the University of Texas in 1974. New York Hospital of Cornell Medical Center established a nutritional support team in 1976 with Barbara Griggs, a surgical critical care nurse, as its nursing coordinator. In the same year another critical care nurse, Loretta Forlaw, joined the nutritional support team at Letterman Army Hospital in San Francisco. One year later a nursing educator, Mary Hoppe, was hired as the first parenteral hyperalimentation nurse at Chicago's St. Mary's Hospital.

These and other pioneers in the area of nutritional support nursing helped to define and develop the nursing role in this new field. As researchers and physicians refined and expanded this form of therapy, parenteral hyperalimentation nurses have applied these advances and this knowledge to the daily care of their patients, broadening and highlighting nursing responsibilities and upgrading nursing skills in the field of nutritional support. They assisted in setting up standards of patient care, writing procedures and protocols, developing the nursing nutritional assessment and various educational materials, and providing practical recommendations for improved patient care.

With increasing experience and knowledge in the field of nutritional support, these nurses in the forefront of this therapy began to communicate their expertise to peers. Articles began to appear in the nursing journals. Early publications introduced the rationale for total intravenous nutritional therapy, described nursing responsibilities, and presented case studies.[53–56] Later articles discussed specific aspects of nutritional support therapy and increasing responsibilities of the nursing care for these patients.[57–59]

Prior to 1970, nursing education courses on the nutritional care of the patient had centered on biochemical and dietary concerns and the rationale and procedures for enteral feedings. In addition to the previously mentioned enhancement of the nutrition curriculum, schools of nursing began to educate nurses in the theory and practice of total nutritional support. Nursing textbooks included sections on parenteral nutrition.[60,61]

THE AWAKENING

A 1974 paper on iatrogenic malnutrition called attention to the plight of malnourished hospitalized patients.[62] Health care providers were urged to focus on the nutritional state of their patients. It was pointed out that new medical technology and advanced therapies could be undermined and nullified by poor wound healing, prolonged recovery, increased susceptibility to infection, and vitamin and mineral deficienices, all of which occur in undernourished patients.

Others also addressed this most serious problem.[63,64] Blackburn reported that one-fourth to one-half of medical and surgical patients hospitalized for two weeks or more developed protein-calorie malnutrition. Attention to proper nutritional support could prevent complications and hasten convalescence, thereby shortening the length of hospital stay and decreasing hospital medical costs. These papers, along with the early successes of total parenteral nutrition, stimulated the nation's physicians, nurses, and dietitians to re-examine the nutritional state of hospitalized patients. Protocols and equipment for extensive nutritional assessment of patients were developed.[65]

Attention was also focused on the nutritional state of the chronically ill. Many patients were not in need of total parenteral nutrition therapy but did require less complete nutritional supplementation. This reawakening of the significance of the patient's nutritional state in concert with the recent advances in liquid diets resulting from the NASA space exploration program[66] opened the door to major developments in the long-neglected field of enteral nutrition. Commercial laboratories began to manufacture a variety of liquid diets to be administered via feeding tube to nutritionally depleted patients. This event in turn sparked the research and development of safer, small bore, more pliant feeding tubes.[67]

A NURSING SPECIALITY

Since its inception in 1967, nutritional support nursing has evolved into a distinctive nursing specialty. Expanded nursing responsibilities, new technology and equipment, and the sharing of knowledge have contributed to the development of this specialty to its present day status.[68,69]

Colley discusses some of the "contrasts and similarities between current and past nursing practice in this speciality," including changes in the areas of nutritional assessment, catheter placement, catheter site and dressing care, and intravenous administration sets as well as the basic responsibilities that have remained constant throughout the development of this specialty.[70]

The scope of nutritional support nursing broadened further with the development of the long-term indwelling intravenous catheters that enabled nutritional support therapy to continue on an outpatient basis.[71,72] However, this advancement, which enabled patients to receive nutritional support at home, presented the nutritional support nurse with additional responsibilities, as described by Baker[56] and Englert.[73] Detailed protocols for catheter dressing care and infusion techniques were developed to meet the needs of this situation. It was imperative that patients and their families fully understood their role in the continuance of nutritional support therapy at home. Nurses devised and taught comprehensive patient-education programs on home nutritional support to patients and their families.

The adaptation of nutritional support therapy to the pediatric patient necessitated the formulation of appropriate nursing care procedures. Pediatric nurses interested in nutritional support gained expertise in the application of this therapy to their patients, adding yet another dimension to this expanding field.

NATIONAL ORGANIZATIONS

Until the mid 1970s there was little opportunity for nurses in this new field to meet. In 1976, however, a group of prominent physicians, biochemists, and researchers in the field of total nutritional support founded the American Society for Parenteral and Enteral Nutrition (ASPEN) to serve as an open forum for the exchange of information by all members of the nutrition team. In addition to medicine and biochemistry, divisions were included for pharmacy, dietetics, and nursing.

This was an occurrence of major import to the new and growing field of nutritional support nursing. It created a common forum for the exploration and discussion of the many issues pertinent to nursing that affected the early practitioners. The first nursing board included Dorothy Godfrey (the representative to ASPEN's Executive Board), DeAnn Englert, Loretta Forlaw, Mary Hoppe, Christine Shaw-Regan, and Marlyn Jerrard.

At yearly clinical conferences, the ASPEN Nursing Committee organized and provided sessions covering a wide range of topics vital to the nutritional support nurse: basic science, nutritional assessment, clinical and metabolic considerations, enteral nutrition, pediatric nutritional support, ethical issues, patient monitoring, and nursing research. June 1984 saw the first independent national nursing seminar entitled "Incorporating Nutritional Support into Nursing Practice" organized by the ASPEN Nursing Committee under its then director, Kathleen Crocker. The 2-day program covered theoretical as well as practical aspects of nutritional support.

In an effort to define the parameters of responsible nursing care for the patient receiving nutritional support therapy, ASPEN nurses formulated the "Nursing Care Standards for Nutritional Support of the Hospitalized Patient" (1984). In addition, the Nursing Committee developed monographs and other publications on nursing care, the most recent being "Nutrition Support Nursing—Core Curriculum" (1984).

The nursing division of ASPEN was the first national organization specifically oriented to nutritional support nursing. The European Society for Parenteral and Enteral Nutrition also initiated a nursing division in 1981. In addition, many parenteral hyperalimentation nurses belong to the National Intravenous Therapy Association (NITA), an international organization of which nutritional support nurses have been active and influential members. The founding of the American Society of Nutritional Support Services (1983) has provided another forum for nurses in the nutritional support field to interact and share information.

As the means to artifically nourish patients with extraordinary nutritional needs have evolved, questions have emerged as to the appropriateness of the initiation and termination of artificial nutrition modalities. The growing concern of the professional, academic, and medical communities over the ethical, as well as legal, issues surrounding the withholding of a dying patient's nutrition and hydration has prompted much discussion, publicity, and legal intervention.

In an effort to examine these complex issues, a multidisciplinary conference was held in May, 1984, under the aegis of the Society for Health and Human Values. The participants included experts in the fields of law, philosophy, religion, medical humanities, biomedical ethics, various medical specialty areas, and nursing. The reader is directed to a published collection of papers from that conference entitled *By No Extraordinary Means: The Choice to Forgo Life-Sustaining Food and Water*, edited by Joanne Lynn, M.D.[74]

The issues most frequently discussed in determining what circumstances warrant withholding nutrition and hydration fall into three major areas. The first addresses the competence or incompetence of the patient to express his or her own choice. The second issue questions whether food and hydration are considered ordinary care (obligatory) or extraordinary medical intervention (optional).[75] The third convtroversial area attempts to differentiate between killing and allowing to die.[76]

Nourishment of the sick and dying has constituted a basic responsibility of the nurse throughout history. Although medical science has given us the tools to fulfill this duty in the highest technical sense, nursing, as well as medicine, now must consider the moral concerns of carrying out this responsibility in certain individual situations.

SUMMARY

The nursing profession can be proud of its role in the development of parenteral hyperalimentation and nutritional support. Nutritional duties of nurses have paralleled general progress in medicine and nursing. The nurse's nutritional responsibilities, one of her primary duties in olden times, were gradually supplanted by technical progress and requirements to administer medications and otherwise to care physically for the patient. The present time has seen the re-emergence of a specialized role for nursing in the areas of parenteral and enteral nutrition. In the few short years since 1967 when the first nurse began work on parenteral hyperalimentation, we have seen the evolution of a highly complex role that requires in-depth knowledge in the area of optimal nutritional support. The parameters of the current role of the nutritional support nurse and a discussion of issues that are of concern to her or him are described in full in the chapters to come.

REFERENCES

1. Dolan J, Fitzpatrick ML, Herrmann E: Nursing in Society: A Historical Perspective (ed 15). Philadelphia, WB Saunders, 1983, pp 1–25
2. Bullough V, Bullough B: The Care of the Sick: Emergence of Modern Nursing. London, Neale Watson Academic Publications, 1979, pp 1–25

3. Dock L, Stewart I: A Short Hx of Nursing. New York, Putnam, 1920, p 26
4. Lonie IM: A structural pattern of Greek dietetics and the early history of Greek medicine. Medical Hx 21:235–260, 1977
5. Guggenheim KY: Nutrition and Nutritional Disease: The Evolution of Concepts. Lexington, MA, Collamore Press, 1981, pp 3–19
6. Rawcliffe C: The hospitals of later Medieval London. Med History 28:1–21, 1984
7. Jelliffe EFP: Nutrition in the nursing curricula: Historical perspectives and present Day Trends. Pediatr Environ Child Health 20:150–181, 1974
8. Drake TGH: Pap and panada. Annals of Medical History 3:289–295, 1931
9. Annan GL: An exhibition on books on the growth of our knowledge of blood transfusion. Bull NY Acad Med 15:622–632, 1939
10. Brown HM: The beginnings of intravenous medication. Ann Med History 1(2):177–197, 1917
11. Cuthbertson D: Historical background to parenteral nutrition. Acta Chir Scand 498(suppl):1–10, 1980
12. Lee HA: Historical reivew of parenteral nutrition, in Lee HA (ed): Parenteral Nutrition in Acute Metabolic Disease. Orlando, FL, Academic Press, 1974, pp 3–10
13. Zimmerman LM, Howell KM: History of Blood Transfusion. Ann Med History 4(5):415–433, 1932
14. Blundell J: Observations on transfusion of blood. Lancet 2:321–326, 1828–1829
15. Todhunter EN: Historical landmarks in nutrition, in Hegsted M (ed): Present Knowledge in Nutrition (ed 4). new York, The Nutrition Foundation, 1976, pp 547–555
16. Olmsted JM, Olmsted EH: Claude Bernard and the Experimental Method in Medicine. New York, Henry Shuman, 1952, pp 35–36, 98–99
17. Hodder EM: Transfusion of milk in cholera. Practitioner 10:14–16, 1873
18. Cooper L: Florence Nightengale's contribution to dietetics. J Amer Dietetic Assoc 30:121–127, 1958
19. Nightengale F: Notes on Nursing: What it is and What it is Not. London, Harrison & Sons, 1859
20. Gilson HE: Some historical notes on the development of diet therapy. J Amer Diet Assoc 23:761–765, 1947
21. Fewell AU: Diet kitchen methods of instruction. Am J Nurs 17(2):105–111, 1916
22. Molleson A: Current comment: Teaching nutrition to student nurses. J Amer Diet Assoc 34:164–171, 1958
23. Hassenplug LW: The teaching dietitian's place in nursing education. J Amer Diet Assoc 36:467–471, 1960
24. Elman R: Parenteral Alimentation in Surgery. New York, Hoeber, 1947, p 6
25. Woodyatt RT, Sansum WD, Wilder RM: Prolonged and accurately timed intravenous injections of sugar. JAMA 65(24):2067–2070, 1915
26. Symposium on intravenous fat emulsions: Clinical experiences with intravenous fat emulsions. Metabolism 6, 1957 (special edition)
27. Rose WC: The significance of amino acids in nutrition. Harvey Lecture 30:49–65, 1934
28. Elman R: Amino acid content of blood following intravenous injection of hydrolyzed casein. Proc Soc Exper Biol Med 37:437–440, 1937
29. Cutherbertson DP: Observations in the disturbance of metabolism produced by injury to the limbs. Q J Med 1:233–246, 1932

30. Thompson WD, Ravdin IS, Frank IL: Effect of hypoproteinemia on wound disruption. Arch Surg 36:500–508, 1938
31. Rhoads JE, Kasinskas W: The influence of hypoproteinemia on the formation of callus in experimental fracture. Surgery 11:38–44, 1942
32. Cannon PR, Wissler RW, Woolridge RL, et al: Relationship of protein deficiency to surgical infection. Ann Surg 120:514–525, 1944
33. Atwater WO, Benedict FG: An experimental inquiry regarding the nutritive value of alcohol. Mem Natn Acad Sci 8:235, 1896
34. Rice Co, Strickler JH: Parenteral nutrition in elderly surgical patients. Geriatrics 7:232–240, 1952
35. Weber CS: Hepatic and Metabolic effects of alcohol. Gastroenterology 50:119–133, 1966
36. Levenson SM, Hopskins BS, Waldron M, et al: Early history of parenteral nutrition. Fed Proc 43(5)1391–1406, 1984
37. Holt LE, Tidwell HC, McNair-Scott TF: The intravenous administration of fat: A practical therapeutic procedure. J Pediatr 6:151–160, 1935
38. Gordon HH, Levine SZ: Respiratory metabolism in infancy and in childhood. XVI. Effects of intravenous infusions of fat on energy exchange of infants. Am J Dis Child 50:894–912, 1935
39. Narat JK: Observations on parenteral administration of fat emulsions. Am J Dig Dis Nutr 4:107–109, 1937
40. Levenson SM, UpJohn HL, Sheehy TW: Two severe reactions following long-term infusion of large amounts of intravenous fat. Metabolism 6:807–814, 1957
41. Waddell WR, Geyer RP, Hurley N, et al: Abnormal carbohydrate metabolism in patients with hypercholesterolemia and hyperlipemia. Metabolism 7:707–1958
42. Rynbergen HJ: Nutrition in the nursing school curriculum. Am J Nurs 50(5):280–283, 1950
43. Betzold KV, Elfert G: New ways to study nutrition. Am J Nurs 52(1):78–79, 1952
44. Brown EF, Lins MD: Are nutrition courses for student nurses up to date? J Am Diet Assoc 31:52–53, 1955
45. Thigpen LW, Mitchell IA: Integrating nutrition into nursing education. J Am Diet Assoc 33:378–380, 1957
46. Grant FW, McCarthy G: Nutrition subject matter in the nursing curriculum. J Am Diet Assoc 58:26–30, 1971
47. Rhoads JE: Diuretics as an adjuvant in disposing of extra water as a vehicle in parenteral hyperalimentation. Fed Proc 21:389, 1962
48. Dudrick SJ, Rhoads JE, Vars HM: Growth of puppies receiving all nutritional requirements by vein. Forschritte der Parenteral Ernahrung 2:16–18, 1967
49. Mogil RA, DeLaurentis DA, Rosemond GP: The infraclavicular puncture. Arch Surg 95:320–324, 1967
50. Dudrick SJ, Wilmore DW, Vars HM, et al: Long-term total parenteral nutrition with growth, development, and positive nitrogen balance. Surgery 64:134–142, 1968
51. Lehr HL, Rosenthal HM, Rawnsley HM, et al: Clinical experience with intravenous fat emulsions. Metabolism 6:666, 1957
52. Riegel C, Koop CE, Drew J, et al: The nutritional requirements for nitrogen balance in surgical patients during the early postoperative period. J Clin Invest 26:18–23, 1947
53. Grant JAN, Moir E, Fago M: Parenteral hyperalimentation. Am J Nurs 69(11):2392–2395, 1969

54. Grant JAN: Patient care in parenteral hyperalimentation. Nurs Clin N Am 8(1):165–181, 1973
55. Colley R, Phillips K: Helping with hyperalimentation. Nursing 73:6–17, 1973
56. Baker DI: Hyperalimentation at home. Am J Nurs 74(10):1826–1829, 1974
57. Heppe C: The new feeding tube sets or your patients are what you feed them. Nursing80 10(3):80–85, 1980
58. Griggs BA: The monitoring and administration of total parenteral nutrition. Natl IV Ther Assoc 4:220–221, 1981
59. Rouflart M: The role of a nurse in a nutritional support team, in Wesdorp R, Soeters PB (eds): Clinical Nutrition '81. New York, Churchill Livingstone, 1982, pp 339–340
60. Luckman J, Sorensan K: Medical Surgical Nursing (ed 2). Philadelphia, WB Saunders, 1980, pp 1404–1407
61. Dugas, Beverly W: Introduction to Patient Care: A Comprehensive Approach to Nursing (ed 4). Philadelphia, WB Saunders, 1983, p 296
62. Butterworth CE: The skeleton in the hospital closet. Nutrition Today 9(2):4–8, 1974
63. Bollet AJ, Owens S: Evaluation of nutritional status of selected hospitalized patients. Am J Clin Nutr 26:931–938, 1973
64. Meiling RL: The Institutional System. Nutrition Today 9(4):34–35, 1974
65. Blackburn GL, Bistrain BR, Maini BS, et al: Nutritional and metabolic assessment of the hospitalized patient. JPEN 1(1):11–22, 1977
66. Thompson WR, Stephens RV, Randall HT, et al: Use of the "space diet" in the management of a patient with extreme short bowel syndrome. Am J Surg 117:449–459, 1969
67. Griggs BA, Hoppe MC: Update: Nasogastric tube feeding. Am J Nurs 7,9(3)481–485, 1979
68. Long J: Guidelines for the nursing care of patients on intravenous hyperalimentation. Am J IV Ther 1:22–25, 1974
69. Englert D: The role of the nurse in intravenous hyperalimentation in the United States. Acta Chir SCand 507(suppl):298–313, 1981
70. Colley R: Total parenteral nutrition in 1981, in Wesdorp R, Soeters P (eds): Clinical Nutrition '81. New York, Churchill Livinstone, 1981, pp 332–338
71. Broviac JW, Cole JJ, Scribner BH: A silicone rubber atrial catheter for prolonged parenteral alimentation. Surg Gynecol Obstet 136:1–5, 1973
72. Broviac JW, Scribner BH: Prolonged parenteral nutrition in the home. Surg Gynecol Obstet 139:14–28, 1974
73. Englert D, Dudrick SJ: Principles of ambulatory home hyperalimentation. Am J IV Ther 5:11–14, 1978
74. Lynn J (ed): By No Extraordinary Means: The Choice to Forgo Life-Sustaining Food and Water. Bloomington, Indiana University Press, 1986
75. Childress J: When is it morally justifiable to discontinue medical nutrition and hydration? in Lynn J (ed): By No Extraordinary Means: The Choice to Forgo Life-Sustaining Food and Water. Bloomington, Indiana University Press, 1986, pp 67–83
76. Brock DW: Forgoing Life-Sustaining Food and Water: Is it killing? in Lynn J (ed): By No Extraordinary Means: The Choice to Forgo Life-Sustaining Food and Water. Bloomington, Indiana University Press, 1986, pp 117–126

Nancy Bergstrom
Jack L. Smith

——— 2 ———————————————————

Basic Principles of Nutrition

Nutrients are required to maintain life, normal functioning, growth, and the repair of tissue. This chapter covers the role and importance of the major nutrients (or *macronutrients*) such as carbohydrates, lipids, and proteins; micronutrients such as calcium, phosphorus, and iron; and vitamins. The major nutrients can be utilized for energy, converted to structural components of cells, or stored as fat, depending upon the level of their supply. The proper utilization of these nutrients requires appropriate concentrations of additional micronutrients, vitamins, minerals, and trace elements. Many of these essential nutrients are required from exogenous sources while some are converted endogenously when adequate supplies of the necessary precursors are present. The nutrient requirements of an individual change throughout the lifespan, in the presence of illness or trauma, and due to interactions of certain drugs.

A basic knowledge of nutritional biochemistry will facilitate an understanding of nutrient absorption, biosynthesis, and utilization. This knowledge enhances the nurses' ability to interpret the findings of clinical assessments, laboratory tests, and anthropometric measures. It is also useful when monitoring patients receiving nutritional supplementation and enteral and parenteral feedings.

CARBOHYDRATES

Dietary carbohydrates are classified either as complex carbohydrates or simple sugars. All carbohydrates are composed of carbon, hydrogen, and oxygen with a generic formula of CH_2O_n. For most carbohydrates, n is either 5, 6, or 7, with 6 being the most common. These carbohydrates are called

NUTRITIONAL SUPPORT IN NURSING
ISBN 0-8089-1889-3

29

pentoses, hexoses, and heptoses, respectively. Chemically, these are polyhydroxy compounds that have either a functional aldehyde or ketone group. They primarily exist as a 5- or 6-member ring with oxygen being one of the elements in the ring.

The simple sugars that are found in the diet are either *monosaccharides*, meaning a one sugar moiety, or *dissaccharides* with two sugar moieties. The major monosaccharides are *glucose* or *fructose*, which occur in some fruits and in honey (Fig. 2-1). *Galactose* and *manose*, two other monosaccharides, occur less frequently. Disaccharides include *sucrose* (table sugar), *maltose*, and *lactose*. Sucrose is composed of glucose and fructose. Maltose contains two glucose units and lactose contains glucose and galactose. When the term *sugar* is used, table sugar or sucrose usually is inferred. Sugars is a generic term, however, referring to all dietary mono- and disaccharides. Sucrose is found naturally in many fruits and is obtained from sugar cane and sugar beets. Lactose or milk sugar is found primarily in milk, and maltose results from the digestion of sugar.

When ingested as monosaccharides, the glucose is actively absorbed in an energy-requiring step. Fructose, however, is absorbed passively, dependent only on its concentration in the intestinal lumen. When disaccharides are ingested,

Monosaccharides	Disaccharides	Polysaccharides

$$C_6H_{12}O_6 + C_6H_{12}O_6 \underset{\text{Hydrolysis}}{\overset{\text{Synthesis}}{\rightleftarrows}} C_{12}H_{22}O_{11} + H_2O$$

Glucose + Fructose $\rightleftarrows$ Socrose + H_2O

Glucose + Galactose $\rightleftarrows$ Lactose + H_2O

Glucose + Glucose $\rightleftarrows$ Maltose + H_2O

Many glucose molecules $\rightleftarrows$ Starch

Many glucose molecules $\rightleftarrows$ Cellulose*

Many glucose molecules $\rightleftarrows$ Pectin*

Many glucose molecules $\rightleftarrows$ Glycogen

* Indigestible

Fig. 2-1.   Monosaccharide composition of sugars.

they are digested by the appropriate disaccharidase (sucrase, maltase, or lactase). Both monosaccharides are absorbed at the same time as they are being hydrolyzed.

Complex carbohydrates found in the diet consist of *starch* and *fiber* from plants and *glycogen* from meat. Starch is a polysaccharide composed of glucose units. Glycogen is also a polysaccharide consisting of glucose units and sometimes is called animal starch. Both are very similar in structure although their glucose units are polymerized. Starch is digested initially by an enzyme in saliva called *amylase*. Digestion is continued by pancreatic amylase in the intestinal tract, further breaking down starch into oligosaccharides and finally into di- and monosaccharides prior to absorption through the intestinal lumen.

Fiber is complex material from plants and consists of several different structures. One term used to quantitate fiber is *crude fiber*, which is the material remaining after the food has been extracted to remove fat, hydrolyzed both in dilute alkali and in dilute acid. The residue remaining is classified as crude fiber. It is crude fiber that is listed in most tables of food composition. Dietary fiber, however, consists of all plant carbohydrates that are not digested by secretions within the small intestine and that are excreted in the stool. Some of these materials actually may be digested by bacteria in the large intestine and may provide some nutrients. The amount of dietary fiber consumed is 3–4 times greater than the amount of crude fiber consumed. This fiber consists of cellulose, pectins, gums, and lignins. Most of the 5- and 7-carbon sugars in the diet are found in the pectin, gums, and lignins.

After absorption, most of the ingested carbohydrate is converted to glucose by the liver. Glucose is the primary carbohydrate used by cells for energy and is used as a basic building block for other carbohydrate-containing material. The glucose molecule can be converted to either liver or muscle glycogen, but first it must be phosphorylated utilizing the energy from adenosine triphosphate (ATP). In muscle, once the glucose is phosphorylated, that is, high energy bonds have been formed, it cannot leave the cell until it has been metabolized to 3-carbon units. This is not true in the liver, as blood glucose levels are maintained by glucose from liver glycogen.

After phosphorylation, the glucose molecule either is polymerized to form glycogen, or metabolized through glycolysis by a series of steps to 3-carbon units (Embden-Meyerhof pathway) (Fig. 2-2). The glycolysis can be either *aerobic* (in the presence of oxygen) or *anaerobic* (in the absence of oxygen). In either case, the process of glycolysis provides energy for the cell and leads to formation of two 3-carbon units. Pyruvic acid is formed in the presence of oxygen; lactic acid in the absence of oxygen.

When glycolysis occurs in the muscle, the pyruvate or lactate can be oxidized by the citric acid cycle [CAC, also known as the Krebs cycle, and the tricarboxylic acid cycle (TCA)] or released to the blood and transported to the liver which converts it back to glucose (Fig. 2-3). The CAC starts with a 4-carbon unit of oxaloacetic acid. Pyruvic acid is converted to a 2-carbon unit which

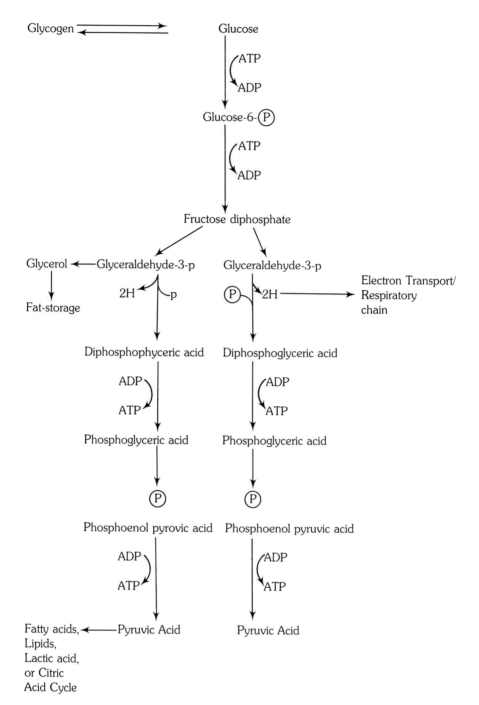

Fig. 2-2. The Embden-Meyerhof Pathway (anabolic glucose catabolism).

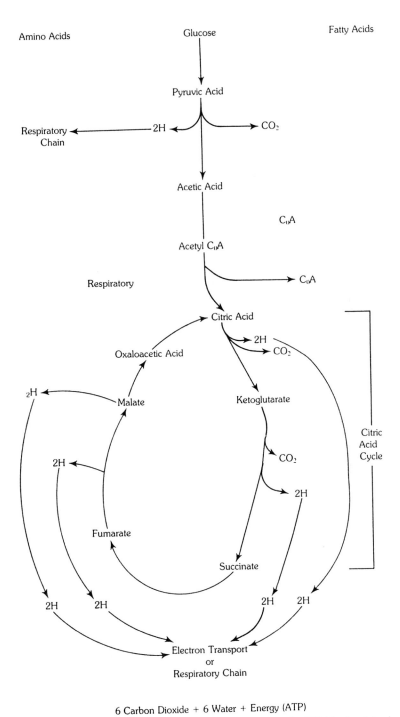

Fig. 2-3. A schematic representation of the citric-acid-cycle (CAC), the tricarboxylic acid cycle (TCA), or the Krebs cycle (aerobic catabolism).

Structure	Name

Saturated Fatty Acids

$CH_3 (CH_2)_{10} COOH$	Laurie
$CH_3 (CH_2)_{12} COOH$	Myristic
$CH_3 (CH_2)_{14} COOH$	Palmitic
$CH_3 (CH_2)_{16} COOH$	Stearic
$CH_3 (CH_2)_{18} COOH$	Arachidic
$CH_3 (CH_2)_{22} COOH$	Lignoceric

Unsturated Fatty Acids

$CH_3 (CH_2)_5 CH === CH (CH_2)_7 COOH$	Palmitoleic
$CH_3 (CH_2)_7 CH === CH (CH_2)_7 COOH$	Oleic
$CH_3 ((CH_2)_4 CH === CH (CH_2)_7 COOH$	Linoleic
$CH_3 cH_2 CH === CH CH_2 CH === CH CH_2 CH === CH$ $(CH_2)_7 COOH$	Linolenic
$CH_3 (CH_2)_4 (CH === CH CH_2)_3 CH === CH (CH_2)_3 COOH$	Arachidonic

Fig. 2-4.   Structure of saturated and unsaturated fatty acids.

combines with a 4-carbon unit to make the 6-carbon citric acid. A series of steps follows during which the 6-carbon citric acid is oxidized causing the removal of the CO_2 molecules in a series of energy-yielding reactions and the formation of the original 4-carbon unit. If a carbohydrate is fully oxidized by the body, the result is the formation of 6 molecules of CO_2 and 6 molecules of H_2O or water (Fig. 2-4).

Interrelationships That Influence Carbohydrate Metabolism

Carbohydrate metabolism is influenced by a number of hormones, vitamins, and minerals. Each will be discussed very briefly.

Hormones

Insulin.   Insulin is synthesized by the beta cells of the pancreas. It permits glucose to enter the cell, a prerequisite for glycolysis. When insulin levels increase, the blood glucose levels generally decrease since glucose leaves the blood and enters the cell.

Glucagon.   Glucagon, secreted by the alpha cells of the pancreas, causes blood glucose levels to increase. Glucagon influences the synthesis of glucose from the glycogen stored in the liver and from lactic acid and amino acids.

Epinephrine and norepinephrine. Epinephrine and norepinephrine are released from the adrenal medulla in response to stress. These hormones cause the breakdown of glycogen from the liver resulting in an increase in blood glucose. Increased levels of epinephrine and norepinephrine also are associated with resistance to insulin that results in an increased level of circulating blood glucose and a decreased availability of glucose for cellular metabolism. These responses are not uncommon in severely ill persons.

Vitamins

As will be discussed later, the primary role of the B vitamins in the body is to form active coenzymes that, in concert with enzymes, are involved in one of several of the metabolic steps required for glucose synthesis (*anabolism*) and degradation (*catabolism*). The overall metabolic reactions of carbohydrates will not occur unless both the coenzyme and the enzyme are present. For the coenzyme to be present, the vitamin must have been consumed in the diet of the individual. The specific vitamins necessary for carbohydrate metabolism are thiamine, riboflavin, niacin, pantothenic acid, biotin, folic acid, and pyridoxine.

Minerals

Several minerals are likewise needed for metabolism, namely, magnesium, chromium, and zinc. The most predominant, magnesium, is involved in most reactions with ATP. Chromium has been shown to be important in the uptake of glucose by the cells and zinc has been shown to be important in the binding of insulin to the cell surface. Glucose intolerance or high levels of glucose in the blood can occur if an individual is deficient in pyridoxine, chromium, or zinc.

Function

One function of carbohydrates is to produce energy. On the average, 1 carbohydrate molecule is able to yield 4 kcal of energy per g of carbohydrate. Note that the average energy requirement for an individual is 1500–2000 kcal/day depending on body size, gender, and activity. In addition, carbohydrates are building blocks for many other compounds particularly as part of glycoproteins and mucopolysaccharides. These complex molecules are important in maintaining the integrity of many cells, particularly the epithelial tissue. If the body takes in more carbohydrates than are needed, any excess is converted to and stored as fat.

LIPIDS

Lipids are composed of carbon, hydrogen, and oxygen with a generic formula of $CH_3\text{-}(CH_2)_n\text{-}COOH$. The lipids are much more reduced, that is, contain less oxygen, than carbohydrates. Because they contain long aliphatic carbon chains, they are not soluble in water and dissolve only in the so-called lipid solvents—ether, benzene, chloroform, and so on. Lipids can be divided into 3 groups: (1) the fatty acids, (2) lipids that contain glycerol, and (3) other lipids that do not contain glycerol.

Fatty acids vary in length from 4 to 22 or more carbon atoms, normally occurring with an even number of carbon atoms. Those with 6–8 carbons are considered short-chain fatty acids; with 8–12 carbons, a medium-chain fatty acid; and with 14 and greater, long-chain fatty acids. Each fatty acid can contain one or more double bonds. Medium- and short-chain fatty acids, however, usually contain only single bonds and are considered fully saturated.

Most lipid in the diet is in the form of triglycerides made up of 3 fatty acids attached to the molecule of glycerol. The properties of triglycerides are determined by their constituent fatty acids. Triglycerides composed of short- and medium-chain fatty acids are more likely to be solid than liquid at body temperatures. Likewise, triglycerides composed of more unsaturated fatty acids are more likely to be liquid than solid at body temperature. Vegetable oils are liquid at room temperature because they are highly unsaturated. In contrast, animal fat such as lard, is made of more saturated and longer-chain fatty acids.

Phospholipid, another form of lipid present in the diet, is also synthesized by the body. Phospholipids are glycerol esters that contain 2 fatty acids with phosphoric acid esterified to the terminal hydroxyl group of glycerol. Ethanol-amine, serine, or choline is esterified on the phosphate. Phospholipids are very prominent in the membranes of the cell and are more likely to contain polyunsaturated fatty acids than saturated fatty acids.

Polyunsaturated fatty acids are essential in the diet. The primary fatty acid in the diet is linoleic acid (18 carbons with 2 double bonds), a precursor to arachidonic acid which is a 20-carbon acid with 4 double bonds. Linoleic acid is considered essential since the body is unable to synthesize it. It is found in the polyunsaturated fatty oils from plant sources and in breast milk.

In addition to the esters of glycerol, some other lipids do not contain glycerol. These lipids are esters of an alcohol called spengosine and are found primarily in tissue of the central nervous system.

Body lipids are either supplied from extraneous sources such as diet or parenteral feeding or are synthesized as needed by the body. Dietary sources of lipids include fats, oils, butter, margarine, meat, nuts, eggs, chocolate, peanut butter, cheeses, ice cream, whole milk and milk products, olives, avocados, and many other foods.

Additional polyunsaturated fatty acids generally are obtained from plant sources such as the oils derived from corn, soy bean, safflower, and cotton seeds. Polyunsaturated fatty acids have been shown to be effective in reducing blood levels of cholesterol and in reducing blood pressure in both normotensive and mildly hypertensive individuals.

Dietary lipids are emulsified by the action of gastric lipase and bile salts in the small intestine. The emulsified tri-, di-, and monoglycerides then are digested by pancreatic and intestinal lipase resulting in di- and monoglycerides, fatty

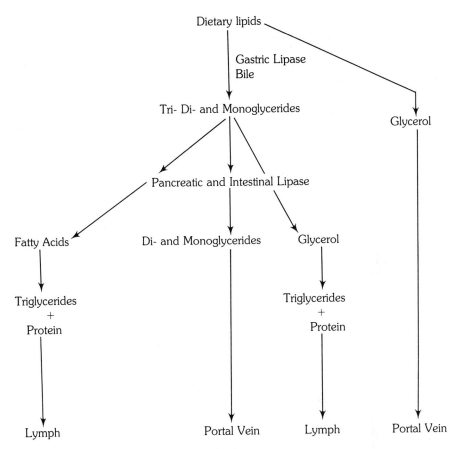

Fig. 2-5. Digestion and absorption of lipids.

acids, and glycerol. These lipid end-products are absorbed from the intestinal lumen into the systemic blood flow with di- and monoglycerides and glycerol being absorbed into the portal vein. Larger fatty acid chains are formed into triglycerides that are absorbed by the lymph and systemic blood (Fig. 2-5).

Dietary lipid usually represents 40–45 percent of the total caloric intake of Americans. The U. S. dietary goals of the Select Committee on Nutrition and Human Needs[1] suggest that fat consumption should be reduced to 30 percent of the total energy intake. Approximately 10 percent of the lipid intake should be polyunsaturated fat.

Lipids function primarily as structural components (in membranes) or as energy stores. Heart and muscle in the resting state use a larger proportion of fat than carbohydrate as energy. Carbohydrate becomes a fuel for tissue only in cases of excess activity.

Structurally, the cell membrane and other portions of the cell that are made of lipids form a nonaqueous part of the cell. They have some unique roles, as far as metabolism is concerned, that require special fat soluble antioxidants such as vitamin E to be maintained.

The other function of lipids is to provide a form for the storage of energy. All excess energy taken into the body that is not immediately utilized is stored as fat. The body stores no protein and very little carbohydrate as reserve energy sources. Any calories, in whatever form, that are not expended are converted to triglycerides by the body and deposited in adipose tissue. These energy stores then can be utilized when needed for energy. In addition to the synthesis of storage lipid, the body also synthesizes steroids such as cholersterol and steroid hormones. Phospholipids and other complex lipids also are synthesized and used as structural lipids.

Interrelationships That Influence Lipid Metabolism

As with carbohydrates and protein, lipids also are influenced by various hormones and vitamins and have many interrelated enzyme reactions with carbohydrates and amino acids.

Hormones

Many hormones influence the metabolism of lipids. Some examples follow.

Insulin. High insulin levels inhibit the release of triglycerides from stored adipose tissue. When insulin levels are high due to high serum glucose levels, fatty acids are not released from adipose tissue since high insulin levels favor fatty acid synthesis. As a result, fatty acids cannot be used for energy needs. This role is particularly important in the parenterally-fed patient receiving high levels of glucose.

Epinephrine. Epinephrine stimulates enzymes involved in clearing chylomicrons and mucoproteins from the blood.

Vitamins

Vitamins known to influence catabolic reactions and lipidogensis are briefly discussed here.

Niacin and riboflavin. Niacin and riboflavin are involved in the oxidation and reduction (both the breakdown and the buildup) of the fatty acid chains. In addition, the coenzymes of these vitamins are involved in the formation of the double bonds of long-chain fatty acids.

Pantothenic acid. Almost all metabolic reactions in the formation of long-chain fatty acids and steroids involve reactions with coenzyme A. Since pantothenic acid is part of coenzyme A, it is essential in all of these reactions.

PROTEINS

Proteins are polymers of amino acids. The individual amino acids contain carbon, hydrogen, oxygen, nitrogen, and sometimes sulphur. Each amino acid has at least one carboxylic acid group (COOH) and one alpha-amino group (NH_2). The alpha indicates that the amino group is on the carbon next to the carboxylic acid. Approximately 21 different amino acids commonly are found in proteins.

In the body, some amino acids can be synthesized by transferring an amino group to the appropriate carbon oxygen skeleton. These amino acids are called *nonessential.* Other amino acids that the body cannot make and that must be obtained from the diet are called *essential* amino acids (see Table 2-1). Essentiality can be due to either a total inability to make the amino acid or, as in the case of young growing children, the inability to make an adequate amount. In either case, additional amino acid must be supplied from the diet.

Each amino acid has its own distinct metabolic pathway that ultimately leads to oxidation to CO_2, water, and ammonia or urea. Urea contains two amino groups, oxygen and 1-carbon. Thus, incomplete oxidation results in obtaining less than the potentially available energy from protein. Protein yields approximately 4 kcal/g of available energy. In addition to the individual metabolic pathways, some amino acids, when they are split, yield carbon structures that can make glucose through a process called *gluconeogenesis.* That is, these carbon structures fit into the glycolytic pathway and therefore are further metabolized as if they are carbohydrate from pyruvate through the CAC to produce energy, or they are resynthesized to form glucose.

Other amino acids are ketogenic, that is, they are metabolized into carbon structures that fit into the lipid metabolic pathways and can form ketone bodies. Ketogenic amino acids are catabolized from acetyl CoA to ketone and cholesterol. These amino acids cannot contribute to the formation of blood glucose. Still other amino acids have branched chains; a portion of their carbon structure is glucogenic and a portion is ketogenic. Branched-chain amino acids are being shown to have an important role in parenteral feeding of hypermetabolic patients.

Dietary protein can be considered to be of different biological quality. Designations consider how efficiently a particular protein can be utilized by the body. Several different criteria are used. The quality of food may be related to the ability to contribute to body protein. A second criterion measures the ratio of essential:nonessential amino acids in the food. This particular property is important in choosing protein to be supplied to young children who need a

Table 2-1
Classifications Used to Describe Amino Acids

Amino Acid	Essential	Nonessential	Glucogenic	Ketogenic	Branched-Chain
Glycine		X	X		
Alanine		X	X		
Methionine	X		X		
Aspartic Acid		X	X		
Glutamic Acid		X	X		
Valine	X		X		X
Leucine	X			X	X
Isoleucine	X		X	X	X
Phenylalanine	X		X	X	
Tyrosine		X	X	X	
Tryptophan	X		X		
Lysine	X			X	
Arginine		X			
Histidine	X		X		
Serine		X	X		
Threonine	X		X		
Proline		X	X		
Asparagine		X	X		
Glutamine		X	X		
Hydroxyproline		X	X		
Arginine		X	X		
Infants and Children Only					
Cystine-Cysteine	X		X		

higher ratio of essential:nonessential amino acids than do adults. The essential amino acids should be present in an "ideal" molar ratio to produce the most efficient utilization. This often is termed the *amino acid pattern* of a protein. What is commonly used as a standard for the "ideal" molar ratio is the ratio of essential amino acids in either whole egg or human serum.

For the dietary amino acids to be utilized in protein synthesis, all amino acids must be present at approximately the same time. Some foods contain different quantities of the essential amino acids than others and may in fact be quite low or limiting in a single amino acid. In general, animal proteins have more essential amino acids in a desired ratio to each other than do plant proteins. They are considered therefore to have a higher biological quality than plant proteins. In addition, plant proteins often are associated with fiber and other carbohydrates that limit their digestibility. If amino acids are not available for absorption, protein is considered of lower quality. For this reason vegetarians must pay attention to the concept of complementarity. Sources of vegetable protein may be rich in many amino acids, but provide poor sources of others. Combining foods of these sources with other foods in the meal that are rich in the deficient amino acid sources complements the quality of protein in the entire meal.

Prior to utilization by the body, amino acids must be denatured and hydrolyzed to at least peptides (molecules containing a limited number of amino acids) or amino acids. The initial denaturation process occurs by cooking, which makes the protein more easily digestible. The first enzymatic step to initiate digestion occurs in the stomach as a result of an enzyme called *pepsin*. Pepsin is an *endopeptidase*; that is, it breaks peptide bonds in the internal structure of the protein to yield large polypeptides. Other endopeptidases, trypsin and chymotrypsin, further hydrolyze the protein after it passes to the duodenum. This is followed by a series of exopeptidases that hydrolyze specific peptide bonds between specific amino acids and yield small peptides often 2–3 amino acids large. The amino acids comprising a peptide are linked by peptide bonds (carboxylic acid linked to an amino group). These bonds can be hydrolyzed to form individual amino acids.

Absorption of Proteins

Absorption occurs when either the free amino acids or small peptides attach to specific sites in the intestinal epithelial cells. If a peptide attaches to the epithelial cell during either the process of absorption or immediately after absorption, it is hydrolyzed to amino acids. Absorption sites exist for neutral, acid, and basic amino acids. The availability of absorption sites limits the quality of amino acids that can be absorbed within a given time. If a tripeptide attaches to the absorption sites, 3 amino acids are absorbed in the same time that 1 amino acid would be absorbed if an individual amino acid was attached to that site. This concept of absorption suggests that, other things being equal, preparations intended for tube feeding or enteral nutrition should contain di- and tripeptides as well as amino acids.

The body is constantly breaking down and building new protein. During growth and in pregnancy, the body is making more protein than it is breaking down and therefore is in what is termed *positive nitrogen balance*—more nitrogen is being retained by the body than is being excreted. When an individual is in nitrogen balance, the amount of nitrogen excreted equals the amount of nitrogen ingested. During other conditions, a person might be in *negative nitrogen balance*—more nitrogen is excreted than is ingested. Negative nitrogen balance commonly occurs during times of restricted food intake, disease, or trauma.

During times of positive nitrogen balance, the body does not store additional protein for future use. Instead, all excess protein is converted to either fat or carbohydrate depending on the metabolic pathway and need. If the total caloric intake is in excess of need, extra calories are stored as fat. The first requirement of the body is the supplying of an adequate amount of calories. In times of limited caloric intake, sufficient fat or carbohydrate calories are not present. Ingested protein will be utilized as calories, and, in this sense, carbohydrate allows the protein ingested to be utilized for the synthesis of new body protein.

All body protein is considered functional; none exists in a storage form. Approximately 80 percent of body weight is made up of muscle; however, in time of need the muscle becomes a large reservoir that can be broken down. The development of muscle mass, however, relates to activity of muscles and not to the amount of protein consumed. This assumes that an adequate amount of protein is available.

Proteins have many functions. Some provide structural elements for cells; others are metabolically active as enzymes or hormones. Still others have transport function (e.g., hemoglobin, transferring retinal binding protein).

Interrelationships That Influence Protein Metabolism

The metabolism of the individual amino acids is related closely to both carbohydrate and lipid metabolism. A portion of the carbon structure of amino acids is converted to either compounds that can fit into the carbohydrate or lipid metabolic pathways. In the formation of nonessential amino acids, carbon structures additionally are primarily derived from either the metabolism of glucose or lipids. The proper metabolism of amino acids requires several vitamins (pyridoxine, folic acid, etc.) and hormones (insulin, growth hormone).

The body needs macronutrients, as previously discussed, and many micronutrients. The availability of micronutrients in food often is used to judge the quality of that food.

MICRONUTRIENTS

Minerals

The essential elements can be classified either as *electrolytes* that are required in larger quantities (sodium, potassium, calcium, magnesium) or as *trace elements* that are required in much smaller quantities. Even though much is known about the requirement of many trace elements, the interrelationships of the trace elements with each other, as well as with vitamins, are just beginning to be understood. Each of the required minerals will be discussed very briefly.

Calcium

Calcium is an essential element of bone with 98 percent of the body calcium being found in bone. The regulation of many cellular functions is dependent, however, on ionic calcium. Calcium is involved in the transmission of nerve impulses, the contraction of muscle cells, and the activity of many hormones. Calcium also is involved in the blood clotting process; the absence of calcium prevents blood clotting. The amount of body calcium is under control from both absorption and excretion. The blood levels of calcium are controlled carefully and are influenced by vitamin D, parathyroid hormone, and calcitonin.

Phosphorus

Phosphorus is the second most prominent mineral in bone and teeth and is found in many cells. As part of phospholipids, phosphorus is present in membranes, and as part of ATP, it is essential for the formation and utilization of energy. A proper ratio between the dietary intake of calcium and phosphorus is essential to ensure the absorption of both elements.

Iodine

Iodine is required in much smaller quantities (micrograms) and is primarily a constituent of thyroid hormones. These hormones are involved in the regulation of metabolic activity of the body.

Iron

The quantity of iron in the body is measured in grams primarily because of the prevalence in hemoglobin in the red blood cell. Other enzymes such as myoglobin in the muscle also carry oxygen and are involved in the oxidative pathways of the body. Iron deficiency is the most common nutritional deficiency in the U.S. population largely due to the needs of women and children.

Magnesium

Magnesium is an intracellular element that is associated with the activity of many enzymes, particularly those enzymes involved with the utilization of ATP. Magnesium is involved in the synthesis of fat, carbohydrate, and protein, as well as nerve transmission and muscle contraction.

Zinc

Interest in zinc nutrition has renewed in the past few years. Zinc has been shown to be required for the synthesis of DNA in protein; hence a zinc deficiency can cause the retardation of growth and the lack of brain development. In addition, insulin and a number of enzymes require zinc for proper function.

Copper

Copper is an element found in many oxidative processes of cells and other oxidative enzymes. It also must be present in adequate amounts for the proper utilization of iron.

Fluoride

Fluoride has been shown to be an essential element in the formation of the crystalline structure of both bone and teeth. Tooth enamel containing fluoride has heightened resistance to tooth decay.

Vitamins

Vitamins must be present for proper metabolism and growth. Vitamins are organic compounds required in the diet that serve catalytic functions with many metabolic processes. In general, the vitamin is converted to a *coenzyme form* that plays an integral role in enzymatic pathways. Vitamins are classified by solubility as either water soluble or fat soluble.

Water Soluble Vitamins

Folacin (folic acid).   Folacin is involved in the synthesis of purines and pyrimidines which are constituents of RNA and DNA. In addition, it is involved in the synthesis of methionine, histidine, serine, and choline. Folacin is important in cell division and cellular growth. If adequate folacin is not present, cells will not thrive. This particularly affects the synthesis of blood cells and the epithelial lining of the intestinal tract. Deficiencies are evidenced by large, immature red cells (megaloblastic anemia) and by small intestinal villae with reduced absorptive capacity.

Niacin.   Niacin is an exception to the general rule that vitamins must be synthesized outside the body. Some niacin can be synthesized from the amino acid tryptophan, if adequate tryptophan is available. The coenzymes of niacin are involved in the oxidation and reduction of carbohydrates and lipids.

Riboflavin.   Riboflavin is a vitamin that is part of the B complex whose coenzymes function in the oxidation and reduction of fat, carbohydrate, and proteins.

Thiamin.   Thiamin is an important part of the oxidative conversion of pyruvic acid and, hence, the CAC. Thiamin also is part of certain nerve cells and is required for proper transmission of nerve impulses.

Pyridoxine (vitamin B_6).   As part of the B complex, pyridoxine is particularly involved in the metabolism of amino acids and the transfer or oxidation of the amino groups.

Cobalamin (vitamin B_{12}).   The coenzymes of B_{12} are involved in metabolism of 1-carbon units and the formation of purines and, therefore, RNA and DNA. This vitamin is required for cell division.

Vitamin C (ascorbic acid).   Ascorbic acid is a water soluble antioxidant. It assists in iron absorption and the conversion of proline to hydroxyproline during the synthesis of collagen. Ascorbic acid is essential for the maintenance of the epithelial cell wall.

Fat Soluble Vitamins

Vitamin A (retinol).   Vitamin A is required in many functions of the body, most prominently in the visual process. Retinol is found in the visual pigments of the eye for both dim light (black and white) vision as well as color vision. In addition, vitamin A is required for the synthesis of certain polysaccharides and is essential in the formation of many membranes of the body. Vitamin A has been found to be needed for proper immune functions, particularly in antigen recognition.

Vitamin D.   Vitamin D is converted to hormones in the body that are directly involved in the regulation of calcium and phosphorus. This regulation includes not only the absorption of calcium, but also the deposition and release of calcium from the bone and teeth. It also appears to be involved in the entrance of calcium into certain cells or cell nuclei.

Vitamin E.   Vitamin E is a fat-soluble antioxidant that protects other organic compounds from being oxidized. In particular, the presence of vitamin E will prevent the oxidation and destruction of vitamin A. It also prevents the rancidity reactions of polyunsaturated fatty acids. The oxidation of unsaturated fatty acids found in membranes causes the membranes to break and results in cellular destruction. This can be prevented by vitamin E.

Vitamin K.   Vitamin K is a fat-soluble vitamin that is involved in blood clotting. It has been shown to be involved in the formation of certain dicarboxylic amino acids that bind calcium.

NUTRITION IN HEALTH

Healthy individuals vary considerably in their need for specific nutrients due in part to gender, age, body size, rate of growth, activity level, metabolic rate, body stores of specific nutrients, climate, and many other factors. Without costly studies, the exact requirement for a specific nutrient in an individual cannot be known.

A number of means are available for healthy individuals, families, and groups to ensure a selection of food that will provide an adequate intake of nutrients and will avoid excesses. The most notable means are (1) the Basic Four based on the USDA Daily Food Guide,[2] (2) Dietary Goals from the Senate Select Committee on Nutrition and Human Needs,[1] (3) USDA Daily Food Guide,[2] and (4) the Recommended Dietary Allowance (RDA) of the Committee on Dietary Allowances of the Food and Nutrition Board.[3]

The Basic Four[2] utilizes the concept of food groups, suggesting the number of servings of food from each group that should be eaten daily. This plan is easy to interpret, but it does not give assurance that all nutrient needs will be met

Table 2-2
Recommended Dietary Allowances, Revised 1980*
Designed for the Maintenance of Good Nutrition of Practically All Healthy People in the U.S.A.

Age and Sex Group	Weight kg	Weight lb	Height cm	Height in	Protein g	Fat-Soluble Vitamins vitamin A µg R.E.†	vitamin D µg‡	vitamin E mg T.E.	Water-Soluble Vitamins vitamin C mgα	thiamine mg	riboflavin mg	niacin mg N.E.§	vitamin B_6 mg	folacin µg	vitamin B_{12} µg	Minerals calcium mg	phosphorus mg	magnesium mg	iron mg	zinc mg	iodine µg
Infants																					
0.0–0.5 yr.	6	13	60	24	kg × 2.2	420	10	3	35	0.3	0.4	6	0.3	30	0.5¶	360	240	50	10	3	40
0.5–1.0 yr.	9	20	71	28	kg × 2.0	400	10	4	35	0.5	0.6	8	0.6	45	1.5	540	360	70	15	5	50
Children																					
1–3 yr.	13	29	90	35	23	400	10	5	45	0.7	0.8	9	0.9	100	2.0	800	800	150	15	10	70
4–6 yr.	20	44	112	44	30	500	10	6	45	0.9	1.0	11	1.3	200	2.5	800	800	200	10	10	90
7–10 yr.	28	62	132	52	34	700	10	7	45	1.2	1.4	16	1.6	300	3.0	800	800	250	10	10	120
Males																					
11–14 yr.	45	99	157	62	45	1000	10	8	50	1.4	1.6	18	1.8	400	3.0	1200	1200	350	18	15	150
15–18 yr.	66	145	176	69	56	1000	10	10	60	1.4	1.7	18	2.0	400	3.0	1200	1200	400	18	15	150
19–22 yr.	70	154	177	70	56	1000	7.5	10	60	1.5	1.7	19	2.2	400	3.0	800	800	350	10	15	150

23–50 yr.	70	154	178	70	56	1000	5	10	60	1.4	1.6	18	2.2	400	3.0	800	800	350	10	15	150
51 + yr.	70	154	178	70	56	1000	5	10	60	1.4	1.6	16	2.2	400	3.0	800	800	350	10	15	150
Females																					
11–14 yr.	46	101	157	62	46	800	10	8	50	1.1	1.3	15	1.8	400	3.0	1200	1200	300	18	15	150
15–18 yr.	55	120	163	64	46	800	10	8	60	1.1	1.3	14	2.0	400	3.0	1200	1200	300	18	15	150
19–22 yr.	55	120	163	64	44	800	7.5	8	60	1.1	1.3	14	2.0	400	3.0	800	800	300	18	15	150
23–50 yr.	55	120	163	64	44	800	5	8	60	1.0	1.2	13	2.0	400	3.0	800	800	300	18	15	150
51 + yr.	55	120	163	64	44	800	5	8	60	1.0	1.2	13	2.0	400	3.0	800	800	300	10	15	150
Pregnancy||					+30	+200	+5	+2	+20	+0.4	+0.3	+2	+0.6	+400	+1.0	+400	+400	+150		+5	+25
Lactation					+20	+400	+5	+3	+40	+0.5	+0.5	+5	+0.5	+100	+1.0	+400	+400	+150		+10	+50

From: Food and Nutrition Board, National Academy of Sciences-National Research Council

*The allowances are intended to provide for individual variations among most normal persons as they live in the United States under usual environmental stresses. Diets should be based on a variety of common foods in order to provide other nutrients for which human requirements have been less well defined.

†Retinol equivalents; 1 retinol equivalent = 1 μg retinol or 6 μg β-carotene.

‡As cholecalciferol: 10 μg cholecalciferol = 400 IU vitamin D.

§α-toco-pherol equivalents: 1 mg d-α-tocopherol × 1αT.E. N.E. (niacin equivalent) = 1 mg niacin or 60 mg dietary tryptophan.

¶The RDA for vitamin B_{12} in infants is based on average concentration of the vitamin in human milk. The allowances after weaning are based on energy intake (as recommended by the American Academy of Pediatrics) and consideration of other factors, such as intestinal absorption.

||The increased requirement during pregnancy cannot be met by the iron content of habitual American diets or by the existing iron stores of many women; therefore, the use of 30 to 60 mg supplemental iron is recommended. Iron needs during lactation are not substantially different from those of non-pregnant women, but continued supplementation of the mother for two to three months is recommended.

since the prevalence of some micronutrients is not known. The Dietary Goals outline specific dietary changes that may produce health benefits. Its focus is on the development of sound eating patterns rather than methods for planning meals and meeting the RDA. The USDA Food Guide[2] assists in planning daily nutrient intake and identifying adequate serving sizes. No assurance exists, however, that all nutrient needs will be met daily. Despite limitations in each of these methods, they can be used effectively to teach patients and families the basics of good nutrition.

Knowledge of the RDA can be important when assessing the adequacy of dietary intake among groups of individuals. The RDA consists of recommendations of average daily nutrients that population groups need in order to meet the requirements of most individuals who are healthy. The estimates for average daily intake have been made to exceed the needs of most persons to ensure safe intake levels for most of the population, even for those who have difficulty with nutrient absorption and utilization. When assessing the dietary intake of individuals, it is important to remember that intakes below 100 percent of the RDA are not necessarily inadequate. Studies of population groups often use dietary intakes of two-thirds or less of the RDA as criteria for evaluating the individual "at risk" for deficiency.

The RDA for major nutrients based on age, gender, height, and weight are presented in Table 2-2. It should be noted that, when using this table to evaluate adequacy of dietary intake, the Food and Nutrition Board,[3] National Academy of Sciences-National Research Council, suggests diets based on a variety of foods since recommendations for all nutrients have not been established.

The RDA for energy intake (Table 2-3) is based on factors that influence energy need such as gender, height for weight, age, and activity level. This table reflects the range of energy needs based on the usual energy output of adults. The decreased metabolic rate of the elderly also has been considered, but alterations in the requirements of the elderly for other nutrients has yet to be addressed.

It is important to recognize that failure to ingest specific nutrients does not immediately result in clinical signs and symptoms of deficiencies. Clinical signs and symptoms are not frequently seen among healthy individuals in the United States who have adequate dietary intake. It is more common to observe deficiencies among persons with decreased intake, chronic illness, malabsorption, acute illness, or acute stress after periods of inadequate intake. A summary of the major nutrients, dietary sources, major body functions, and effects of inadequate or excess intake are presented in Table 2-4.[4]

ALTERATIONS DURING ILLNESS

Disease states produce varying levels of stress on individuals. Stress results in neurohumoral responses that alter metabolism thereby influencing energy requirements and the biosynthesis of carbohydrates, fat, and protein.

Table 2-3
RDA Recommended Energy Intake[*]

Category	Age (years)	Weight (kg)	Weight (lb)	Height (cm)	Height (in)	(kcal)	Energy Needs (With Range)	(MJ)
Infants	0.0–0.5	6	13	60	24	kg × 115	(95–145)	kg × 0.48
	0.5–1.0	9	20	71	28	kg × 105	(80–135)	kg × 0.44
Children	1–3	13	29	90	35	1300	(900–1800)	5.5
	4–6	20	44	122	44	1700	(1300–2300)	7.1
	7–10	28	62	132	52	2400	(1650–3300)	10.1
Males	11–14	45	99	157	62	2700	(2300–3700)	11.3
	15–18	66	145	176	69	2800	(2100–3900)	11.8
	19–22	70	154	177	70	2900	(2500–3300)	12.2
	23–50	70	154	178	70	2700	(2300–3100)	11.3
	51–75	70	154	178	70	2400	(2000–2800)	10.1
	76+	70	154	178	70	2050	(1650–2450)	8.6
Females	11–14	46	101	157	62	2200	(1500–3000)	9.2
	15–18	55	120	163	64	2100	(1200–3000)	8.8
	19–22	55	120	163	64	2100	(1700–2500)	8.8
	23–50	55	120	163	64	2000	(1600–2400)	8.4
	51–75	55	120	163	64	1800	(1400–2200)	7.6
	76+	55	120	163	64	1600	(1200–2000)	6.7
Pregnancy						+300		
Lactation						+500		

From Recommended Dietary Allowances, Food and Nutrition Board, National Academy of Sciences-National Research Council, Washington, DC, Revised 1980, p 23.
*The energy allowances for the young adults are for men and women doing light work. The allowances for the two older age groups represent mean energy needs over these spans, allowing for a 2 percent decrease in basal (resting) metabolic rate per decade and a reduction in activity of 200 kcal/day for men and women between 51 and 75 years; 500 kcal for men over 75 years and 400 kcal for women over 75. The customary range of daily energy output is shown for adults in parentheses and is based on a variation in energy needs of + 400 kcal at any one age, emphasizing the wide range of energy intakes appropriate for any group of people.

Energy allowances for children through age 18 are based on median energy intakes of children these ages followed in longitudinal growth studies. The values in parentheses are 10th and 90th percentiles of energy intake, to indicate the range of energy consumption among children of these ages.

The level of stress has been related to the amount of urinary nitrogen excretion, plasma glucose, glucagon, insulin, and lactate levels, and to oxygen consumption.[5] The levels of stress, rated from zero for unstressed fasting states to three for septic and hypermetabolic states, are useful in understanding nutrient requirements in a variety of patient conditions.

In stress states, levels of norepenephrine, epinephrine, and cortisol are

(Text continues p. 54)

Table 2-4
Major Nutrients, Dietary Sources, Bodily Functions, and Signs and Symptoms of Inadequacy or Excess

Nutrient	Dietary Sources	Major Body Functions	Effects of Inadequacy*	Effects of Excess
Protein	meat, poultry, fish, dried beans and peas, lentils, egg, cheese, milk, legumes, nuts, seeds	provides the building material (amino acids) for growth, repair and maintenance of every cell; regulates fluid balance between blood and cells; supplies energy at 4 kcal/g	kwashiorkor (loss of weight and muscle mass), decreased immune response, increased susceptibility to infection, edema	reduced calcium retention, weight gain and obesity
Carbohydrate	cereal grains, pastas, bread, fruits, vegetables, potato milk, corn, dried peas and beans, sugar, jelly, candy	provides energy for body processes and physical activity; aids in utilization of fat and spares protein; supplies 4 kcal/g	marasmus, weight loss, growth retardation	weight gain and obesity
Fat	butter, margarine, shortening, oil, lard, salad dressing, cream, egg yolk, meat and the fat surrounding it, whole milk, cheese, fried food, peanut butter	supplies energy in a concentrated form; carrier of fat-soluble vitamins, supplies essential fatty acids; insulates the body and promotes the maintenance of normal body temperature; supplies 9 kcal/g	flaky and scaly skin, diarrhea, poor growth, loss of hair, increased susceptibility to infection	increased levels of triglycerides and cholestrol in the blood, accumulation of adipose, tissue, weight gain and obesity
Fat-Soluble Vitamins: Vitamin A (Retinol equivalents, mcg)	liver, carrots, sweet potato, dark green leafy vegetables, broccoli, winter squash, apricots, cantaloupe, peaches, milk, fish liver oil	important component in visual process of the eye including adaptation to dark; assists in formation and maintenance of skin, mucous membranes, bones, teeth	xerophthalmia (an eye condition leading to blindness), night blindness, permanent blindness, poor growth	yellow pigmentation of skin, loss of appetite, vomiting

Nutrient	Important Sources	Some Major Physiological Functions	Some Deficiency Symptoms	Some Toxicity Symptoms
Vitamin D (mcg)	salt water fish and their oils, fortified milk and margarine, eggs, liver, butter (can be synthesized with skin exposure to sunlight)	promotes mineralization of bones and teeth; necessary in absorption and regulation of calcium and phosphorus	rickets (bone deformation), osteomalacia (softening of bones)	poor growth, weight loss, vomiting, poor appetite, calcium deposition in soft tissues
Vitamin E (mcg)	seeds, fats, and polyunsaturated oils of vegetable products, whole grains	allows vitamin A unsaturated fatty acids to perform their specific functions; protects red blood cells from oxidation	anemia in premature infants, no other deficiency syndrome cited for man	none reported
Water-Soluble Vitamins:				
Ascorbic Acid (Vitamin C) (mg)	citrus fruits, strawberries, cantaloupe, cabbage, broccoli, dark green leafy vegetables, green pepper, tomato	assists in maintaining collagen (supportive material) which gives structure to cells; promotes iron absorption; helps in wound healing	scurvy, easy bruising, slow wound healing, fatigue, muscle ache, swollen joints degeneration of skin, teeth, gums, and blood vessels	increased requirement for vitamin C, kidney stone, interference with anticoagulant therapy and glycosuric tests
Folacin (Folic Acid) (mcg)	dark green leafy vegetables, liver, dried beans and peas, nuts, whole grain or fortified cereals, seeds	assists in red blood cell formation; helps enzymes and other biochemical systems function	anemia, GI disturbances	none reported

Table 2-4 (continued)

Nutrient	Dietary Sources	Major Body Functions	Effects of Inadequacy[*]	Effects of Excess
Niacin (Niacin Equivalents) (mg)	meat, poultry, fish, liver, whole grain or fortified cereal products, cereal brans	key component of coenzymes necessary to release food energy; aids digestion; promotes normal appetite	pellagra, skin and GI lesions, diarrhea, depression, anxiety	flushing, burning, and tingling around the neck and hands
Riboflavin (mg)	milk, milk products, liver, dark green leafy vegetables	functions as part of coenzymes that assist in energy release; component in protein, carbohydrate, and fat metabolism	cheilosis (cracks at corners of the mouth), soreness of lips, redness of tongue, poor growth, increased blood vessels in eye	none reported
Thiamin (mg)	pork and liver, cashews, whole grain or fortified cereal products, dried peas and beans	functions as part of coenzyme in the metabolism of carbohydrates and fat; promotes growth, good appetite, and muscle tone	beriberi; peripheral nerve changes, edema, heart failure, loss of appetite, depression, muscle tenderness, low blood pressure	none reported
Vitamin B-6 (Pyridoxine) (mg)	liver, poultry, meat, vegetables, whole grain or fortified cereals, seeds, bananas	involved in metabolism of protein and amino acids	anemia, irritability, convulsions, skin lesions, peripheral nerve changes, cracks at corners of the mouth	none reported
Vitamin B-12 (mcg)	meat, fish, poultry, eggs, milk, and dairy products (not present in plant foods)	assists in maintenance of nerve tissue and normal blood formation	pernicious anemia, neurologic disorders	none reported

Minerals:

Mineral	Sources	Functions	Deficiency Symptoms	Excess Symptoms
Calcium (mg)	milk, milk products, dark green leafy vegetables, fish with small edible bones	needed for bone and tooth formation, blood clotting, nerve transmission	facial paresthesia (abnormal sensation), osteoporosis (abnormal porosity of bone), rickets, bone deformation, stunted growth	heart irregularities
Phosphorus (mg)	milk, milk products, meat, fish, poultry, eggs, legumes, nuts	needed for bone and tooth formation, acid-base balance, assists cells use energy	paresthesia of hands and feet (abnormal sensation), weakness, demineralization of bone, seizures	erosion of jaw
Iodine (mcg)	salt water fish, shell-fish, iodized salt	constituent of thyroid hormone, thyroxin, that regulates metabolic rate	goiter (enlargement of thyroid gland)	depressed thyroid activity
Iron (mg)	liver, beef, pork, nuts, dried beans and peas, enriched or fortified cereals and breads, dark green leafy vegetables	constituent of hemoglobin and enzymes involved in energy metabolism	iron deficiency anemia, fatigue	siderosis, cirrhosis of liver
Magnesium (mg)	fortified cereals, whole grains, dark green leafy vegetables, legumes, nuts	activates enzymes, involved in protein synthesis, helps nerves and muscles work	growth failure, behavioral disturbances, tremor spasms	diarrhea
Zinc (mg)	oysters, beef, pork, liver, dried peas and beans, whole grain or fortified cereals, nuts	constituent of several enzymes and of insulin	delayed wound healing, retarded sexual and physical development, hair loss, severe rash similar to acne, loss of taste acuity, depression, skin lesions	fever, nausea, vomiting, diarrhea

From Basic Nutrition Facts. Michigan Department of Public Health, Lansing, 1980.
*Although nutrient deficiency diseases (kwashiorkor, marasmus, xeropthalmia, rickets, scurvy, pellagra, beriberi) may be rare, the effects of inadequate nutrient intake may be evident in a variety of less well-defined signs. These effects of inadequacy are also often associated with malabsorption problems or other metabolic diseases.

increased. These increases are accompanied by increased plasma glucagon and insulin levels.[5] The glucagon: insulin ratio increases as does insulin resistance; high levels of plasma glucose persist despite high levels of plasma insulin. Despite the increased plasma glucose pool in this hypermetabolic state, the peripheral utilization of glucose decreases. Clinically, the plasma glucose level would be expected to increase moderately (in individuals without a history of diabetes) following general elective surgery or multiple trauma (plasma glucose level of approximately 150 ± 25 mg/dl). Sepsis and hypermetabolic states are characterized by markedly elevated plasma glucose (plasma glucose approximately 250 ± 50 mg/dl).

Decreased peripheral utilization of glucose is accompanied by fat mobilization to meet the energy requirements.[5] Triglyceride levels may increase markedly, rising nearly twofold in the acute septic patient when compared with nonseptic general surgery patients.

The metabolic response to stress is reflected by increased protein catabolism and increased utilization of amino acids for energy. Amino acids, particularly branched-chain amino acids (leucine, isoleucine, valine), are utilized as a source of energy.[5,6] The catabolic state results in increased nitrogen loss exceeding 15 g/day in hypermetabolic states, compared with 5–10 g/day following general elective surgery.[5]

Energy Requirements

Energy requirements have been measured during a variety of patient activities.[7] Caloric expenditures were calculated by measuring oxygen consumption, carbon dioxide production, and urinary nitrogen losses. The average normal man (70 kg) uses approximately 23 kcal/kg of body weight per day just lying awake in bed. This energy requirement is increased by 20 percent when average hospital activity is added to this resting need.

Resting energy expenditure increases as a result of stress (Table 2-5). Elective surgery results in very small increases in the expenditure of resting energy, but more major trauma or illness has been shown to produce hypermetabolic stress states increasing energy requirements by nearly 200 percent. The activity of hospitalized patients generally is considered to increase energy needs by 20 percent.[7]

MALNUTRITION

Body Composition

The net result of dietary intake is reflected in the composition and functioning of the human body. Total body mass is composed of fat stores, lean body mass (whole body minus nonessential lipids), and body cell mass (cellular elements that are concerned with physical and chemical work, respiration, and mitosis).

Table 2-5
The Influence of Surgery and Trauma on Energy Requirements

Diagnosis	Energy Requirements (kcal/kg body weight [70 kg man])	Total (kcal)
Normal subject		
(bed rest)	23	1600
(hospital activity)	30	2100
Elective surgery		1900
Multiple skeletal trauma		
(bed rest)	28–30	1960–2100
(activity)	36	2500
Sepsis		
(bed rest)	35	
(activity)	42	
Major burn		
(bed rest)	45	
(activity)	50–55	3500–4000

Data from Long CL, Blakemore WS: Energy and protein requirements in the hospitalized patient. JPEN 3:69–71, 1979.

Fat stores are highly variable, influenced to a great extent by caloric requirements, dietary intake, physical activity and/or training, and metabolic efficiency. As much as 25 percent of the "normal" weight for height of an individual may be fatty stores. These stores can be mobilized and used for energy when dietary intake decreases below the level needed to meet the demand for energy. Anthropometric measurements such as height, weight, and tricep and/or other skin fold thicknesses facilitate the assessment of stored body fat when used in connection with tables of norms or standard values. Changes in body weight occurring over a brief time span may be reflective of acute conditions that cause the body to rely on stored fat for adequate energy.

Lean body mass (LBM) accounts for approximately 75 percent of total body mass. The skin and skeleton comprise approximately 10 percent of the total mass. The skeleton is particularly sensitive to nutritional status during fetal development, from infancy through early adulthood, during pregnancy, and after menopause. The skeletal mass of women at age 30 or 40 may influence the skeletal integrity of the postmenopausal woman, with women of larger skeletal mass retaining more mass than smaller boned women as they age.[8] The bone density of postmenopausal women is influenced by nutrition, particularly the balance between dietary calcium, phosphorus, and protein.

Skin and muscle membranes reflect nutritional status at all stages of life. Deficiencies of a number of nutrients may be implicated in the development of mucous membrane and skin lesions (Table 2-4). Among hospitalized patients, deficiencies may result in delayed wound healing, the development or delayed healing of pressure sores and stasis ulcers, and the development of skin and mucous membrane lesions.

Body cell mass (BCM) is comprised of cells that are dependent on respiration and cellular metabolism to provide energy for work and reproduction. BCM, a component of LBM (35–45 percent of body weight for males; 30–50 percent of body weight for females), is composed of two major types of tissues: somatic and visceral. Somatic tissue, skeletal and smooth muscle, functions intermittently (contracting and relaxing) and is concerned primarily with work. The viscera or parenchymal cells function continuously to meet oxidative and metabolic needs. The muscle mass varies according to use, physical training, and state of health; nevertheless, it remains fairly constant in healthy individuals.

Arm muscle circumference and creatinine height index used in connection with tables of norms are measures of somatic protein stores and are used commonly in nutritional assessments. Serum iron binding capacity and serum transferrin (calculated from serum iron binding capacity) are indicators of visceral protein status. Proteins and serum albumin synthesized by the liver are influenced by nutritional status. The amount of plasma protein is influenced by dietary intake of protein, nutrient absorption, and the balance between protein synthesis and catabolism.

Immunocompetence can also be related to nutritional status. For example, the total lymphocyte count (TLC) and presence of the delayed hypersensitivity response may reflect adequacy of protein, calorie, and micronutrient stores.

Nutrient Depletions and Dietary Deficiencies

Nutrient depletion caused by starvation, decreased levels of dietary intake, or deficiencies resulting from prolonged inadequate intake may produce lesions that may be observed clinically. The length of time from decreased dietary intake of a nutrient or from total starvation to the development of clinically observable lesions varies to a great extent depending on initial body stores, basal metabolic rate, absorption and synthesis of nutrients, and the rate of nutrient turnover. In persons with adequate fat stores, fat-soluble vitamins are depleted over a period of one to several months; proteins, minerals, and water-soluble vitamins are depleted much more rapidly, requiring only hours in the case of certain minerals (sodium, potassium, and chlorides).

Dietary deficiencies resulting from insufficient intake over prolonged periods of time often are not observed in the general population of the United States. In third world countries, malnourished states are more common, resulting in kwashiorkor, marasmus, protein-calorie malnutrition, rickets, blindness, and other infirmities. In infants and children these deficiencies result in stunted growth, increased susceptibility to infection, morbidity and mortality from a variety of causes, malformed bones, and poor dentition. An increased infant mortality rate also is associated with poor maternal nutrition.

Malnutrition, frequently observed among hospitalized patients, occurs among individuals who are unable to ingest food or who ingest inadequate quantities to meet metabolic requirements. A negative nitrogen balance, when the body must use nitrogen for energy, results from inadequate intake of proteins or calories and is related to muscle atrophy or wasting, fever, infection, stress, and anxiety.[9] Negative nitrogen balance may begin within hours of the last nutrient intake or the beginning of a stressor. Protein malnutrition may begin with a short time when available protein is insufficient to support synthesis of protein of protein for muscle or visceral tissue.

Stored fat is used for energy whenever dietary intake is insufficient to supply energy. Fat stores are highly mobile and are quickly responsive to the metabolic needs of the body. During fasting states, these stores are used to produce energy.

Malnourished States

Kwashiorkor, marasmus, and mixed kwashiorkor/marasmus have been reported among hospitalized patients.[10,11] Kwashiorkor is a syndrome resulting primarily from protein malnutrition, while marasmus is the result of decreased energy intake. When total food intake is decreased, vitamin and mineral deficiencies also may be present.

Kwashiorkor, uncomplicated by marasmus, is the result of decreased intake of amino acids for protein synthesis, evidenced clinically by a decrease in plasma proteins, anemia, decreased muscle mass, changes in hair texture and pigment, fatty liver, and diarrhea with loss of electrolytes. Decreased plasma proteins can be reflected further by decreased immune responses with increased susceptibility to infection, and by edema secondary to fluid shifts resulting from changes in osmotic pressure.

While patients with kwashiorkor have deficiencies in visceral proteins, they may have adequate somatic proteins and fat. Indeed, the height for weight that reflects somatic protein may be normal or above normal. Triceps skinfold and arm muscle circumference measures also will be adequate, although the creatinine/height index may be impaired. Visceral protein deficiency will be reflected by mild to moderate decline in serum albumin, serum transferrin, and total lymphocytes. Anergy or impaired immunity is likely to be present.

Marasmus, occurring when total calorie intake is inadequate or nearly inadequate, is characterized by decreased body stores of fat and muscle wasting as body proteins are used for energy. Plasma proteins may be normal or slightly low. In children, growth will be retarded depending on the rate of protein synthesis.

In contrast to kwashiorkor, marasmus is evidenced by a decrease in somatic proteins in the presence of adequate visceral proteins. The somatic protein deficits are clinically evident as weight for height is decreased, and triceps, skinfolds, and arm muscle circumference are below standards. Immunity may also be impaired.

Protein-calorie malnutrition is characterized clinically by deficits in both visceral and somatic proteins. The clinical picture combines the features of kwashiorkor and marasmus previously described.

The Relationship Between Nutritional Status and Patient Outcomes

Protein-calorie malnutrition has been shown to exist in one-third to one-half of adult medical-surgical patients,[10,11] in nearly 20 percent of pediatric intensive care patients,[12] and in 85 percent of nursing home residents.[13] This alarmingly high prevalence of malnutrition has been shown to occur in all age groups and among patients with a wide variety of diagnoses.

The consequences of protein-calorie malnutrition, reflected by increased morbidity and mortality rates, have received much attention. Numerous authors have attempted to identify the nutritional parameters that are most predictive of complications among hospitalized patients. One of the most frequently reported methods of prediction is based on the instant nutritional assessment, a method that utilizes two indicators of visceral protein stores, serum albumin (SALB) and TLC, as indicators of "at risk" nutritional status.[14] SALB levels below 3.5 mg% and TLCs less than 1500/mm^3 have been associated with a higher incidence of morbidity and mortality among medical and surgical patients than would be expected if these indices were within normal limits.[14,15] Similar increases in morbidity and mortality have been reported among elective surgery patients,[16] burn patients,[17] patients having surgery for colorectal cancer,[18] and a cross-section of hospitalized patients.[19] The details of these studies are summarized in Table 2-6.

SALB levels are related positively to morbidity and mortality in epidemiologic studies, yet many individuals with levels below 3.5 mg percent do not develop complications, and some individuals with levels above 3.5 percent do develop complications. Complications also are influenced by factors such as severity of illness, presence of infection or sepsis, clotting factors, coexisting physical conditions, and emotional state. SALB, however, is influenced by activity level, hydration, malabsorption, liver failure, surgical stress, burns, open wounds, and neoplastic disease.[20] A positive significant relationship exists between BCM, serum total protein, and SALB, thus justifying the selection of these parameters as predictors; nevertheless, they are imperfect predictors of changes in nutritional status.[21]

The value of other measures of nutritional status as predictors of morbidity and mortality have also received the attention of investigators. A study of the relative value of anthropometric, immunologic, and biochemical measurements of nutritional status demonstrated that only a small percentage of elective

(Text continues p. 61)

Table 2-6
Altered Serum Albumin (ALB) and Total Lymphocyte Counts (TLC) as a Risk Factor for Increased Morbidity and Mortality

Reference	Subjects	Criteria for Diagnosis		Total #	Subjects %	Predictive Value Complications #	%	Deaths #	%
15	500 consecutive general hospital admissions	ALB	>3.5g%	462	(92.4)	20	(4.3)	6	(1.3)
			<3.5g%	38	(7.6)	7	(18.0)	3	(7.9)
		TLC	>1500/mm³	349	(69.8)	15	(4.3)	3	(0.9)
			<1500/mm³	151	(30.2)	12	(7.9)	6	(4.0)
		ALB > 3.5 g% + TLC	>1500/mm³	328	(65.6)	10	(3.0)	3	(0.9)
		ALB > 3.5 + TLC	<1500/mm³	134	(26.8)	10	(7.5)	3	(2.2)
		ALB < 3.5 g% + TLC	>1500/mm³	21	(4.2)	5	(23.8)	0	(0)
		ALB < 3.5 g + TLC	<1500/mm³	17	(3.4)	2	(11.8)	3	(17.6)
15	130 surgical ICU patients	ALB	>3.5g%	94	(72.3)	47	(50.0)	13	(13.8)
			<3.5g%	36	(27.7)	23	(63.9)	10	(27.8)
		TLC	>1500/mm³	55	(42.3)	25	(45.5)	4	(7.2)
			<1500/mm³	75	(57.7)	45	(60.0)	19	(25.3)
		ALB < 3.5g% + TLC	<1500/mm³	28	(21.5)	19	(67.9)	10	(35.7)
		Both normal		47	(36.1)	19	(40.4)	4	(8.5)

16	120 elective abdominal surgery patients	ALB	>3.5g%	101	(84.2)	36	(36)	not listed
			<3.5g%	19	(15.8)	12	(63)	
17	62 consecutive burn patients (day 10 postburn measurements)	ALB	>3.5g%	43	(69.4)	0	(0)	mortality rate 11%
			<3.5g%	19	(30.6)	15	(79)	
		TLC	>1500/mm^3	44	(70.9)	3	(7)	
			<1500/mm^3	18	(29.1)	12	(67)	
18	83 patients operated on for colorectal cancer	ALB > 3.5g%		65	(78)	20	(31)	3 (4.6)
		< 3.5g%		18	(22)	11	(61)	5 (28)
		Body Weight	>120%IBW*	28	(33)	13	(46)	4 (14)
			IBW	37	(45)	7	(19)	1 (3)
			<IBW	18	(22)	11	(61)	3 (17)
19	2060 hospitalized patients	ALB > 3.5g%		1551	(75)	—	—	27 (1.7)
		3.4–3.1g%		221	(11)	—	—	22 (9.9)
		3.0–2.6g%		156	(7.6)	—	—	37 (23.7)
		2.5–2.1g%		82	(4.0)	—	—	35 (42.7)
		< 2.0		50	(2.4)	—	—	31 (62.0)

*IBW = ideal body weight.

surgery patients (3 percent of 64 patients) were free of all signs of malnutrition and that the majority (97 percent) of the patients have one or more abnormalities.[22] Only SALB, serum transferrin, and delayed hypersensitivity, however, produced statistically significant predictive values. Additional patient evaluations by these investigators[22] resulted in the development of the Prognostic Nutritional Index (PNI). The PNI assigns relative weights to four measurements resulting in a score as follows:

$$PNI = 158 - 16.6 \text{ (albumin)} - 0.78 \text{ (triceps skinfold)} - .20 \text{ (transferrin)} - 5.8 \text{ (delayed hypersensitivity)}$$

The risk of morbidity and mortality, using the PNI, has been divided into three categories: low risk (PNI < 40); intermediate risk (PNI = 40–49); high risk (PNI ≥ 50).[23]

The accuracy of the PNI in predicting morbidity and mortality of individuals was evaluated using 100 consecutive patients having major gastrointestinal surgery. The model (PNI) effectively predicted 89 percent of the patients who ultimately developed complications. Of the 38 patients who were judged at low risk, 3 developed complications. Among the patients rated at high risk, 46 percent of the 39 patients developed complications.[23] The details of these studies are summarized in Table 2-7.

Recent weight change, triceps skinfold, mid-upper air circumference, albumin, serum transferrin, and TLC were used by Debonis et al.[24] as indicators of malnutrition in 90 general surgery patients. The values obtained were scored on a scale of 0 to 12 according to the degree of abnormality. Of the 90 patients, 12 (13.3 percent) were classified as well-nourished (a total score of 0), 38 (32.3% percent) were classified as malnourished (scores of 3–12), and 49 (54.4 percent) were at risk for malnutrition (scores of 1–2). Triceps skinfold and mid-upper arm circumference were the parameters most often abnormal in lesser degrees of malnutrition while body weight, albumin, and TLC abnormalities were more indicative of severe malnutrition.

Forse et al.,[21] however, found the TLC to be a poor indicator of the nutritional state. Of 153 patients receiving total parenteral nutrition (TPN), the TLC had a false-positive rate of 34 percent and a false-negative rate of 50 percent when predicting nutritional status. The TLC correlated poorly with both the body cell mass and the Na_e to K_e ratio, a sensitive measure of nutritional status.

A multitude of other measures of nutritional status and the efficiency of these measures, alone or in combination, have been investigated for predictive power. The following assessment factors related to nutritional status are examples of some variables that have been shown to have useful, but less than perfect, predictive ability: absolute weight loss,[18,25,26,27] clinical evaluation,[28] and skin testing.[27,29]

Each method of assessing nutritional status and/or predicting morbidity or

Table 2-7
Altered Nutrition as a Risk Factor for Morbidity and Mortality

Author	Subjects	Variable	Criteria for Diagnosis of Malnutrition Level	Total #	Subjects %	No Complications #	No Complications %	Complications #	Complications %	Deaths #	Deaths %
Mullen et al. (1979)	64 consecutively admitted elective surgery patients	Serum albumin	>3.0g/dl	49	(84)	39	(79)	10	(21)	5	(8)
			<3.0g/dl	9	(16)	4	(45)	5	(55)		
		Serum transferrin	>220mg/dl	28	(50)	26	(92)	2	(8)		
			<220mg/dl	28	(50)	17	(59)	11	(41)		
		Delayed hypersensitivity	reactive	abn = 25	(62)	35	(86)	5	(14)		
			anergic	n = 15	(38)	27	(67)	13	(33)		
Buzby et al. (1980)	Phase II 100 major nonemergency gastrointestinal surgery (assessed on admission and 48 hours before surgery)	Low risk	*PNI = <40	38	(38)	35	(92)	3	(8)	1	(3)
		Intermediate risk	PNI: 40-49	23	(23)	16	(70)	7	(30)	1	(4.3)
		High risk	PNI = >50	39	(39)	21	(54)	18	(46)	13	(33)

*PNI = 158 − 16.6(Alb) − 0.78(TSF) − 0.20(TFN) − 5.8(DH), where Alb is serum albumin, TSF is triceps skinfold, TFN is serum transferrin, and DH is cutaneous delayed hypersensitivity.

mortality has major conceptual weaknesses and imperfect predictive power. Further investigations are warranted to improve clinical methods for identifying patients in need of nutritional support. Despite current predictive imperfections, the high incidence of complications and deaths related to altered nutritional status justifies meticulous attention to the needs of patients for nutritional support.

REFERENCES

1. U. S. Government Printing Office, Washington, DC, U. S. Senate Select Committee on Nutrition and Human Needs. Dietary Goals for the United States (ed 2), (No. 052-070-043376-8), 1977
2. Agriculture Research Service, Washington, DC, U. S. Department of Agriculture, Food for Fitness - A Daily Food Guide, Leaflet No. 424, September, 1977
3. National Academy of Sciences, Washington, DC, Food and Nutrition Board, National Research Council. *Recommended Dietary Allowances* (ed 9), 1980
4. Michigan Department of Public Health, Lansing, MI. Basic Nutrition Facts, 1980
5. Siegel JH, Cerra FB, Coleman B, et al: Physiological and metabolic correlations in human sepsis. Surgery 86:163–193, 1979
6. Cerra FB, Upson D, Angelico R, et al: Branched chains support postoperative protein synthesis. Surgery 92:192–198, 1982
7. Long CL, Blakemore WS: Energy and protein requirements in the hospitalized patient. JPEN 3:69–71, 1979
8. Matkovic V, Kostial K, Simonovic I, et al: Bone status and fracture rates in two regions of Yugoslavia. Am J Clin Nutr 32:540–549, 1979
9. Reed PB: Nutrition: An Applied Science. St. Paul, West Publishing Company, 1980
10. Bistrian BR, Blackburn GL, Hallowell E, et al: Protein status of general medical patients. JAMA 230:858–860, 1974
11. Bistrian BR, Blackburn GL, Vitale J, et al: Prevalence of malnutrition in general medical patients. JAMA 235:1567–1570
12. Pollack MM, Wiley JS, Kanter R, et al: Malnutrition in critically ill infants and children. JPEN 6:20–24, 1982
13. Shaver HJ, Loper JA, Lutes RA: Nutritional status of nursing home patients. JPEN 4:367–370, 1980
14. Seltzer MH, Bastidas A, Cooper DM, et al: Instant nutritional assessment. JPEN 3:157–159, 1979
15. Seltzer MH, Fletcher HS, Slocum GA, et al: Instant nutritional assessment in the intensive care unit. JPEN 5:70–72, 1981
16. Klidjian AM, Archer TJ, Foster KJ, et al: Detection of dangerous malnutrition. JPEN 6:119–121, 1982
17. Morath MA, Miller, SF, Finley, RK: Nutritional indicators of postburn bacteremic sepsis. JPEN 5:488–491, 1981
18. Hickman DM, Miller RA, Rombeau JR, et al: Serum albumin and body weight as predictors of postoperative course in colorectal cancer. JPEN 4:314–316, 1980
19. Reinhardt GF, Myscofski JW, Wilken DB, et al: Incidence and mortality of hypoalbumenemic patients in hospitalized veterans. JPEN 4:357–359, 1980

20. Rothschild MA, Oratz M, Schreider SS: Albumin synthesis. N Engl J Med 286:749–751, 816–821

21. Forse RA, Skizgal HM: Serum albumin and nutritional status. JPEN 4:450–454, 1980

22. Mullen JL, Gertner MH, Buzby GP, et al: Implications of malnutrition in the surgical patient. Arch Surg 114:121–125, 1979

23. Buzby GP, Mullen JL, Matthews DC, et al: Prognostic nutritional index in gastrointestinal surgery. Am J Surg 139:160–166, 1980

24. Debonis D, Pizzolato M, Zamboni M, et al: Quantitative nutritional assessment of 102 consecutive patients admitted to a general surgery ward in Buenos Aires, Argentina. Nutr Int 2:168–171, 1986

25. Seltzer MH, Slocum BA, Cataldi-Betcher EL, et al: Instant nutritional assessment: Absolute weight loss and surgical mortality. JPEN 6:218–221, 1982

26. DeWys DM: Nutritional care of the cancer patient. JAMA 224:374–376, 1980

27. Daly JM, Dudrich SJ, Copeland EM: Evaluation of nutritional indices as prognostic indicators in cancer patients. Cancer 43:925–931, 1979

28. Baker JP, Detsky AS, Wessen DE, et al: Nutritional assessment: A comparison of clinical judgement and objective measures. Med Intell 306:969–972, 1982

29. Twomey P, Ziegler D, Rombeau J: Utility of skin testing in nutritional assessment: A critical review. JPEN 6:50–58, 1982

Barbara A. Griggs

3

Indications for Nutritional Support in the Adult Patient

It is now well recognized that the disease process contributes to an increased metabolic demand and a decreased by-mouth intake that results in predictable degrees of protein-calorie malnutrition (PCM). The question is no longer if but which form of parenteral or enteral nutritional support should be given.

The manner and degree of nutritional intervention should be directly related to the patient's nutritional state at onset of illness, the specific disease process, and the anticipated or planned treatment modality. A nutritional assessment should be an essential component of every patient's initial workup (see Chapter 4). The ideal method of consuming nutrients is by mouth, with supplemental feedings added to regularly scheduled meals or between meals as desired or necessary. If the patient is unable or unwilling to eat and has a normally functioning gastrointestinal (GI) tract, however, tube feeding should be considered. Patients with nonfunctioning GI tracts or GI tract disorders will require parenteral feeding by either the central or peripheral route. Deciding on a route or method of administration, however, will depend on the organs affected by disease. This chapter briefly describes the disease entities that may disrupt or alter normal organ function.

GENERAL INDICATIONS

Data have conclusively documented widespread, significant protein-calorie malnutrition among hospitalized patients.[1-6] Each patient's nutritional status should be determined on admission to the hospital. A diet history obtained from the patient or a family member should include past weight loss and recent

NUTRITIONAL SUPPORT IN NURSING
ISBN 0-8089-1889-3

alterations in eating patterns. A recent or gradual weight loss of as little as 10% is considered significant for increased morbidity and mortality.[7] Routine admission laboratory data also provide information relative to nutritional status. All patients should have a specific dietary plan incorporated into their overall therapeutic plan.

Patients who are taking in minimal calories or nothing by mouth (NPO) for 5–10 days or longer are candidates for specialized nutritional support. For these patients, parenteral or enteral feeding methods should be considered. The method of feeding will depend on the reason that by-mouth intake is contraindicated or inadequate, for example, diagnostic tests, recent stroke, endotracheal intubation, gastric outlet obstruction, ileus, and so on. Patients undergoing preoperative bowel preps need no longer be limited to empty calories in the form of clear liquids. Instead, a low-residue formula that provides 1 kcal/ml can be given by mouth.[8]

Today it is widely accepted that malnourished patients should receive nutritional support preoperatively. A classic publication from 1936 states that a preoperative weight loss of 20 percent or above was associated with a postoperative mortality rate of $33\frac{1}{3}$ percent in patients with chronic peptic ulcer disease.[9] Multiple studies have shown that there are increased surgical risks associated with malnutrition.[10–16]

Perioperative nutritional support should also be considered as it may reduce operative morbidity and mortality in the malnourished operative candidate.[17–20] A combination of nutritional therapies is frequently indicated for patients throughout their hospitalization.

THE GI TRACT—FUNCTION AND DYSFUNCTION

The GI tract is approximately 30 feet long and includes the mouth, esophagus, stomach, gallbladder, liver, pancreas, and the small and large intestines. Absorption of fluids and nutrients is the main function of the GI tract.

Digestion starts in the mouth and continues in the stomach, aided by specific enzymes. The stomach acts as a reservoir, holding and releasing small amounts of partially digested food at specific intervals to the duodenum, the first section of the small intestine. Once in the small intestine, food substances are further broken down by bile and pancreatic enzymes to complete the digestive process. As the emulsion moves along, nutrients are absorbed through the microvilli of the intestines into the blood stream and lymphatic system. Finally, the emulsion passes into the large intestine, where water and electrolytes are reabsorbed and the end products collect to be eventually expelled. Because this normal process follows a sequence of events, any disease or injury that affects sections of the GI tract can disrupt the process and have a profound effect on the patient's ability to ingest and/or assimilate nutrients properly and in sufficient quantities.

GI dysfunction occurs when disease processes result in: (1) malabsorption, (2) obstruction, (3) strictures, (4) fistulas, or (5) surgical excision of absorptive surfaces. A dysfunction of the GI tract is the primary indication for parenteral nutritional support.[21] Enteral alimentation, however, has been successfully used in selected patients.

Inadequate absorption of nutrients in the small and large intestines results from a variety of acute and chronic diseases. For example, Crohn's disease, short-gut syndrome, radiation enteritis, nontropical sprue, and scleroderma affect the small intestine. Ulcerative colitis, intestinal parasites, and infectious diarrhea, on the other hand, primarily affect the large intestine. Parenteral nutritional support is the preferred method during acute stages of these diseases when bowel rest is necessary to promote healing and decrease mucosal trauma caused by food and the persistent caustic effect of gastric secretions. For most patients, parenteral therapy will be temporary; once the acute episode has resolved, the goal should be to reuse the GI tract. Some patients will be able to take food by mouth while others may require a longer transitional stage with tube feedings.

Patients with Crohn's disease or nonspecific regional enteritis experience intermittent flare-ups of pain and diarrhea that necessitate hospitalization and, frequently, TPN therapy. The intestinal picture is further complicated in these patients because of fibrosis that results in strictures, mucosal damage, and fistula formation. Most patients with Crohn's disease live in a state of nutritional depletion. TPN can therefore provide needed nutrients during periods of exacerbation. In addition, bowel rest with adequate nutritional support will allow spontaneous remission without surgery for some patients.[22-29] For those patients requiring surgery, preoperative TPN should decrease their operative risk. Elemental diets have also been utilized in patients with acute inflammatory bowel disease.[30-32]

Obstructions and strictures can occur at various places along the GI tract. Tumors of the head and neck or ingestion of a caustic substance such as lye interfere with the intake of normal food.[33-34] Gastric outlet obstruction, GI bleeding, and nausea and vomiting caused by disease or its treatment (chemotherapy/radiation therapy) all contribute to a decreased or absent food intake.[35-38] Small bowel obstructions due to tumor or a prolonged paralytic ileus postoperatively may also prevent usage of the GI tract for necessary nutritional support. Parenteral nutritional support is the feeding method of choice for most of these conditions, at least initially. However, tube feedings and elemental diets (rapid absorption/minimal digestion) have also been used successfully.[39-43]

Another incapacitating disease of the GI tract is intestinal pseudo-obstruction.[44] Although the cause is unknown, the disorder presents with all the signs and symptoms of bowel obstruction in the absence of an occluding lesion. It can be an acute or chronic condition. Patients who suffer from chronic intestinal pseudo-obstruction are plagued with distention and diarrhea. Enteral diets can be tolerated by some patients. Others ultimately go home on parenteral nutritional support.[45-46]

TPN can relieve or lessen symptoms of GI dysfunction through bowel rest; however, TPN cannot eliminate symptoms. It is a suppportive therapeutic modality to be used on an individual basis.

Aggressive nutritional support has had a significant impact on GI fistulas and should be a primary therapy for these patients. Prior to 1960 a review of patients with GI-cutaneous fistulas noted a mortality rate of 61 percent, dependent on location and etiology of the fistula.[47] The introduction of TPN allowed GI tract rest that resulted in decreased fistula drainage, increased spontaneous closure, and a significant drop in mortality rate.[48-51] Esophageal, duodenal, pancreatitic, and colonic fistulas tend to close spontaneously after 4–6 weeks on parenteral nutrtitional support.[52-53] Jejunal and ileal fistulas, however, are less likely to close spontaneously.[49,50,53] Fistulas requiring surgical closure have an associated decrease in morbidity and mortality if patients have received preoperative nutritional support.

Oral intake is contraindicated because it is not absorbed well and it increases fistula output leading to fluid and electrolyte imbalances and impaired wound healing. The aim of therapy should be to correct imbalances and sepsis and to increase wound healing, immunocompetence, and overall nutritional status.

Parenteral nutritional support is the primary choice, particularly with high output fistulas. Tube feedings with elemental formulas have been used with low ileal, colonic, or very proximal fistulas.[54-55]

Patients with short-gut syndrome resulting from surgical resection for ischemia, Crohn's disease, trauma, or malignant infiltration require TPN for longer periods of time.[56] The amount of nutritional support needed depends on the extent and location of the resected bowel. Some of these patients continue to receive parenteral nutrition at home (see Chapter 10). This may be temporary, taking up to several years until the remaining bowel can adapt and absorb sufficient nutrients for daily maintenance, or it may be permanent.[57-62]

Pancreatic Disease

The pancreas produces and secretes enzymes into the duodenum to aid in the metabolism of protein, carbohydrates, and fat. Within the pancreas are the islands of Langerhans, a group of differentiated cells that produce insulin and glucagon for glucose metabolism and serum glucose regulation. Diseases such as pancreatitis and diabetes mellitus result in digestive and metabolic abnormalities.

Pancreatitis may be acute or chronic. Patients with acute episodes experience severe epigastric pain, fever, nausea, and vomiting. Some causes of acute pancreatitis are biliary disease, trauma, postabdominal surgery, high fat foods, and excessive alcohol intake.

The initial treatment for acute pancreatitis is total restriction of all oral intake and abdominal decompression via continuous nasogastric drainage. The nasogastric tube may remain in place 7–10 days. For some patients, it may take 4–6 weeks for the inflammation to subside sufficiently to enable normal eating. Nutritional support is indicated and beneficial in these patients because morbidity and mortality are affected by malnutrition. In addition, it has been reported that GI tract secretions in fistula patients are reduced during parenteral nutritional support, which is beneficial to pancreatic response.[49,63–64]

Both parenteral nutrition and enteral nutrition have been used successfully for patients with pancreatitis.[65–74] Patients with chronic pancreatitis suffer repeated attacks, frequently precipitated by excessive alcohol ingestion. The treatment is the same as for acute pancreatitis during the acute episode. Additional attention must be given to the nutritional repletion of these patients because many are malnourished secondary to alcoholism and inadequate nutrient intake.[75]

Some patients develop pancreatic pseudocysts or abscesses that require surgical intervention. A pseudocyst requires about 6 weeks to mature prior to surgery. During this time, patients usually receive parenteral nutritional support with dextrose-amino acid solutions. Fat emulsions are administered selectively. An abscess, however, requires immediate surgical drainage.

Parenteral nutritional support is temporary for most patients with pancreatitis. Once inflammation has subsided, enteral feeeding should be restarted slowly. Some patients need to avoid rich and spicy foods, caffeine, and alcohol. In addition, some patients will require supplemental pancreatic enzymes and bile salts to aid digestion. Proper dietary counseling is a necessity for these patients.

Patients with insulin-dependent diabetes mellitus also require dietary counseling. When diabetic patients are hospitalized for complications of their disease, special care must be taken with nutritional support, particularly when surgery is necessary. Enteral alimentation is the feeding of choice.

Contrary to the opinion of some clinicians, the high dextrose in TPN formulations can be given safely with exogenous insulin and careful monitoring.[76] The degree and stability of the diabetes will affect the type, amount, and method of administration of exogenous insulin. Some patients require modification of the hypertonic dextrose with a higher percentage of calories from fat (see Chapter 7). In most diabetic patients, TPN is a temporary therapy, primarily related to surgical intervention. Resumption of an oral diet is usually accomplished as soon as possible.

Hepatic Failure

The liver plays a vital role in the metabolism of carbohydrates, protein, and fat. It secretes bile that is stored in the gallbladder where it is released to the duodenum to aid in digestion.

The primary diseases of the liver include hepatitis and cirrhosis. Hepatitis, an inflammation of the liver, is generally an acute condition that resolves with proper medical attention and time. Cirrhosis, on the other hand, results in irreversible damage and eventual death for many patients. It is a degenerative disease leading to progressive loss of function.

Adequate nutrition is essential to maintain the liver's function and, over time, to aid cellular regeneration. Patients with liver impairment or failure thus present a special nutritional challenge. The inability of a damaged liver to properly synthesize proteins necessitates moderate to severe protein restriction. The exact amount of protein allowed will depend on the degree of damage and whether the patient has encephalopathy, an advanced sign of liver failure. When protein is broken down in the gut, ammonia production is increased; therefore, parenteral administration of protein as a part of a balanced intravenous nutritional regimen may be more effective than oral intake. Certainly the formulation will have to be individualized based on the patient's condition and therapeutic response. Most clinicians currently use a standard combination of essential and nonessential amino acids for patients with mild to moderate liver failure and minimal encephalopathy.[77-79] This combination, however, has a less positive response in patients with severe liver failure and encephalopathy. A favorable response has been shown in patients with marked hepatic encephalopathy when selected amino acids that maximize the branched-chain amino acids (valine, leucine, and isoleucine) and minimize the aromatic amino acids (phenylalanine, tyrosine, glutamate, aspartate, and methionine) are used.[80-90] Special formulas have been developed for both parenteral and enteral administration that are commercially available (see Chapter 7).

RENAL FAILURE

The kidneys maintain fluid and electrolyte balance by selective reabsorption and excretion of water and metabolic waste products.

Renal failure occurs when blood flow is obstructed or the functioning unit is damaged, resulting in accumulation of fluid, electrolytes, and waste products. Acute renal failure (ARF) may develop after surgery, trauma, or thermal injury and is caused by hypotension, shock, and/or sepsis.[91-95] ARF can also be related to drug ingestion and dye infusion such as the dye used in the diagnostic intravenous pyelogram. ARF may resolve itself or progress to necessitate dialysis.

Patients with specific diseases of the kidneys that result in chronic renal failure (CRF) such as chronic glomerulonephritis, pyelonephritis, and polycystic disease must cope with a constant fluid, metabolic, and protein imbalance. These patients require routine dialysis.

Malnutrition is common in advanced renal failure. The primary focus of nutritional therapy for the renal patient includes: (1) stabilization of the catabolic process by providing adquate nutrients, (2) maintenance of fluid balance, avoiding both under- and overhydration, (3) maintenance of a metabolic balance, and (4) weight gain with a sense of well-being.

The choice of diet and feeding method depends on the etiology and extent of renal failure, the use of and/or type of dialysis, and the functioning ability of the GI tract. Although enteral nutrition is the feeding of choice, most patients with renal disease have some degree of GI dysfunction, particularly nausea and vomiting. In these patients, or during those episodes, parenteral nutrition is the method of choice.

Specialized TPN formulations can be prepared for renal failure patients. These formulations contain concentrated dextrose, limited protein, and vitamins in a restricted volume. Patients need protein to decrease or reverse catabolism, but their protein intake is restricted to prevent the accumulation of waste products (see Chapter 7).

Controversy persists regarding the use of essential amino acids (EAA) versus a combination of essential and nonessential amino acids (NEAA) for patients with renal disease. Original studies showed improved survival and wound healing, weight gain, and stabilization of blood urea nitrogen (BUN) in patients with ARF receiving only EAA solutions.[96–104] Later studies, however, showed no advantage of EAA when compared with a reduced or normal concentration of both EAA and NEAA.[105–107] When a decision is made to avoid or delay dialysis, parenteral formulations using only EAA may aid in preventing or minimizing the frequency of dialysis. For those patients undergoing regular dialysis to replace protein losses, higher protein intake is necessary and a balance of EAA and NEAA is more desirable.

The preferred method of nutritional support is by mouth with supplemental feedings. Enteral formulas, specific for patients with renal disease, have been developed that can be given by tube feeding or taken orally (see Chapter 7). Tube feedings may be instituted during the transition from parenteral to enteral feedings and until the patient is well enough or able to eat. Comprehensive dietary counseling is essential to ensure compliance with the necessary fluid and nutrient restrictions.

HEART DISEASE

Although the heart does not play a direct role in digestion and metabolism, cardiac disease impairs the perfusion of nutrients.

The most frequent cause of valvular heart disease is rheumatic fever. The mitral and aortic valves are usually affected, although there can also be damage to the tricuspid valve. Damage of these valves leads to blood engorgement in the lungs causing fluid to leak from the pulmonary tissues and alveoli. The result is pulmonary edema and progressive heart failure. Patients with early, mild congestive failure may show no significant abnormalities at rest because of reserve cardiac function. Increased activity compromises that reserve, however, and patients experience fatigue and shortness of breath. In some patients the cardiac reserve ultimately becomes inadequate to supply normal amounts of blood even at rest, and the patient becomes bedridden.

Cardiac cachexia,[108–109] also called protein-calorie undernutrition,[110] is a syndrome of malnutrition that often accompanies chronic congestive heart failure. Cardiac cachexia occurs most frequently in patients with chronic valvular disease. Starvation results in wasting of cardiac muscle that eventually depresses myocardial function.

Coronary artery disease progresses silently until the diminished coronary blood flow leads to an infarction and myocardial damage.

The two major types of heart disease, valvular and coronary artery disease, affect different patient groups in terms of nutritional status. Patients with coronary artery disease often appear healthy and may in fact seem overnourished because they are overweight, a condition probably contributing to their disease. Patients with valvular disease who have longstanding congestive failure, on the other hand, are often weak and malnourished. Actual weight may not have changed significantly because of edema, but other signs of malnutrition may be present (see Chapter 4).

When surgery is necessary for malnourished patients with valvular disease, preoperative nutritional support should be considered. The feeding method of choice may be oral or intravenous. Studies have demonstrated that preoperative nutritional support will improve morbidity and mortality.[111–112] TPN should also be considered postoperatively until the patient is able to take an adequate oral diet to minimize potential complications.[111,113] Special TPN formulations are available for the cardiac patient that limit sodium and increase the dextrose concentration to restrict total fluid volume (see Chapter 7).

Patients undergoing cardiac surgery are at risk for postoperative complications such as renal dysfunction[93] and ARF.[95,114] If the patient is unable to eat normally for more than 3–4 days postoperatively, parenteral or tube feedings should be initiated.[115]

Parenteral nutrition is temporary in cardiac patients and is directly related to surgical intervention. Enteral alimentation is initiated as soon as possible postoperatively. Some patients benefit by supplemental tube feeding until they are strong enough or have sufficient appetite to consume enough calories for basic maintenance. When refeeding patients with severe cardiac cachexia, a very important point to remember is that one must proceed slowly in order to prevent cardiac overload and its associated complications.[116] Slow, steady repletion is the ideal (see Chapter 2).

PULMONARY DISEASE

The lungs oxygenate blood and remove carbon dioxide. Diseases of the lungs interfere with this balance and can create a life-threatening situation.

Acute episodes of respiratory distress may be associated with an exacerbation of a chronic problem or a postoperative complication. Acute episodes usually require intubation and mechanical ventilation. In acute respiratory distress syndrome (ARDS), positive end expiratory pressure (PEEP) is also required to increase functional residual capacity of the lungs.

Patients with long-term respiratory conditions such as emphysema, chronic bronchitis, and chronic obstructive pulmonary disease may also require periodic ventilatory support. Any of these conditions can cause atrophy of the respiratory muscles and muscle breakdown to meet metabolic requirements. In a study of patients receiving mechanical ventilation, 92 percent of the patients receiving optimal nutritional support were successfully weaned from the ventilator as opposed to 54 percent of the patients receiving regular intravenous therapy.[117]

The nutritional requirements of the ventilator-dependent patient can be met by parenteral or enteral therapy; however, the carbohydrate content of the formulas usually needs to be modified because excessive dextrose contributes to an increased PCO_2 and ventilatory insufficiency.[118–122] A combination of low carbohydrate and high fat as the nonprotein calorie source has been successful for patient management (see Chapter 2).[123–124]

Tube feedings, primarily into the duodenum or jejunum, can be administered safely to intubated patients being mechanically ventilated. The risk of aspiration is minimized but not eliminated by the presence of a cuffed endotracheal or tracheostomy tube. Once patients have been weaned from the ventilator and are stable, oral feedings can be started. Breathing tends to take precedence over eating in most patients with chronic respiratory problems. These patients therefore require careful monitoring and home followup to be certain that they are eating adequately to prevent further muscle breakdown and increasing difficulty breathing.

NEUROLOGIC DISORDERS

Conscious and unconscious, voluntary and involuntary actions are controlled by the central nervous system (CNS). Diseases of the CNS have a profound effect on the patient's ability to control nutritional intake.[125–126] Patients with strokes, dysphagia, and coma require careful evaluation and appropriate nutritional intervention.

A stroke that causes one-sided paralysis directly affects a patient's ability to swallow. While not used extensively, TPN may play an important role during the initial phase of recovery when oral intake is contraindicated because of an absent gag reflex and increased risk of aspiration. Use of TPN may depend on the nutritional status of the patient at the time of injury and the anticipated time of refeeding. Many of these patients have functioning GI tracts; thus, enteral alimentation is the feeding method of choice. In some hospitals, occupational therapists specializing in swallowing disorders are available to evaluate and retrain patients.[127] They also work closely with family members to teach them how to properly feed the patient.

Semisolid foods precede liquids for the stroke patient. Once tolerated, liquids can slowly be added. Liquids are more difficult for patients to swallow without aspiration. Proper patient preparation and supervision will minimize complications. Important nursing considerations to remember include positioning, mouth care, suctioning, choice of foods, constant attendance, and education of the patient and family.[128]

For those patients unable to start feedings by mouth within 5 days, tube feedings can provide adequate nutrients to maintain energy levels until the patient is ready to start a refeeding or training program. Nasally inserted feeding tubes should be removed prior to starting oral feedings because the tube interferes with the patient's ability to swallow. Peripheral parenteral nutrition (PPN) can be particularly useful for selected patients during the training period. If the patient is moderately depleted, or if 7–10 days are necessary for retraining, PPN can provide additional nutrients.[128] Renal and cardiac status, plus the availability of peripheral veins, must be taken into consideration, however, because of the types and volumes of PPN formulations (see Chapter 7).

Dysphagia (difficulty swallowing) caused by tumors or strictures requires aggressive nutritional intervention. On admission, many patients present with gradual but progressive weight loss and protein-calorie malnutrition. If surgery is indicated, preoperative TPN is usually the feeding method of choice. TPN is also indicated during a course of radiation therapy when swallowing becomes even more difficult because of mucosal inflammation and edema.

Comatose patients are in need of repletion and maintenance nutritional support. The cause of the coma and the presence of other related medical problems will influence the method of nutritional support. TPN is frequently indicated for the acutely ill patient with metabolic complications, for example, the head-injured patient.[129] Tube feedings are indicated for less complicated, more stable patients. Jejunal tube feedings are preferred over gastric tube feedings to minimize the possiblity of aspiration.

The inability to tolerate oral feedings over the long term necessitates alternative use of the GI tract. A feeding gastrostomy or jejunostomy is usually selected for patient or family management at home or for nursing home placement (see Chapter 10).

HYPERCATABOLIC STATES

Of all patient indications for nutritional support, hypercatabolic states are undisputed. Patients with sepsis, trauma, and thermal injury require aggressive nutritional repletion and maintenance. When to start feeding depends only on hemodynamic stability. The metabolic demands of these patients are such that a combination of nutritional therapies is frequently used.

Sepsis

Sepsis is often a complication of surgery. In a patient already stressed by increased metabolic requirements, sepsis further increases the patient's needs. Sepsis can be localized or systemic. Ongoing bacteremias and generalized sepsis compromise patient stability and interfere with the body's ability to appropriately metabolize infused nutrients.[130–132]

TPN is usually necessary to meet the increased caloric requirements because the GI tract may not be functioning normally. Parenteral formulation modification will be required based on the cardiac and metabolic stability of the patient.[131,133–135]

Thermal Injury

Patients with thermal injuries have increased energy expenditure[136–137] and caloric requirements related to the percentage of total body surface area that is burned.[138–139] Most burn patients receive nutritional support within 48 hours of admission. TPN may be necessary for some patients; however, because of increased risk of sepsis and problems of vascular access, tube feedings are preferred.[139–141] Patients with extensive burns are more prone to paralytic ileus. This often resolves during the resuscitation period, enabling enteral alimentation to be started.[142] Although volumes are advanced quickly, caloric intake may be supplemented with PPN or fat emulsions until the desired enteral volume is reached.[143] Aggressive nutritional support has been shown to significantly affect morbidity and mortality of the thermally injured patient.[142,144]

Trauma

Patients with multiple injuries have significantly increased metabolic requirements.[145–146] A temporary nonfunctioning GI tract is common for trauma patients; thus TPN becomes the feeding method of choice. Early nutritional intervention is vital in hypercatabolic patients because they are prone to multiple complications such as wound dehiscence, abscess, hepatorenal syndrome, acute respiratory distress syndrome, and GI bleeding. Trauma patients present a nutritional challenge to provide essential nutrients while maintaining hemodynamic stability. Patients may require several weeks of parenteral nutritional support. Some patients are able to tolerate oral feedings during the transitional phase as they are weaned from TPN. Other trauma patients require a transitional period with tube feedings.

CANCER

Patients with carcinomas often have multiple nutritional problems. Cancer is associated with anorexia and body store depletion, known as cancer cachexia.[147–148] Carcinomas of the GI tract directly interfere with adequate intake and absorption of nutrients. Weight loss is frequently one of the first signs that something is wrong. Treatment modalities such as radiation and chemotherapy further aggravate and contribute to a negative nutritional state.

Most clinicians believe that patients who are receiving aggressive treatment for their carcinoma should receive aggressive nutritional support simultaneously. Some studies have shown positive responses in patients to radiation and chemotherapy given in conjunction with nutritional support.[149-156]

The method of feeding is dependent on the type and extent of the carcinoma. Enteral alimentation remains the method of choice, provided the patient is not vomiting, can absorb the nutrients, and is not obstructed. Many cancer patients have little if any appetite; consequently, tube feedings are sometimes necessary to meet daily caloric requirements. Patients who are able to eat and drink small amounts should continue to do so, in addition to what is given via tube feeding. Elemental diets have been used successfully both preoperatively and postoperatively.[157]

For those patients with nonfunctioning GI tracts, parenteral nutritional support is indicated.[158] Strict aseptic technique is essential in these immunosuppressed patients who are at risk of sepsis.

Many cancer patients being treated on an outpatient basis also receive TPN or tube feedings at home (see Chapter 10).

ANOREXIA NERVOSA

Anorexia nervosa is an eating disorder manifested by severe undernutrition resulting from prolonged dieting to the point of starvation.[159-161] Anorexia nervosa primarily affects young women.[162-163] The control they achieve over their body becomes exhilarating; however, their perception is distorted and they are unable to see what is happening to them. Anorexics tend to equate weight loss with personal achievement and have feelings of helplessness, anger, and guilt if they are somehow forced to eat. There seems to be a correlation between a diminished physical self and an increased inner self. They reject the risks associated with severe weight loss. Patients with anorexia nervosa and their families need psychological support (see Chapter 9). In addition to psychiatric therapy, nutritional therapy is essential.[164-165]

Parenteral or enteral nutritional support can be given.[166-171] TPN is frequently more effective in the initial stages of refeeding because it is less like food and can be more readily accepted. Occasionally patients will interfere with their central line, causing sepsis and the discontinuation of parenteral therapy. Tube feedings can be successful if the patient will cooperate by not pulling out the tube. Psychiatric and nutritional support therapies must be provided simultaneously. One often will not work without the other. It is important to remember, particularly with severely depleted patients, to initiate refeeding slowly to prevent possible electrolyte imbalances and ventricular arrhythmias or congestive heart failure.[171–173]

OBESITY

It has been stated that "88 million Americans are overweight and 40 million are considered clinically obese."[174] One classification scheme divides obesity into three categories: mild, moderate, and severe. Mild is up to 30 percent above ideal body weight, moderate is 30–100 percent above ideal body weight, and severe is greater than 100 percent above ideal body weight.[175–176]

Obesity is a major health problem associated with diabetes mellitus, hypertension, cardiovascular disease, and decreased longevity.[177–180] While overeating is the most prevalent and commonly believed cause, investigation into obesity has shown that there are more complicated and some unknown causes of this distressing condition.[181–182]

Treatment of obesity has included very low-calorie diets, fasting and supplemented fasting, behavior modification, exercise, and surgery, including gastric and jejunoileal bypass and gastric stapling.[183–192] Many of these treatments have failed over the long term. In addition, bypass surgery has resulted in significant complications.[193–197] It may be that successful weight loss and weight maintenance for many patients will be dependent on a balanced diet in conjunction with moderate exercise and behavioral modification that become a way of life.

Of note is that aggressive nutritional support should not be denied to the hospitalized obese patient. Their needs are the same as a thinner patient.[198] While weight loss results from increased metabolic demands of the disease process and its treatment, weight reduction should not be a goal during injury or illness.

CONTRAINDICATIONS

TPN

While many hospitalized patients are candidates for TPN, there are situations in which it is of limited value or should not be used. The following is derived from guidelines established by the American Society for Parenteral and Enteral Nutrition.[199]

TPN is of limited value when the GI tract is usable within 7–10 days in a well-nourished patient with minimal stress and trauma or in the immediate postoperative or poststress period. It is also considered of limited value if the patient is in an untreatable disease state such as widely metastatic malignancy with no known effective therapy. Decisions to initiate or withdraw TPN should be made on an individual basis after full discussion with the patient and family.

TPN should not be used in patients with a functional and usable GI tract; rather, enteral feeding is preferred. It should also not be used when sole dependence will be far less than 5 days or to delay an urgently needed operation. Two issues that must be addressed in accordance with hospital policy and existing law include when aggressive nutritional support is not desired by the patient or legal guardian and when the patient's prognosis does not warrant it. Finally, TPN should not be used when the risks exceed the potential benefits.

PPN

PPN utilizing fat as the major nonprotein calorie source should not be used in patients with abnormal fat metabolism or acute myocardial ischemia.[200] PPN probably should not be used in patients who are fluid restricted or have limited peripheral venous access.[201–202]

Tube Feedings

Tube feedings are of limited value if the patient is able to take adequate nutrients by mouth.[203]

Nasoenteric tube feedings should not be used in patients with complete gastric or intestinal obstruction and probably should not be used in patients with incomplete intestinal or partial gastric outlet obstruction and severe gastroesophageal reflux and ileus.[204]

Nasogastric feedings should probably not be used for intubated patients, particularly when PEEP is necessary, because of the risk of aspiration. Similarly, patients with an absent or diminished gag reflex or decreased mental status should preferentially be fed into the jejunum.[205]

As with TPN, legal and ethical issues for not initiating or withdrawing tube feedings must be addressed with the patient and family in accordance with hospital policy and existing law (see Chapters 1 and 2). Finally, tube feedings should not be used when the risks exceed the potential benefits.

SUMMARY

Nutritional support should not be considered an option; rather, it should be an integral part of the care plan for every patient. The method of feeding should be individual, depending on the patient's present state of nutrition, the disease entity, and the anticipated treatment plan. Nutritional evaluation on admission and reevaluation every 2–3 weeks throughout the patient's hospitalization is necessary to select the nutritional therapy indicated at each step of treatment. Indications for nutritional support therapy change; our responsiblity is to keep up with those changes to best serve our patients.

REFERENCES

1. Bollet AJ, Owens S: Evaluation of nutritional status of selected hospitalized patients. Am J Clin Nutr 26:931–938, 1973
2. Bistrian BR, Blackburn GL, Hallowell E, et al: Protein status of general surgical patients. JAMA 230:858–860, 1974
3. Butterworth C: The skeleton in the hospital closet. Nutrition Today (March/April):4–8, 1974
4. Bistrian BR, Blackburn GL, Vitale J, et al: Prevalence of malnutrition in general medical patients. JAMA 235:1567–1570, 1976
5. Hill GL, Pickford I, Young GA, et al: Malnutrition in surgical patients. An unrecognized problem. Lancet 1:681–692, 1977
6. Jensen JE, Jensen TG, Dudrick SJ: Nutrition and orthopedic surgery. Nutri Supp Serv 4:27–37, 1984
7. Blackburn GL, Bistrian BR, Maini BS, et al: Nutritional and metabolic assessment of the hospitalized patient. JPEN 1:11–22, 1977
8. Crossland SS, Geelhoed GW, Guy DG, et al: Preoperative nutritional support for bowel surgery patients. Contemporary Surgery 16:37–47, 1980
9. Studley HO: Percentage of weight loss, a basic indicator of surgical risk in patients with chronic peptic ulcer. JAMA 106:458–460, 1936
10. Williams RH, Heatley RV, Lewis MH: Proceedings: A randomized controlled trial of preoperative intravenous nutrition in patients with stomach cancer. Br J Surg 63:667–671, 1976
11. Meakins JL, Pietsch JB, Bubenick O, et al: Delayed hypersensitivity: Indicator of acquired failure of host defenses in sepsis and trauma. Ann Surg 186:241–250, 1977
12. Buzby GP, Mullen JL, Matthews DC, et al: Prognostic nutritional index in gastrointestinal surgery. Am J Surg 139:160–167, 1980
13. Hickman DM, Miller RA, Rombeau JL, et al: Serum albumin and body weight as predictors of postoperative course in colorectal cancer. JPEN 4:314–316, 1980
14. Mullen JL, Buzby GP, Matthews DC, et al: Reduction of operative morbidity and mortality by combined preoperative and postoperative nutritional support. Ann Surg 192:604–613, 1980
15. Muller JM, Brenner U, Dienst C, et al: Preoperative parenteral feeding in patients with gastrointestinal carcinoma. Lancet 1:68–71, 1982
16. Starker PM, LaSala PA, Askanazi J, et al: The influence of preoperative total parenteral nutrition upon morbidity and mortality. Surg Gynecol Obstet 162:569–574, 1986
17. Abel RM, Fischer JE, Buckley MJ, et al: Malnutrition in cardiac surgical patients. Results of a prospective, randomized evaluation of early postoperative parenteral nutrition. Arch Surg 111:45–50, 1976
18. Holler AR, Fischer JE: The effect of perioperative hyperalimentation on complications in patients with carcinoma and weight loss. J Surg Res 23:31–34, 1977
19. Mullen JL, Gertner MH, Buzby GP, et al: Implications of malnutrition in the surgical patient. Arch Surg 114:121–125, 1979
20. Pittam MR, Janes E, Palmer BV: Postoperative enteral tube feeding in patients with squamous carcinoma of the head and neck. Nutri Supp Serv 2:6–13, 1982
21. Dudrick S, Wilmore D, Vars H, et al: Can intravenous feeding as the sole means

of nutrition support growth in the child and restore weight loss in an adult? An affirmative answer. Ann Surg 169:974–984, 1969

22. Steiger E, Wilmore DM, Dudrick SJ, et al: Total intravenous nutrition in the management of inflammmatory disease of the intestinal tract. Fed Proc 28:808, 1969

23. Fischer JE, Foster GS, Abel RM, et al: Hyperalimentation as primary therapy for inflammatory bowel disease. Am J Surg 125:165–175, 1973

24. Dudrick SJ, MacFayden BV, Daly JM: The management of inflammatory bowel disease with parenteral hyperalimentation, in Clearfield HR, Dinoso VP (eds): Gastrointestinal Emergencies. Orlando, FL, Grune & Stratton, Inc, 1976, pp 193–199

25. Reilly J: Inflammatory bowel disease in total parenteral nutrition, in Fischer JE (ed): Total Parenteral Nutrition. Boston, Little, Brown, 1976, pp 187–202

26. Driscoll RH, Rosenberg IH: Total parenteral nutrition in inflammatory bowel disease. Med Clin N Am 62:185, 1978

27. Mullen JL, Hargrove WC, Dudrick SJ, et al: Ten years' experience with intravenous hyperalimentation and inflammatory bowel disease. Ann Surg 187:523–529, 1978

28. Elson CO, Layden TJ, Nemchausky BA, et al: An evaluation of total parenteral nutrition in the management of inflammatory bowel disease. Dig Dis Sci 25:42–48, 1980

29. Meryn S, Lochs H, Pamperl K, et al: Influence of parenteral nutrition on serum levels of proteins in patients with Crohn's disease. JPEN 7:553–556, 1983

30. Bury KD, Turnier E, Randall HT: Nutritional management of granulomatous colitis with perineal ulceration. Can J Surg 15:1, 1972

31. Voitk AJ, Eschave V, Feller JH, et al: Experience with elemental diets in the treatment of inflammatory bowel disease. Is this primary therapy? Arch Surg 107:329–333, 1973

32. Rocchio MA, Cha CS, Haas KF, et al: Use of chemically defined diets in the management of patients with acute inflammatory bowel disease. Am J Surg 127:469–475, 1974

33. Johnston CA, Keane TJ, Prudo SM: Weight loss in patients receiving radical radiation therapy for head and neck cancer: A prospective study. JPEN 6:399–402, 1982

34. Groher ME: Mechanical disorders of swallowing, in Groher ME (ed): Dysphagia. Boston, Butterworths, 1984, pp 61–84

35. Cohen AM, Ottinger LW: Delayed gastric emptying after gastric surgery. Ann Surg 184:689, 1976

36. Donaldson SS: Nutritional consequences of radiotherapy. Cancer Res 37:2407–2413, 1977

37. Shils ME: Nutritional problems associated with gastrointestinal and genitourinary cancer. Cancer Res 37:2366–2372, 1977

38. Welch D: Nutritional compromise in radiation therapy patients experiencing treatment-related emesis. JPEN 5:57–60, 1981

39. Bounous G, Gentile JM, Hugon J: Elemental diet in the management of the intestinal lesion produced by 5-fluorouracil in man. Can J Surg 14:312–324, 1971

40. Hadda H, Bounous G, Tahan WT, et al: Long-term nutrition with an elemental diet following intensive abdominal irradiation: Report of a case. Dis Colon Rectum 17:373–376, 1974

41. Dobbie RP, Butterick OD: Continuous pump/tube enteric hyperalimentation—use in esophageal cancer. JPEN 1:100–104, 1977

42. Block JH, Chlebowski RT, Herrold JN: Continuous enteric alimentation with a blenderized formula in cancer cachexia. Clin Oncol 7:93–98, 1981

43. Bloch AS: Nutritional considerations, in Groher ME (ed): Dysphagia. Boston, Butterworths, 1984, pp 175–193

44. Schuffler MD: Chronic intestinal pseudo-obstruction syndromes (Symposium on motility disorders). Med Clin N Am 65:1331–1358, 1981

45. Schuffler MD, Rohrmann CA, Chaffee RG, et al: Chronic intestinal pseudo-obstruction: A report of 27 cases and review of the literature. Medicine 60:173–196, 1981

46. Warner E, Jeejeebhoy KN: Successful management of chronic intestinal pseudo-obstruction with home parenteral nutrition. JPEN 9:173–178, 1985

47. Edmunds LH, Williams GM, Welch LE: External fistulas arising from the gastro-intestinal tract. Ann Surg 152:445, 1960

48. Sheldon GF, Gardiner BN, Way LE, et al: Management of gastrointestinal fistulas. Surg Gynecol Obstet 133:385–389, 1971

49. MacFayden BV, Dudrick SJ, Ruberg RL: Management of gastrointestinal fistulas with parenteral hyperalimentation. Surg 74:100–105, 1973

50. Aguirre A, Fischer JE, Welch CE: Role of surgery and hyperalimentation in therapy of gastrointestinal-cutaneous fistulas. Ann Surg 180:393–401, 1974

51. Deitel M: Nutritional management of external gastrointestinal fistulas. Can J Surg 19:505–511, 1976

52. Long JM, Steiger E, Dudrick SJ, et al: Total parenteral nutrition in the management of esophagocutaneous fistulas. Fed Proc 30:300, 1971

53. Aguirre A, Fischer JE: Intestinal Fistulas, in Fischer JE (ed): Total Parenteral Nutrition. Boston, Little, Brown, 1976, pp 203–218

54. Voitk AJ, Echave V, Brown RA, et al: Elemental diet in the treatment of fistulas of the alimentary tract. Surg Gynecol Obstet 137:68–72, 1973

55. Rocchio MA, Cha CM, Haas KF, et al: Use of chemically defined diets in the management of patients with high output gastrointestinal cutaneous fistulas. Am J Surg 127:148, 1974

56. Wright HK, Olson MD: The short gut syndrome, pathology and treatment. Curr Probl Surg (June):3–51, 1971

57. Scribner BH, Cole JJ, Christopher TG, et al: Long-term total parenteral nutrition. JAMA 212:457, 1970

58. Wilmore DW, Dudrick SJ, Daly JM, et al: The role of nutrition in the adaptation of the small intestine after massive resection. Surg Gynecol Obstet 132:673, 1971

59. Voitk A, Echave V, Brown R, et al: Use of an elemental diet during the adaptive stage of short gut syndrome. Gastroenterology 65:419, 1973

60. Broviac JW, Scribner BH: Prolonged parenteral nutrition in the home. Surg Gynecol Obstet 139:24, 1974

61. Scheflan M, Galli SJ, Perrotto J, et al: Intestinal adaptation after extensive

resection of the small intestine and prolonged administration of parenteral nutrition. Surg Gynecol Obstet 143:757–762, 1976

62. MacFayden BV: The use of intravenous hyperalimentation in gastrointestinal diseases. Nutri Supp Serv 2:6–10, 1982

63. Dudrick SJ, Wilmore DW, Steiger E, et al: Spontaneous closure of traumatic pancreatoduodenal fistulas with total parenteral nutrition. J Trauma 10:542–552, 1970

64. Weisz GM, Moss GS, Folk FA: Parenteral hyperalimentation in management of gastrointestinal fistulas. Can J Surg 15:310–313, 1972

65. Ragins H, Levenson SM, Signer R, et al: Intrajejunal administration of an elemental diet at neutral pH avoids pancreatic stimulation. Am J Surg 125:223–227, 1973

66. Voitk A, Brown RA, Echave V, et al: Use of an elemental diet in the treatment of complicated pancreatitis. Am J Surg 125:223–227, 1973

67. Feller JH, Brown RA, Toussaint GP, et al: Changing methods in the treatment of severe pancreatitis. Am J Surg 127:196–201, 1974

68. Blackburn GL, Williams LF, Bistrian BR, et al: New approaches to the management of severe acute pancreatitis. Am J Surg 131:114–124, 1976

69. White TT, Heimbach DM: Sequestrectomy and hyperalimentation in the treatment of hemorrhagic pancreatitis. Am J Surg 132:270–275, 1976

70. Goodgame JT, Fischer JE: Parenteral nutrition in the treatment of acute pancreatitis: Effect on complications and mortality. Ann Surg 186:651–658, 1977

71. Copeland EM, Dudrick SJ: Intravenous hyperalimentation in IBD, pancreatitis and cancer. Surg Annu 12:83–101, 1980

72. Grundfest S, Steiger E, Selinkoff P, et al: The effect of intravenous fat emulsions in patients with pancreatic fistula. JPEN 4:27–31, 1980

73. Silberman H, Dixon N, Eisenberg D: The safety and efficacy of a lipid-based system of parenteral nutrition in acute pancreatitis. Am J Gastroenterol 77:494–497, 1982

74. Grant JP, James S, Grabowski V, et al: Total parenteral nutrition in pancreatic disease. Ann Surg 200:627–631, 1984

75. Floch MH: Pancreatic diseases, in Nutrition and Diet Therapy in Gastrointestinal Disease. New York, Plenum, 1981, pp 203–221

76. Mascioli EA, Bistrian BR: TPN in the patient with diabetes. Nutri Supp Serv 3:12–16, 1983

77. Fischer JE, Bower RH: Nutritional support in liver disease. Surg Clin N Am 61:653–660, 1981

78. Jacobs DO, Boraas MC, Rombeau JL: Enteral nutrition and liver disease, in Rombeau JL, Caldwell MD (eds): Clinical Nutrition, Volume 1, Enteral and Tube Feeding. Philadelphia, WB Saunders, 1984, pp 376–402

79. Bower RH, Fischer JE: Hepatic indications for parenteral nutrition, in Rombeau JL, Caldwell MD (eds): Clinical Nutrition, Volume 2, Parenteral Nutrition. Philadelphia, WB Saunders, 1986, pp 602–614

80. Fischer JE, Rosen HM, Ebeid AM, et al: The effect of normalization of plasma amino acids on hepatic encephalopathy in man. Surgery 80:77–91, 1976

81. Okada A, Ikeda Y, Itakura T, et al: Treatment of hepatic encephalopathy with a new parenteral amino acid mixture (Abstract). JPEN 2:218, 1978

82. Freund H, Yoshimura N, Fischer JE: Chronic hepatic encephalopathy: Long term

therapy with a branched-chain amino-acid-enriched elemental diet. JAMA 242:347–349, 1979

83. Streibel JP, Holm E, Lutz H, et al: Parenteral nutrition and coma therapy with amino acids in hepatic failure. JPEN 3:240–246, 1979

84. Cerra FB, Cheung NK, Fischer JE, et al: A multi-center trial of branched-chain enriched amino acid infusion (F080) in hepatic encephalopathy. (Abstract). Hepatology 2:699, 1982

85. Freund H, Dienstag J, Lehrick J, et al: Infusion of branched-chain amino acid solution in patients with hepatic encephalopathy. Ann Surg 196:209–220, 1982

86. Rossi-Fanelli F, Riggio O, Cangiano C, et al: Branched-chain amino acids vs lactulose in the treatment of hepatic coma: A controlled study. Dig Dis Sci 27:929–935, 1982

87. Egberts EH, Schomerus H, Hamster W, et al: Effective treatment of latent portosystemic encephalopathy with oral branched chain amino acids, in Capocaccia L, Fischer JE, Rossi-Fanelli F (eds): Hepatic Encephalopathy in Chronic Liver Failure. New York, Plenum Press, 1984, pp 351–357

88. Fiaccadori F, Ghinelli F, Pedretti, et al: Branched-chain amino-enriched solutions in hepatic encephalopathy: A controlled trial, in Capocaccia L, Fischer JE, Rossi-Fanelli F (eds): Hepatic Encephalopathy in Chronic Liver Failure. New York, Plenum Press, 1984, pp 311–321

89. Horst D, Grace N, Conn HO, et al: Comparison of dietary protein with an oral, branched chain-enriched amino acid supplement in chronic portal-systemic encephalopathy: A randomized controlled trial. Hepatology 4:279–287, 1984

90. Cerra FB, Cheung NK, Fischer JE, et al: Disease-specific amino acid infusion (F080) in hepatic encophalopathy: A prospective, randomized double-blind controlled trial. JPEN 9:288–295, 1985

91. Doberneck RC, Reiser MP, Lillehei CW: Acute renal failure after open-heart surgery utilizing extracorporeal circulation and total body perfusion. J Thorac Cardiovasc Surg 43:444–452, 1962

92. Porter GA, Kloster FE, Herr RJ, et al: Renal complications associated with valve replacement surgery. J Thorac Cardiovasc Surg 53:145–152, 1967

93. Abel RM, Wick J, Beck CH, et al: Renal dysfunction following open-heart operations. Arch Surg 108:175–177, 1974

94. Abbott WM, Abel RM, Beck CH, et al: Renal failure after ruptured aneurysm. Arch Surg 110:1110–1112, 1975

95. Abel RM, Buckley MJ, Austen WG, et al: Acute postoperative renal failure in cardiac surgical patients. J Surg Res 20:341–348, 1976

96. Wilmore DW, Dudrick SJ: Treatment of acute renal failure with intravenous essential L-amino acids. Arch Surg 99:669–673, 1969

97. Dudrick SJ, Steiger E, Long JM: Renal failure in surgical patients. Treatment with intravenous essential amino acids and hypertonic dextrose. Surgery 68:180, 1970

98. Abbott WM, Abel RM, Fischer JE: Treatment of acute renal insufficiency after aortoiliac surgery. Arch Surg 103:590–594, 1971

99. Abel RM, Abbott WM, Fischer JE: Acute renal failure treatment without dialysis by total parenteral nutrition. Arch Surg 103:513–514, 1971

100. Abel RM, Abbott WM, Fischer JE: Intravenous essential L-amino acids and hypertonic dextrose in patients with acute renal failure. Am J Surg 123:632–638, 1972

101. Abel RM, Beck CH, Abbott WM, et al: Treatment of acute renal failure with intravenous administration of essential amino acids and glucose. Surg Forum 23:77, 1972

102. Abel RM, Beck CH, Abbott WM, et al: Improved survival from acute renal failure after treatment with intravenous essential L-amino acids and glucose: Results of a prospective, double-blind study. N Engl J Med 288:695, 1973

103. Abel RM, Shih VE, Abbott WM, et al: Amino acid metabolism in acute renal failure: Influence of intravenous essential L-amino acid hyperalimentation therapy. Ann Surg 180:350–355, 1974

104. Leonard CD, Luke RG, Siegel RR: Parenteral essential amino acids in acute renal failure. Urology 6:154–157, 1975

105. Blackburn GL, Etter G, Mackenzie T: Criteria for choosing amino acid therapy in acute renal failure. Am J Clin Nutr 31:1841–1853, 1978

106. Feinstein EI, Blumenkrantz MJ, Healy M, et al: Clinical and metabolic responses to parenteral nutrition in acute renal failure: A controlled double-blind study. JPEN 60:124–137, 1981

107. Mirtallo JM, Schneider PJ, Mavko K, et al: A comparison of essential and general amino acid infusions in the nutritional support of patients with compromised renal function. JPEN 6:109–113, 1982

108. Pittman JG, Ghen P: The pathogenesis of cardiac cachexia. Part I. N Engl J Med 271:403–409, 1964

109. Pittman JG, Ghen P: The pathogenesis of cardiac cachexia. Part II. N Engl J Med 271:453–460, 1964

110. Heymsfield SB, Nutter DO: The heart in protein-calorie undernutrition, in Hurst JW (ed): Update I: The Heart. New York, McGraw-Hill, 1979, pp 191–209

111. Gibbons GW, Blackburn GL, Harken DE, et al: Pre- and postoperative hyperalimentation in the treatment of cardiac cachexia. J Surg Res 20:439–444, 1976

112. Wanibuchi Y, Ino T, Aoki K, et al: Recent results and problems in the surgical treatment of acquired valvular heart disease. Jpn Circ J 47:1106–1111, 1983

113. Abel RM, Fischer JE, Buckley MJ, et al: Hyperalimentation in cardiac surgery. J Thorac Cardiovasc Surg 67:294–300, 1974

114. Abel RM, Buckley MJ, Austen WG: Etiology, incidence, and prognosis of renal failure following cardiac operations: Results of a prospective analysis of 500 consecutive patients. J Thorac Cardiovasc Surg 71:323–333, 1976

115. Abel RM: Nutritional support and the cardiac patient, in Rombeau JL, Caldwell MD (eds): Clinical Nutrition, Volume 2, Parenteral Nutrition. Philadelphia, WB Saunders, 1986, pp 575–585

116. Heymsfield SB, Smith J, Redd S, et al: Nutritional support in cardiac failure. Surg Clin N Am 61:635–652, 1981

117. Bassili HR, Deitel M: Effect of nutritional support on weaning patients off mechanical ventilators. JPEN 5:161–163, 1981

118. Askanazi J, Elwyn DH, Silverberg PA, et al: Respiratory distress secondary to a high carbohydrate load: A case report. Surgery 87:596–598, 1980

119. Askanazi J, Rosenbaum SH, Hyman AI, et al: Respiratory changes induced by the large glucose loads of total parenteral nutrition. JAMA 243:1444–1447, 1980

120. Askanazi J, Nordenstrom J, Rosenbaum SH, et al: Nutrition for the patient with respiratory failure: Glucose vs fat. Anesthesiology 54:373–377, 1981

121. Covelli HD, Black JW, Olsen MD, et al: Respiratory failure precipitated by high carbohydrate loads. Ann Intern Med 95:579–581, 1981

122. Rodriguez J, Weissman C, Askanazi J, et al: Metabolic and respiratory effects of glucose infusion. Anesthesiology 57(suppl):119, 1982

123. Askanazi J, Weissman MD, Rosenbaum SH, et al: Nutrition and the respiratory system. Crit Care Med 10:163–172, 1982

124. Garfinkel F, Robinson S, Price CS: Replacing carbohydrate calories with fat calories in enteral feeding for patients with impaired respiratory function. JPEN 9:106, 1985

125. Morrell RM: Neurologic disorders of swallowing in Groher ME (ed): Dysphagia. Boston, Butterworths, 1984, pp 37–59

126. Twomey PL, St. John JN: The neurologic patient, in Rombeau JL, Caldwell MD (eds): Clinical Nutrition, Volume 1, Enteral and Tube Feeding. Philadelphia, WB Saunders, 1984, pp 292–302

127. Asher IE: Management of neurologic disorders—the first feeding session, in Groher ME (ed): Dysphagia. Boston, Butterworths, 1984, pp 133–155

128. Griggs BA: Nursing management of swallowing disorders, in Groher ME (ed): Dysphagia. Boston, Butterworths, 1984, pp 195–218

129. Rapp RP, Young B, Twyman D, et al: The favorable effect of early parenteral feeding on survival in head-injured patients. J Neurosurg 58:906–912, 1983

130. Siegel JH, Cerra FB, Coleman B, et al: Physiological and metabolic correlations in human sepsis. Surgery 86:163–193, 1979

131. Freund HR: Parenteral nutrition in the septic patient, in Rombeau JL, Caldwell MD (eds): Clinical Nutrition, Volume 2, Parenteral Nutrition. Philadelphia, WB Saunders, 1986, pp 533–554

132. Siegel JH: Physiologic and nutritional implications of abnormal hormone-substrate relations and altered protein metabolism in human sepsis, in Rombeau JL, Caldwell MD (eds): Clinical Nutrition, Volume 2, Parenteral Nutrition. Philadelphia, WB Saunders, 1986, pp 555–574

133. Freund HR, Ryan JA, Fischer JE: Amino acid derangements in patients with sepsis: Treatment with branched chain amino acid rich infusions. Ann Surg 188:423–430, 1978

134. Blackburn GL, Moldawer LL, Usai S, et al: Branched chain amino acid administration and metabolism during starvation, injury and infection. Surgery 60:307, 1979

135. Nanni G, Siegel JH, Coleman B, et al: Increased lipid fuel dependence in the critically ill septic patient. J Trauma 24:14, 1984

136. Soroff HS, Pearson E, Arney GK, et al: Metabolism of burned patients, in Artz CP (ed): Research on Burns. Washington, American Institute of Biological Sciences, 1962, pp 126–136

137. Wilmore DW, Curreri PW, Spitzer KW, et al: Supranormal dietary intake in thermally injured hypermetabolic patients. Surg Gynecol Obstet 132:881–886, 1971

138. Curreri PW, Richmond D, Marvin JA, et al: Dietary requirements of patients with major burns. J Am Diet Assoc 65:415–417, 1974

139. Stein JM, Pruitt BA: Suppurative thrombophlebitis, a lethal, atrogenic disease. N Engl J Med 282:1452, 1970

140. Larkin JM, Moylan JA: Complete enteral support of thermally injured patients. Am J Surg 131:722–724, 1976
141. Solem LD: Enteral elemental nutrition in burn patients. Contemp Surg 28:36–41, 1986
142. Wilmore DW, Pruitt BA: Parenteral nutrition in burn patients, in Fischer JE (ed): Total Parenteral Nutrition. Boston, Little, Brown, 1976, pp 231–252
143. Wilmore DW, Moylan JA, Helmkamp GM, et al: Clinical evaluation of a 10% intravenous fat emulsion for parenteral nutrition in thermally injured patients. Ann Surg 178:503–513, 1973
144. Alexander JW, MacMillan BG, Stinnett JD, et al: Beneficial effects of aggressive protein feeding in severely burned children. Ann Surg 192:505, 1980
145. Kinney JM, Long CL, Duke JH: Carbohydrate and nitrogen metabolism after injury, in Porter R, Knight J (eds): Energy Metabolism in Trauma. Ciba Foundation Symposium. London, Churchill Livingstone, 1970, pp 103–126
146. Ruderman RL, Pollard A: Basic principles of surgical nutrition, in Deitel M (ed): Nutrition in Clinical Surgery. Baltimore, Williams & Wilkins, 1980, pp 13–18
147. Costa G: Cachexia: The metabolic component of neoplastic diseases. Prog Exp Tum Res 3:321, 1963
148. Theologides A: Pathogenesis of cachexia and cancer, a review and hypothesis. Cancer 29:484, 1972
149. Schwartz GF, Green HL, Bendon ML, et al: Combined parenteral hyperalimentation and chemotherapy in treatment of disseminated solid tumors. Am J Surg 121:169–173, 1971
150. Haddah H, Bounous G, Tahan W, et al: Long-term nutrition with an elemental diet following intensive abdominal irradiation: Report of a case. Dis Colon Rectum 17:373–376, 1974
151. Bounous G, LeBel E, Shuster J, et al: Dietary protection during radiation therapy. Strahlen Therapie 149:476–483, 1975
152. Copeland EM, MacFadyen BV, Lanzotti V, et al: Intravenous hyperalimentation as an adjunct to cancer chemotherapy. Am J Surg 129:167–173, 1975
153. Lanzotti VC, Copeland EM, George SL, et al: Cancer chemotherapeutic response and intravenous hyperalimentation. Cancer Chemother Rep 59:437–439, 1975
154. Copeland EM, Souchon EA, MacFadyen BV, et al: Intravenous hyperalimentation as an adjunct to radiation therapy. Cancer 39:609–616, 1977
155. Issell BF, Valdivieso M, Zaren HA, et al: Protection against chemotherapy toxicity by IV hyperalimentation. Cancer Treat Rep 62:1139–1143, 1978
156. Valdivieso M, Bodey GP, Benjamin RS: Role of hyperalimentation as an adjunct to intensive chemotherapy for small cell bronchogenic carcinoma. Cancer Treat Rep 65:145–151, 1981
157. Girtanner RE: Preop and postop nutritional support. Contemp Obstet Gynecol 25:153–173, 1985
158. Copeland EM, Daly JM, Dudrick SJ: Nutrition as an adjunct to cancer treatment in the adult. Cancer Res 37:2451–2456, 1977
159. Feighner JP, Robins E, Guze SB, et al: Diagnostic criteria for use in psychiatric research. Arch Gen Psychiatry 26:57–63, 1972
160. Kanis JA, Brown P, Fitzpatrick K, et al: Anorexia nervosa: A clinical, psychiatric, and laboratory study. Q J Med 43:321–338, 1974

161. Crisp AH, Hsa LKG, Harding B, et al: Clinical features of anorexia nervosa. J Psychosom Res 24:179–191, 1980
162. Drossman DA, Ontjes DA, Heizer WD: Anorexia nervosa. Gastroenterology 77:1115–1131, 1979
163. Schwabe AD, Lippe BM, Chang RJ, et al: Anorexia nervosa. Ann Intern Med 94:371–381, 1981
164. Russell GFM: The current treatment of anorexia nervosa. Br J Psychiatry 138:164–166, 1981
165. Bruch H: Treatment in anorexia nervosa. Int J Psychoanal Psychother 9:303–312, 1982–1983
166. Akamatsu K, Nishizaki T, Endo H, et al: A case of anorexia nervosa improvement following intravenous administration of fat emulsion (intralipid) combined with tube feeding. Nippon Naika Gakkal Zasshi 61:274–281, 1972
167. Finkelstein BA: Parenteral hyperalimentation in anorexia nervosa. Letter to editor. JAMA 219:217, 1972
168. Hirschmann GH, Rao DD, Chan JCM: Anorexia nervosa with acute tubular necrosis treated with parenteral nutrition. Nutr Metab 21:341–348, 1977
169. Maloney MJ, Farrell MK: Treatment of severe weight loss in anorexia nervosa with hyperalimentation and psychotherapy. Am J Psychiatry 137:310–314, 1980
170. Pertschuk MJ, Forester J, Buzby G, et al: The treatment of anorexia nervosa with total parenteral nutrition. Biol Psychol 16:539–550, 1981
171. Forester J: The use of total parenteral nutrition in the treatment of anorexia nervosa, in Rombeau JL, Caldwell MD (eds): Clinical Nutrition, Volume 2, Parenteral Nutrition. Philadelphia, WB Saunders, 1986, pp 520–532
172. Gottdiener JS, Gross HA, Henry WL, et al: Effects of self-induced starvation on cardiac size and function in anorexia nervosa. Circulation 58:425–433, 1978
173. Powers PS: Heart failure during treatment of anorexia nervosa. Am J Psychiatry 139:1167–1170, 1982
174. Schroeder LA: Weight control—fad, fact or fiction? Nutr International 2:281–289, 1986
175. Garrow JS: Treat Obesity Seriously: A Clinical Manual. London, Churchill Livingstone, 1981, pp 1–7
176. Stunkard AJ: The current status of treatment for obesity in adults, in Stunkard AJ, Stellar E (eds): Eating and Its Disorders. New York, Raven Press, 1984, pp 157–174
177. Gordon T, Kannel WB: Obesity and cardiovascular disease: The Framingham study, in Clinics in Endocrinolgy and Metabolism. Philadelphia, WB Saunders, 1976, pp 367–375
178. Hubert HB, Feinleib M, McNamara PM, et al: Obesity as an independent risk factor for cardiovascular disease: A 26 year followup of participants in the Framingham heart study. Circulation 67:968, 1983
179. National Institutes of Health Consensus Development Panel: Health implications of obesity. Ann Intern Med 103:1073–1077, 1985
180. Van Itallie TB: Health implications of overweight and obesity in the United States. Ann Int Med 103 (6, Part II) (suppl):983–988, 1985
181. Keesey RE: A set point theory of obesity, in Brownell KD, Foreyt JP (eds): Handbook of Eating Disorders: Physiology, Psychology and Treatment. New York, Basic Books, 1986, pp 63–87

182. Stunkard AJ, Sorensen TIA, Hanis C, et al: An adoption study of human obesity. N Engl J Med 314:193–198, 1986

183. Abramson EE: A review of behavioral approaches to weight control. Behav Res Ther 11:547–556, 1973

184. Horton ES: The role of exercise in the prevention and treatment of obesity, in Bray GA (ed): Obesity in Perspective. Bethesda, MD, National Institute of Health, 1973, pp 62–66

185. Brightwell DR, Clancy J: Self-training of new eating behavior for weight reduction. Diseases of the Nervous System 37:85–89, 1976

186. Lindner PG, Blackburn GL: Multidisciplinary approach to obesity utilizing fasting modified by protein-sparing therapy. Obesity and Bariatric Medicine, 5:198, 1976

187. Alden JF: Gastric and jejunoileal bypass: A comparison in the treatment of morbid obesity. Arch Surg 112:799–806, 1977

188. Bray GA, Benfield JR: Intestinal bypass for obesity: A summary and perspective. Am J Clin Nutr 30:121–127, 1977

189. Currey H, Malcolm R, Riddle E, et al: Behavioral treatment of obesity: Limitations and results with the chronically obese. JAMA 237:2829–2831, 1977

190. Vertes V, Genuth SM, Hazelton IM: Supplemented fasting as a large-scale outpatient program. JAMA 238:2151–2153, 1977

191. Bistrian BR, Sherman M: Results of the treatment of obesity with a protein-sparing modified diet. Int J Obes 2:143, 1978

192. Joffe SN: A review: Surgery for morbid obesity. J Surg Res 33:74–88, 1982

193. Moxley RT, Prozefsky T, Lockwood DH: Protein nutrition and liver disease after jejunoileal bypass for morbid obesity. N Engl J Med 290:921, 1974

194. Printen KJ, Mason EE: Peripheral neuropathy following gastric bypass for treatment of morbid obesity. Obesity and Bariatric Medicine 6:185, 1977

195. Shizgal HM, Forse RA, Spanier AH, et al: Protein malnutrition following intestinal bypass for morbid obesity. Surgery 86:60, 1979

196. Halverson JD, Scheff RJ, Gentry K, et al: Jejunoileal bypass: Late metabolic sequelae and weight gain. Am J Surg 140:347, 1980

197. Undergraff TA, Neufeld NJ: Protein, iron and folate status of patients prior to and following surgery for morbid obesity. J Am Diet Assoc 80:437, 1982

198. Grant JP: Patient selection, in Grant JP (ed): Handbook of Total Parenteral Nutrition. Philadelphia, WB Saunders, 1980, pp 7–46

199. A.S.P.E.N. Board of Directors: Guidelines for use of total parenteral nutrition in the hospitalized adult patient. JPEN 10:441–445, 1986

200. Silberman H: Total parenteral nutrition by peripheral vein: Current status of fat emulsions. Nutr International 2:145–149, 1986

201. Walters J, Freeman JB: Parenteral nutrition by peripheral vein, in Mullen J, Crosby L, Rombeau JL (eds): The Surgical Clinics of North America: Symposium on Surgical Nutrition. Philadelphia, WB Saunders, 1981, pp 593–594

202. Freeman JB, Fairfull-Smith RJ: Physiologic approach to peripheral parenteral nutrition, in Fischer JE (ed): Surgical Nutrition. Boston, Little, Brown, 1983, pp 703–717

203. Matarese LE: Enteral alimentation, in Fischer JE (ed): Surgical Nutrition. Boston, Little, Brown, 1983, pp 719–755

204. Rombeau JL, Jacobs DO: Nasoenteric tube feeding, in Rombeau JL, Caldwell ME

(eds): Clinical Nutrition, Volume I, Enteral and Tube Feeding. Philadelphia, WB Saunders, 1984, pp 261–274

205. Gustke RF, Varma RR, Soergel KH: Gastric reflux during perfusion of the proximal small bowel. Gastroenterology 59:890–895, 1970

Loretta Forlaw

4

Nutritional Assessment*

A heightened awareness of the nutritional needs of hospitalized patients has evolved in conjunction with the development of parenteral nutrition and improved methods for delivery of enternal nutrition. Moderate to severe malnutrition has been reported to affect approximately 30–50 percent of hospitalized patients.[1,2] Inadequate nutrition may affect the patient's strength, general sense of well being, ability to heal wounds, resistance to infection, and length of hospital stay.

An understanding of the signs, symptoms, and diagnostic procedures that identify the patient with a potential for or actual malnutrition enhances the nurse's ability to provide optimal nursing care and seek appropriate consultation with other disciplines.

MALNUTRITION OF HOSPITALIZED PATIENTS

The classic types of malnutrition that occur in hospitalized patients are *marasmus, kwashiorkor, and marasmic-kwashiorkor.*

Marasmus (protein-calorie deprivation) is characterized by gradual weight loss and fat and muscle wasting due to protein-calorie deprivation. It is most likely to develop in the mild to moderately stressed patient who cannot maintain an adequate oral intake and is in a state of semi-starvation. These individuals are generally underweight and emaciated. Visceral protein status may be relatively

---

* The opinions or assertions contained herein are the private views of the author and are not to be construed as official or as reflecting the view of the Department of the Army or the Department of Defense.

NUTRITIONAL SUPPORT IN NURSING
ISBN 0-8089-1889-3

normal; arm muscle circumference and skinfold thicknesses, however, are substantially below normal standards.[3]

Kwashiorkor is characterized by decreased visceral proteins. It is most likely to develop in the patient whose intake has consisted mainly of carbohydrate and little if any protein. The patient may appear well nourished or even obese. Arm muscle circumference and skinfold thicknesses are at or above normal standards.[3]

Marasmic-kwashiorkor (protein-calorie-malnutrition) is characterized by skeletal muscle wasting, depletion of fat stores, and depressed visceral proteins. These patients generally have suffered an acute catabolic state in conjunction with prior starvation. They are often cachectic in appearance. The markedly obese patient may have interosseus muscle wasting. Arm circumference and skinfold thickness are at or below normal standards (Table 4-1).[4]

NUTRITIONAL ASSESSMENT

Each member of a multidisciplinary nutritional support service contributes to optimal nutritional assessment of the hospitalized patient. The nurse may be

Table 4-1
Protein–Calorie Malnutrition

	Marasmus	Kwashiorkor
Clinical setting	Lack of calories	Lack of protein + stress
Time course to develop	Months–years Starved appearance Weight/height <80 percent std Triceps skinfold <3 mm Midarm muscle circumference <15 cm	Weeks–months Well nourished appearance Hair easily pluckable Edema
Laboratory findings	Serum albumin >2.8 gm/100 ml	Serum albumin <2.8 gm/100 ml Lymphocytes 1200 cells/cu mm Nonreactive skin tests
Clinical course	Reasonably preserved responsiveness to short-term stress	↓ Wound healing ↓ Immunocompetence ↑ Infections/other complication
Mortality rate	Low (unless related to underlying disease process)	High

From Butterworth CE, Weinsier, RL: Malnutrition in hospital patients: Assessment and treatment, *in* Goodhart RS, Shils ME (eds): Modern Nutrition in Health and Disease. Philadelphia, Lea and Febiger, 1980, p. 670. With permission.

responsible for performing many of the components of a nutritional assessment and so should understand their relevance to determining and monitoring the patient's nutritional status. The information obtained should be incorporated into the patient's care plan. Suggested goals of nutritional assessment include the following:

1. To identify nutritional states and deficiencies that adversely affect health.
2. To obtain specific information to assist in planning and delivery of nutritional support.
3. To evaluate the efficacy of nutritional support and to modify the patient's care plan as needed to obtain the desired result.[5]

Dietary History

A good dietary history should attempt to define the eating patterns of an individual in an effort to identify possible dietary deficiencies.[3] An additional inquiry into social habits such as improper diets, vitamin usage, and alcohol intake should be elicited since these findings may identify whether an individual's lifestyle is an important factor in the development of nutritional deficiencies. A brief nutritional history should document the patient's usual and current intake. This will indicate whether a more in-depth nutritional history with the aid of a clinical dietitian is necessary. This short history may be obtained by a 24-hour recall, food records, or food frequency questionnaires. The 24-hour dietary history documents simply what the patient recalls eating over the past 24 hours. The 24-hour period should be representative of the patient's usual eating patterns. An additional method is a dietary intake record for a period of 3–7 days. This is valuable in hospitalized patients who are suspected of having poor oral intake. Calorie counts can be performed with the nurse's documentation of the food consumed. These studies provide only an estimate of an individual's intake, however, since many patients may alter their food consumption as a result of their inability to tolerate a hospital diet. These factors must be kept in mind when interpreting the data. Questionnaires are also available for dietary analysis; from these a clinical dietitian can interpret nutrient intake in order to define specific nutrient deficiencies. Ambulatory or home patients can document their baseline food intake by recording their diet for a full week.

Anthropometric Measurements

An anthropometer or stature scale on the balance beam should be used for determining the patient's actual height. Height recall may not be accurate. Height decreases after age 50, with the effect being more pronounced in men than women.[6] If the patient is unable to stand, length from heel to top of the head can be measured with a flexible tape measure, while the patient lies flat in bed with arms folded across the chest.[6] The ideal weight for height is usually

Table 4-2
Rules of Fives and Sixes of Determination of Ideal Body Weight

Frame size	Men	Women
Medium	Allow 106 lb for first 5 feet of height, plus 6 lb for each additional inch	Allow 100 lb for first 5 feet of height, plus 5 lbs for each additional inch
Small	Subtract 10 percent	Subtract 10 percent
Large	Add 10 percent	Add 10 percent

Adapted from American Diabetic Association, A guide for professionals: the effective application of exchange lists for meal planning, New York American Diabetic Association, 1977, page 17. With permission.

determined from standard tables such as the 1983 Metropolitan Height and Weight Tables that use the elbow breadth for determination of frame size.[7] A quick method for estimating ideal weight is presented in Table 4-2.[8]

A balance beam scale should be used for patients able to stand unassisted. Litter-, chair-, or sling-type scales are available for patients who cannot stand unassisted. The same calibrated scale should be used for each weighing. To enhance accuracy, weight should be obtained at approximately the same time of day with the patient wearing the same amount of clothing.

The fat content of subcutaneous tissue can be estimated by caliper measurement of skinfold thickness at one or more sites (most common in the triceps, suprailiac, and subscapular). The tricep skinfold (TSF) is the most common and easily measured area. The TSF is measured by pinching a lengthwise double fold of skin and fat between the thumb and forefinger about 1 cm above patient's freely hanging arm. Calipers are then placed over the fold and 3 separate readings in millimeters are taken. The average of the readings is the TSF.[3] Errors in measurement are most often related to observer technique, measurement site, subject position, and equipment.[9]

A similar technique is used to measure other skinfolds. In fact, use of more than 1 skinfold (the sum of the triceps and subscapula skinfold thickness) has been shown to correlate well with weight change. Table 4-3 provides the reference standards used for the sum of the triceps and subscapular skinfolds.[10] Generally, fat stores less than the 35th percentile suggest moderate depletion, and those less than the 25th percentile indicate severe depletion.

Midarm muscle circumference (MAMC) is an estimation of skeletal muscle mass and can be calculated from the midarm circumference (MAC) and TSF measurements using the following equation:

$$MAMC = MAC - (TSF \times 0.314)$$

Table 4-4 lists standards for men and women by age.[10]

Table 4-3
Reference Standards for Sum of Triceps and Subscapular Skinfold*

Age Group (yr)	Percentile						
	5	10	25	50	75	90	95
American Men							
18–74	11.5†	13.5	19.0	26.0	34.5	44.0	51.0
18–24	10.0	12.0	15.0	21.0	30.0	41.0	51.0
25–34	11.5	13.5	19.0	26.0	35.5	45.0	54.0
35–44	12.0	15.0	21.0	28.0	36.0	44.0	48.5
45–54	13.0	15.0	21.0	28.0	37.0	46.0	53.0
55–64	12.0	14.0	20.0	26.0	34.0	44.0	48.0
65–74	11.5	14.0	19.5	26.0	34.0	42.5	49.0
American Women							
18–74	18.5	22.0	28.5	39.0	53.0	65.0	73.0
18–24	17.0	19.0	24.0	31.0	41.5	54.5	64.0
25–34	18.5	20.5	26.5	35.0	48.0	64.0	73.0
35–44	20.0	23.0	30.0	40.5	55.0	68.0	75.0
45–54	22.0	25.0	33.5	45.0	58.0	69.5	78.5
55–64	19.0	25.0	33.0	46.0	58.0	68.0	73.0
65–74	20.0	25.0	32.0	41.0	52.2	63.0	70.0

From Buzby GT, Mullen JL: Nutritional assessment, in Rombeau JL, Caldwell MD (eds): Clinical Nutrition, Volume I: Enteral and Tube Feeding, Philadelphia, WB Saunders, 1984, page 127–147. With permission.
*Developed from data collected during the Health and Nutrition examination Survey of 1971–1974.
†Values are in mm.

Arm muscle area (AMA) reflects skeletal muscle mass and is determined by using the following formula:

$$AMA = \frac{(MAC - TSF)^2}{4\pi}$$

Nomograms for both MAMC and AMA are available.[3]

Standard arm measurements for males and females have been compiled. Intra-observer and inter-observer variation can limit the value of these measurements, however, and it is recommended that serial measurements be performed by the same person to avoid inter-observer variation and minimize inappropriate techniques.[10]

Measurement of Immune Function

Alterations in the immune system are influenced by stress, specific disease states, and malnutrition. The methods most commonly used for assessment of immunocompetence are total lymphocyte count (TLC) and response to skin test antigens.[3]

Table 4-4
Reference Standards for Midarm Muscle Circumference*

Age Group (yr)	Percentile						
	5	10	25	50	75	90	95
American Men							
18–74	26.4†	27.6	29.6	31.7	33.9	36.0	37.3
18–24	25.7	27.1	28.7	30.7	32.9	35.5	37.4
25–34	27.0	28.2	30.0	32.0	34.4	36.5	37.6
35–44	27.8	28.7	30.7	32.7	34.8	36.3	37.1
45–54	26.7	27.8	30.0	32.0	34.2	36.2	37.6
55–64	25.6	27.3	29.6	31.7	33.4	35.2	36.6
65–74	25.3	26.5	28.5	30.7	32.4	34.4	35.5
American Women							
18–74	23.2	24.3	26.2	28.7	31.9	35.2	37.8
18–24	22.1	23.0	24.5	26.4	28.8	31.7	34.4
25–34	23.3	24.2	25.7	27.8	30.4	34.1	37.2
35–44	24.1	25.2	26.8	29.2	32.2	36.2	38.5
45–54	24.3	25.7	27.5	30.3	32.9	36.8	39.3
55–64	23.9	25.1	27.7	30.2	33.3	36.3	38.2
65–74	23.8	25.2	27.4	29.9	32.5	35.3	37.2

From Buzby GT, Mullen JL: Nutritional assessment, in Rombeau JL, Caldwell MD (eds): Clinical Nutrition, Volume I: Enteral and Tube Feeding, Philadelphia, WB Saunders, 1984, page 127–147. With permission.
*Developed from data collected during the Health and Nutrition examination Survey of 1971–1974.
†Values are in cm.

The formula for determining total lymphocyte count is:

$$TLC = \frac{\% \text{ lymphocytes} \times \text{white blood cell count (WBC)}}{100}$$

A TLC less than 2000/mm³ is considered suggestive of impaired immunocompetence.[3]

Evaluation of cell-mediated immunity is reflected in delayed cutaneous hypersensitivity in response to intradermal injection of common antigens. Generally, 3 or more antigens are injected subcutaneously, and reactions are evaluated at 24, 48, and 72 hours for area of induration and erythema.

In general, results are classified as anergic if no reaction is observed, relative anergic if reactions of 1–5 mm are observed, and reactive if reactions greater than 5 mm occur. The patient's ability to respond to one or more of the antigens is usually considered a normal result.[3]

This remains a very controversial area. An excellent review by Twomey et al.[11] outlines the numerous nonnutritional factors and the lack of standardization in the performance and evaluation of skin tests, which must be considered when evaluating skin tests in conjunction with other assessments such as weight and nitrogen balance.

Physiologic Measurements

An indirect measurement of muscle mass depletion is the creatinine-height index (CHI). A 24-hour urine collection is required. The results are expressed as a percentage of the actual milligrams of creatinine excreted for the 24-hour period to the predicted creatinine excretion based on height.

$$CHI = \frac{measured \ urinary \ creatinine \times 100}{ideal \ urinary \ creatinine}$$

To obtain accurate results, careful 24-hour collections of urine must be done. This includes having the patient void and discard the urine immediately before the collection begins, and void and include the last specimen at the end of the urine collection. One missed void invalidates the results; careful explanations to the patient including reminder signs in the bathroom that a 24-hour urine collection is in progress are recommended. An average of three serial 24-hour collections gives the most accurate results. Another limitation of the CHI is that body frame size and musculature of individuals and changes in creatinine excretion with age are not taken into account by the established norms. Table 4-5 provides reference standards for 24-hour urinary creatinine excretion.[10]

Serum concentrations of transport proteins synthesized by the liver are often used to estimate visceral protein status. The most commonly measured serum proteins are albumin and transferrin. Transferrin can be measured directly by radial immunodiffusion or indirectly from total iron binding capacity (TIBC) using a conversion equation. Multiple equations for conversion of TIBC to transferrin are available. If the indirect method is used, each hospital should develop its own standards for conversion in accordance with individual laboratories.[10]

Serum albumin, with a relatively long half-life of approximately 21 days, changes slowly with poor dietary protein intake. Transferrin, having a much shorter half-life of 8–10 days, reflects changes in visceral protein status more acutely. It should be kept in mind that transferrin values determined from TIBC can be altered by iron deficiency, causing the obtained value to reflect both protein and iron deficiencies. The state of hydration and the presence of stress or trauma also may significantly alter serum values of both proteins.[10]

Retinol binding protein and prealbumin, with extremely short half-lives of 10 hours and 1–2 days respectively, are extremely sensitive indicators of visceral protein status. Serum concentration of these proteins changes acutely with minor stress, however, and therefore may be misleading as a nutritional indicator in such situations.[10] Anthropometrics and serum albumin are most useful in

Table 4-5
Reference Standards for 24-Hour Urinary Creatinine Excretion

Men*		Women†	
Height (cm)	Ideal Creatinine (mg)	Height (cm)	Ideal Creatinine (mg)
157.5	1288	147.3	830
160.0	1325	149.9	851
162.6	1359	152.4	875
165.1	1386	154.9	900
167.6	1426	157.5	925
170.2	1467	160.0	949
172.7	1513	162.6	977
175.3	1555	165.1	1006
177.8	1596	167.6	1044
180.3	1642	170.2	1076
182.9	1691	172.7	1109
185.4	1739	175.3	1141
188.0	1785	177.8	1174
190.5	1831	180.3	1206
193.0	1891	182.9	1240

From Buzby GT, Mullen JL: Nutritional assessment, in Rombeau JL, Caldwell MD (eds): Clinical Nutrition, Volume I: Enteral and Tube Feeding, Philadelphia, WB Saunders, 1984, page 127–147. With permission.
*Creatinine coefficient = 23 mg/kg of ideal body weight.
†Creatinine coefficient = 18 mg/kg of ideal body weight.

following patients who are markedly depleted and require long-term nutritional repletion. Anthropometrics provide an assessment of the efficacy of nutritional therapy and exercise in repletion of lean muscle versus excessive deposition of fat.

Nitrogen balance is an objective measure of the adequacy of calorie and protein intake. It remains the clinical method of choice for monitoring short-term changes in body protein stores. Urinary nitrogen losses can be obtained from a 24-hour urine collection utilizing the Kjeldahl method or can be estimated by measuring urinary urea nitrogen.[12] Nitrogen balance using urinary urea nitrogen can be calculated as follows:

nitrogen balance = nitrogen intake − nitrogen output

Nitrogen balance calculations are as follows:

1. To convert protein to nitrogen, divide g of protein by 6.4 for intravenous amino acids and 6.25 for enteral formulations. Example:

1000 cc/day of 85% amino acids provide 85 g protein or 13.2 g nitrogen.

2. Multiply reported urine urea nitrogen (UUN) value by 20 percent to account for nonurea nitrogen. Example:

$$UUN - 490 \text{ mg\%} \times 20\% = 588 \text{ mg\%}$$

3. Multiply UUN (mg/100 ml) value by urine volume in liters/day (Urine volume = 2000 cc). Example:

$$\frac{588 \text{ mgm/100ml} \times 2 \text{ liters/day}}{100} = 11.76 \text{ g}$$

4. Subtract nitrogen out from nitrogen in.

$$\begin{array}{l} 13.2 \text{ g nitrogen in} \\ \underline{11.8 \text{ g nitrogen out}} \\ +1.4 \text{ g nitrogen} \end{array}$$

5. If patient is having stool, fistula, or other losses, add +2–4 g to nitrogen out.

$$\begin{array}{l} 13.2 \text{ g nitrogen in} \\ \underline{13.8 \text{ g nitrogen out}} \\ -.6 \text{ g nitrogen} \end{array}$$

Ideally, the patient should have 2–3 g positive nitrogen balance for anabolism.

Basal energy expenditure (BEE) can be estimated from the Harris-Benedict equations which take into account age, sex, height, and weight of the patient.

$$BEE \text{ (Men)} = [66.47 + (13.75W) + (5.0H)] - (6.76A)]$$
$$BEE \text{ (Women)} = [655.10 + (9.56W) + (1.85W)] - (4.68A)]$$

where W = weight in kg, H = height in cm, and A = age in years.[13] The rules of five and sixes can be used to determine the patient's ideal weight, which can be used in the Harris-Benedict equation if the patient has experienced significant weight loss (Table 4-2).

Energy expenditure can be measured by direct or indirect calorimetry. Direct calorimetry measures heat production from the body. This requires a stationary closed chamber, a situation not practical for many hospitalized patients.[12,14] Indirect calorimetry is the measurement of oxygen consumption, carbon dioxide production, and nitrogen excretion from which heat production can be calculated.[12,14] Indirect calorimetry also has the advantages of being relatively portable and permits the calculation of the total respiratory quotient (RQ) as follows:

$$\text{Total RQ} = \frac{VCO_2}{VO_2}$$

The RQ reflects net substrate oxidation. In clinical practice the contribution of protein oxidation to gas exchange is calculated as follows:

$$\text{Nonprotein RQ} = \frac{VCO_2 - 4.754 \text{ (urinary nitrogen)}}{VO_2 - 5.923 \text{ (urinary nitrogen)}}$$

This adjustment allows for calculation of the relative quantity of energy produced from carbohydrate, protein, and fat.[14] Thus a nonprotein RQ of .7 indicates net fat oxidation, a nonprotein RQ of 1 reflects net carbohydrate oxidation, and a nonprotein RQ of 0.85 suggests equal oxidation of fat and carbohydrate.[14] Nonprotein RQs greater than 1 are only seen in patients who are hyperventilating or during excessive intravenous carbohydrate delivery.[14] A nonprotein RQ of 1.01–1.25 in a patient who is not hyperventilating is indicative of the synthesis of adipose tissue from carbohydrate, suggesting the need to decrease carbohydrate delivery in order to prevent development of fatty liver and its consequences.[14]

Using total RQ when 24-hour urinary nitrogen collections are not feasible results in less than a 2 percent error in calculations.[14]

The most commonly used instrument for determination of indirect calorimetry in the clinical setting is the metabolic measurement cart (MMC). MMCs are portable systems that have the capability to measure energy expenditure in nonintubated patients and those requiring mechanical ventilation. Most MMCs have a canopy system for long-term continuous measurements, along with a fully automatic calibration and computerized data system. Resting energy expenditure (REE) generally reflects 75–100 percent of daily energy expendi-

Table 4-6
Estimated Energy Requirements for Postoperative Patient
with Minor Surgery

Patient's age:	69 years
Height:	178 cm
Current weight:	69 kg
Ideal weight:	70 kg*
Sex:	male

Harris-Benedict Equation
BEE(men) = [[66.47 + 13.75(70 kg) + 5.0(178)] − 69(6.76)]
                   [(66.47 + 962.5 + 890) − 466.44]
                                BEE = 1452.57
Activity factor = 30% − ambulatory
Injury factor = 20% − minor operation
Estimated daily requirements = 2266 kcal/day

*If patient were below ideal weight and needed to gain weight, you would add 500 kcal/day to promote one pound weight gain/week.

ture.[14] This value must then be adjusted to meet the energy costs of physical activity, injury, and/or illness. The most common multiples used with estimated or measured energy requirements are those derived by Long and coworkers,[15] which provide a 20–30 percent increase above REE for activities such as sitting in a chair or short walks, 20 percent increase above REE for minor surgery, 30 percent for major surgery, 35 percent for long bone fractures, and 60 percent for sepsis. Ongoing studies continue to provide additional data on appropriate multiples for patients with cancer, head injuries, and other disease states (see Table 4-6).

Indirect calorimetry or estimation of energy requirements and nitrogen balance provide a base from which to minimize inappropriate composition of nutritional solutions and to optimize maintenance or repletion of normal body composition in hospitalized patients.

New Approaches

Total body potassium quantification, a measurement of the body's naturally occurring radioactive potassium (40_k), is currently being performed in research settings to determine body cell mass. This technique is based on the assumption that the ratio of potassium:nitrogen in the body is constant. Research findings have documented that in certain patient populations (e.g., cancer cachexia and obesity), this ratio is not constant. Clinical applicability is therefore limited.[16,17]

Another method for assessing body cell mass used primarily for research purposes is 42_k dilutional technique. An indirect technique for determining 42_k has been developed utilizing the following equation:

$$k_e - R \times TBW - Na_e$$

where K_e = total exchangeable potassium, R = ratio of the sum of Na content and potassium content divided by the water content of blood sample, TBW = total body water, and NaI_e = quantity of total exchangeable sodium.[17,18]

The radiographic measurement of midarm provides a quantitative assessment of subcutaneous fat, muscle, and bone in the upperarm. The current value of this test is in the research area to help establish more precise standards for arm anthropometric measurement.[19] For morbidly obese patients where standard anthropometric measurements are difficult to perform and imprecise, this radiographic technique may be useful in the measurement of body composition as the patient loses weight.[19]

Computerized tomography has advantages over conventional radiography. It provides a sharp delineation of the characteristic density difference between fat, lean tissues, and bone. Images are three dimensional rather than the two-dimensional information provided by traditional x-ray images. Data from computerized tomography can define changes in visceral organ mass associated with undernutrition, measure regional muscle mass, define the relationship of subcutaneous to internal fat, establish bone density, and diagnose fatty liver. A major limitation of computerized tomography for routine nutritional elevations is radiation exposure, particularly for repeated observation and cost.[20]

PHYSICAL ASSESSMENT

The patient's therapeutic modalities may alter blood values. Factors such as fluid status can influence biochemical results and anthropometric measurements. The data collected through nutritional assessment techniques thus must be viewed in the context of the patient's overall medical condition and therapeutic plan. Physical assessment provides information that can further identify nutritional alterations in the depleted patient.

Physical examination of the patient with malnutrition or the potential for developing malnutrition is an essential part of the standard nutritional assessment and is often best performed by the nurse on the support service team. The physical examination is conducted with special emphasis on signs reflecting nutritional deficiencies.[4] Signs of nutritional deficiencies are observed most commonly during examination of the skin, hair, eyes, and mouth. Less commonly affected are the glands and nervous system.

The physical examination also provides information pertinent to the choice of feeding regimens for the patient requiring nutritional support. For example, a comatose patient or one with seizures may initially require nasoduodenal rather than nasogastric feeding or even total parenteral nutrition to reduce the risk of aspiration pneumonia. A patient whose level of consciousness improves could be converted to enteral or oral feeding. The patient with signs of fluid overload will require a more concentrated formula to meet energy and nitrogen requirements. Patients with amputations will need to have the mass of the missing limb considered when calculating substrate requirements. Physical examination of the skin, hair, glands, skeleton, eyes, and face will often reveal signs of the majority of nutrient deficiencies (Tables 4-7 and 4-8).[5] See Appendix A for definitions. One must keep in mind that physical signs of nutritional deficiencies occur only after significant body nutrition depletion. It is also important to relate symptoms to the patient's diet history and medical history; for example, poorly fitting dentures can produce angular stomatitis.

The patient should be followed at least weekly for physical signs of nutrient deficiency while acutely ill. A flow sheet helps in monitoring the patient's progress. Tables 4-7 and 4-8 can be used as a guide for completing the physical examination flow sheet.

Knowledge of specific nutrient functions can provide a basis for correlation and recognition of the significance of nutritional deficiency states.

(Text continues p. 106)

Table 4-7
Physical Examination—Signs and Symptoms of Nutritional Deficiencies

Area of Examination	Water/Fat Soluble Vitamins	Protein/Calorie	Essential Fatty Acids
Hair		Lack of luster Easy pluckability Sparse	Alopecia
Skin	Follicular hyperkeratosis (Vitamin A) Petechia (Vitamin C) Purpura (Vitamin C, K) Pellagrous dermatitis (Niacin)	Subcutaneous fat loss	Scaly dermatitis
Face Eyes	Nasolabial Seborrhea (Riboflavin) Xerosis of conjuctivae (Vitamin A) Keratomalacia (Riboflavin) Corneal vascularization (Riboflavin) Blepharitis (B-Complex, Biotin) Bitot's spots (Vitamin A) "Spectacle eye" (Biotin)		
Lips	Cheilosis (Vitamin B$_6$, Iron, Riboflavin) Angular stomatitis (Riboflavin, Iron)		Cheilosis

Tongue	Bald (Niacin, Vitamin B_{12})	Edema
	Glossitis (Vitamin B_6, Iron, Riboflavin, Folic Acid)	
Nails	Brittle, lined, rigid (Nonspecific)	
Glands		Parotid enlargement
Muscles, Extremities		Interosseous muscle
		Wasting temporal muscle
		Wasting intercostal
		Muscle wasting calf
		Muscle wasting edema
Neurologic	Pain calves, weak thighs (Thiamin)	Edema
	Edema (Thiamin)	
	Absent vibratory sense in the feet (B_{12})	
	Hyporeflexia (Thiamin)	
	Decreased position sense (B_{12})	
	Confabulation, disorientation (B_{12})	
	Weakness, paresthesia of legs (Thiamin, Pyridoxine, Panthothenic Acid, B_{12})	

From Forlaw L, Bayer L: Introduction to Nutritional and Physical Assessment of the Adult Patient for The Nurse. American Society of Parenteral and Enteral Nutrition. Washington, DC, 1983, p 1–22. With permission.

Table 4-8
Physical Examination—Signs and Symptoms of Mineral and Trace
Element Deficiencies

Area of Examination		Minerals and Trace Elements
Hair	Decreased pigmentation	Copper
	Alopecia	Zinc
Skin	Dilated superficial veins	Copper
	Pallor superficial	Copper
Face	Seborrhea dermatitis	Zinc
Lips	Angular stomatitis	Iron
Nails	Thin, brittle, flattened Spoon-shaped	Iron
Glands	Thyroid enlargement	Iodine
Muscles,	Weakness	Potassium, Magnesium
Extremities,	Lethargy	Potassium, Calcium, Iron
Neurologic	Confusion	Magnesium, Phosphorus
	Flaccid paralysis	Potassium
	Irritability	Potassium, Calcium, Magnesium
	Convulsions	Calcium

From Forlaw L, Bayer L: Introduction to Nutritional and Physical Assessment of the Adult Patient for The Nurse. Washington, DC, American Society of Parenteral and Enteral Nutrition, 1983, p 1–22. With permission.

Table 4-9
Nursing Diagnosis

Nursing Diagnosis	Goal	Nursing Intervention/Orders
Potential for altered nutritional status due to illness or associated with hospitalization.	Maintenance or repletion of nutritional status. Patient will maintain weight or gain 1–2 lbs/week.	Height and weight on admission. Daily weight when loss is 5 percent or greater of usual ideal body weight. History on admission Anthoprometric measurements by dietitian or nutrition support nurse. Estimation of nutrition requirements.
	Patient will take and utilize estimated nutrients.	Documentation of nutrition intake by dietician or nutrition support nurse.
	Patient will not exhibit signs and symptoms of nutrient deficiency.	Physical examination for signs and symptoms suggestive of or related nutrient deficiency.

SUMMARY

The nursing process is useful in documenting the nutritional evaluation and needs of the patient. Table 4-9 provides an example of utilizing nursing diagnosis for specific problem identification and nursing intervention.

Nutritional and physical assessment of the patient who is malnourished or potentially malnourished is essential to prevent, detect, and reverse complications related to nutritional deficiency states. The nurse can play a key role in collecting, coordinating, and analyzing this information with other members of the nutritional support service.

REFERENCES

1. Mullen JL, Buzby GP, Weldman TF, et al: Prediction of operative morbidity and mortality by preoperative nutritional assessment. Surg Forum 30:80–82, 1979
2. Mullen JL: Consequences of malnutrition in the surgical patient. Surg Clin N Am 61:465–487, 1981
3. Grant JP, Custer PB, Thurlow J: Current techniques of nutritional assessment. Surg Clin N Am 61:437–463, 1981
4. Butterworth CE, Weinsier RL: Malnutrition in hospitalized patients: Assessment and treatment, in Goodhart RS, Shils MD (eds): Modern Nutrition in Health and Disease. Philadelphia, Lea and Febiger, 1980, pp 667–684
5. Forlaw L, Bayer L: Introduction to nutritional and physical assessment for the nurse. Washington, DC, American Society of Parenteral and Enteral Nutrition, 1983, pp 1–22
6. Linder P, Linder D: How to assess degrees of fatness. Cambridge, MA, Cambridge Scientific Industries, 1973
7. 1979 Build Study, Society Actuaries and Association of Life Insurance Medical Directors of America, 1983
8. A Guide for Professionals: The Effective of Exchange Lists for Meal Planning. New York American Diabetic Association, 1977, p 17
9. Butterworth CE, Blackburn CL: Hospital malnutrition. Nutrition Today 10:8–17, 1975
10. Buzby GL, Mullen JL: Nutritional assessment, in Rombeau JL, Caldwell MD (eds): Clinical Nutrition, Volume I: Enteral and Tube Feeding. Philadelphia, WB Saunders, 1984, pp 127–147
11. Twomey P, Ziegler MA, Rombeau J: Utility of skin testing in nutritional assessment: A critical review. JPEN 6:50–58, 1982
12. Wilmore DW: The Metabolic Management of the Critically Ill. New York, Plenum, 1977
13. Harris JA, Benedict FG: A Biometric Study of Basal Metabolism in Man. Washington, DC, Carnegie Institute of Washington, Publication No. 279, 1919
14. Feurer ID, Mullen JL: Measurement of energy expenditure, in Rombeau JL, Caldwell MD (eds): Clinical Nutrition, Volume II: Parenteral Nutrition. Philadelphia, WB Saumders, 1986, pp 224–235
15. Long CL, Schaffel N, Geiger JW, et al: Metabolic response to injury and illness:

Estimation of energy and protein needs from indirect calorimetry and nitrogen balance. JPEN 3:452–459, 1979

16. Crosby LO: New Horizons. Surg Clin N Am 61:743–753, 1981
17. Shizgal HM: Total body potassium and nutritional status. Surg Clin N Am 56:1185–1194, 1976
18. Kenna RA: Assessment of malnutrition using body composition analysis. Clin Consul Nutri Supp January, 9, 1981
19. Heymsfield SB, Olafson RP, Kutner MH, et al: A radiographic method of quantifying protein-calorie undernutrition. Am J Clin Nutr 32:693–702, 1979
20. Heymsfield, SB: Clinical Assessment of Lean Tissues, in Roche AF (ed): Body Composition in Youths and Adults. Columbus, OH, Ross Laboratories, 1985

APPENDIX A

Glossary of Nutritional Terms*

Angular stomatitis: Also called angular cheilosis. Superficial erosions and fissuring of the commissures of the lips. And overclosure of an endentulous mouth or excess salivation with drooling at all corner of the lips.

Bald tongue: Characterized by absence of papillae.

Blepharitis: Inflammation of the eyelids.

Bitot's spots: Superficial, foamy gray, triangular spots on the conjunctiva, consisting of keratinized epithelium.

Cheilosis: A condition marked by fissuring and dry scaling of the vermilion surface of the lips and angles of the mouth.

Follicular hyperkeratosis: Hypertrophy of the corneous layer of the skin.

Glossitis: Inflammation of the tongue.

Intercostal muscles: Muscles situated between the ribs.

Interosseous muscles: Muscles between bones.

Keratomalacia: A usually bilateral condition associated with vitamin A deficiency. It begins with xerotic spots (Bitot's spots) on the conjunctiva, while the cornea becomes xerotic and insensitive, the haze increases until finally the entire cornea becomes soft and necrosis occurs.

Magenta tongue: Reddish/purple colored tongue; seen with riboflavin deficiency.

Pellagrous dermatitis: Scaly dermatitis appearing on parts of the body exposed to light trauma.

Petechiae: Small punctate hemorrhages.

Purpura: Characterized by purplish or brownish/red discoloration easily visible through the epidermis, caused by hemorrhage into the tissue.

"Spectacle eye":   Periorbital dermatitis seen with biotin deficiency.

---

* From Dorland Illustrated Medical Dictionary, 26th Edition. Philadelphia, W.B. Saunders, Co., 1981. With permission.

Xerophthalmia: Dryness of the conjunctiva and cornea due to vitamin A
   deficiency. The conditions begins with night blindness and conjunctival xerosis
   and progresses to corneal xerosis and in the late stages, to keratomalacia.
Xerosis conjunctivae: Dryness of the conjunctiva.

Rhonda S. Patterson

5

Enteral Nutrition Delivery Systems

Nonvolitional enteral nutrition is utilized when the patient cannot or will not take in adequate oral nutrients. The ingestion of whole food, semisolid food, or liquids by the enteral route is preferable to the more invasive procedures involved in parenteral nutrition. Enteral feedings offer a safe, effective, economical alternative to parenteral nutrition.

The various techniques of enteral feeding, including both operative and nonoperative access to the gastrointestinal (GI) tract, are reviewed in this chapter. Nursing care as related to the specific route of access is also discussed.

ROUTE OF ACCESS

Selection of the route of access for enteral feedings depends on multiple factors. Each patient must be evaluated as to the functional status of the GI tract, the anticipated length of feeding, and whether the patient is an operative candidate. For clarity, this discussion of enteral feeding techniques is divided into operative and nonoperative methods of access.

OPERATIVE ACCESS

Cervical Pharyngostomy and Esophagostomy

Cervical pharyngostomy or esophagostomy may be performed as a primary head and neck operation. This type of operative access is well tolerated. Tolerance and comfort are enhanced when small gauge feeding catheters are

NUTRITIONAL SUPPORT IN NURSING
ISBN 0-8089-1889-3

used; the tubes can easily be concealed under clothing, thus allowing the patient to carry out daily activities.

Indications for cervical pharyngostomy or esophagostomy include tumors or traumas to the head and neck that require surgical intervention. Patients with obstructive lesions below the area of the cervical esophagus would not be candidates.

Reyster et al. described a simplified technique for cervical pharyngostomy in the 1960s.[1] A curved clamp is introduced through the mouth into the contralateral pyriform fossa so that it may be palpated below the lateral corner of the hyoid bone. A small incision is made through the skin over the tip of the clamp, and the instrument is bluntly dissected through the soft tissue to emerge through the skin. The tip of the feeding catheter is grasped by the clamp, pulled into the pharynx, and redirected down the esophagus and into the stomach. This type of pharyngostomy depends on the presence of a tube to maintain patency of the stoma. Possible complications of the procedure include bleeding, injury to local cervical structures, and infection.

Cervical esophagostomy as described by Ware et al. is another technique that may be performed at the time of head and neck surgery or independently (Fig. 5-1).[2] Feeding via esophagostomy is comfortable for the patient because it eliminates irritation of the nose and throat. Preferably the esophagostomy is placed on the left side of the esophagus since it tends to lie to the left of the midline. If, however, the esophagostomy is performed at the time of a radical neck dissection, the esophagostomy should be placed on the side opposite the dissection.

A silicone feeding tube is preferred to minimize irritation. The initial tube should remain in place for the first 7–10 days while the stoma heals.

Nursing Care

In the immediate postoperative period, a pressure dressing is applied to reduce edema. The stoma should be cleaned and dressed daily using the following procedure:

- Clean stoma site with H_2O_2 and sterile cotton tip swabs
- Remove H_2O_2 with sterile water
- Pat dry with sterile gauze
- Apply sterile gauze pressure dressing and tape securely
- Chart observations of stoma site to determine possible infection or necrosis

The silicone feeding tube should be taped securely to avoid accidental tube dislodgement. If the tube becomes dislodged, the physician should be notified and a new tube inserted as soon as possible. Once the stoma has healed, dressings may not be necessary, but daily cleansing of site is continued. Feedings are usually initiated after the second or third postoperative day.

If intermittent catheterization is planned, the patient is taught to insert and

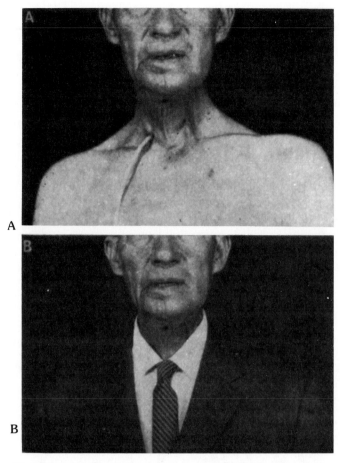

Fig. 5-1. (A) Cervical esophagostomy. (B) Easily concealed under clothing. (From Ware L, et al: Cervical esophagostomy: A simplified technique. Ann Surg 165:142–144, 1967. With permission.)

remove the tube. A small dressing should be placed over the stoma site to collect secretions.

Gastrostomy

Gastrostomy is frequently used in patients with mechanical or functional obstructing lesions of the head and neck or esophagus and in neurologically-impaired patients. The gastrostomy can be used for short- or long-term feeding. The risk of aspiration is greater with intragastric feedings than with intrajejunal feeding; however, there appears to be fewer pulmonary problems with gastrostomy feeding than nasoenteric feedings.[3]

There are three common types of gastrostomies: Stamm, Witzel, and Janeway. Local, regional, or general anesthesia is used for insertion depending on the patient's clinical condition.

Stamm Gastrostomy

The Stamm gastrostomy is the simplest to perform and is generally done if the patient is a poor surgical risk or if the need for tube feeding is only temporary. A small incision is made in the left upper quadrant of the abdomen. The stomach is elevated through the incision with Babcock clamps. A small incision is made through the body of the stomach and dilated with Kelly clamps. A Foley, mushroom, or Malicot catheter is inserted into the stomach through the incision and directed toward the pylorus. Several pursestring sutures are inserted at $\frac{1}{2}$-inch intervals and tied down to invaginate the stomach around the tube. Several interrupted sutures are used to fix the stomach to the abdominal wall at the catheter site, and a nonabsorbable suture is used to secure the catheter to the skin (Fig. 5-2).[4]

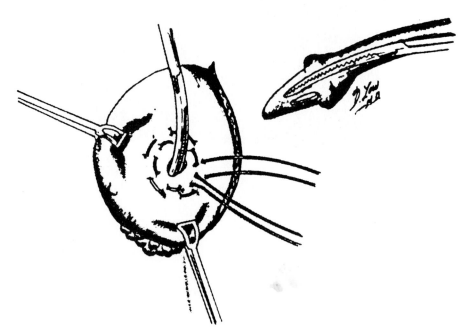

Fig. 5-2. Stamm temporary gastrostomy. A folley or mushroom catheter may be used. (From Rombeau JL, et al: Feeding by Tube Enterostomy (Enteral and Tube Feeding). Philadelphia, WB Saunders, 1984, p 277. With permission.)

The advantages of the Stamm gastrostomy include simplicity of insertion and ease of closure. Once the gastrostomy is no longer needed, the removal of the tube is simple and is generally followed by prompt closure.

Potential complications associated with the Stamm gastrostomy include surgical wound infection, peritonitis from leakage of gastric contents or the spilling of formula into the peritoneal cavity, and tube dislodgement. Inadvertent removal of the tube is followed by rapid shrinkage of the cutaneous orifice in a few hours. To preserve the gastrostomy, a tube must promptly be reinserted. Once the new tube has been reinserted, water-soluble contrast material is injected and x-rays taken to check placement of the tube and to ensure there is no intra-abdominal leakage.

Witzel Gastrostomy

A Witzel gastrostomy is similar to a Stamm gastrostomy in that a tube is inerted into the stomach in a similar fashion. Before the tube is brought through the omentum and exited from the abdomen, however, a seromuscular tunnel is made in the stomach around the tube for 4–6 cm (Fig. 5-3). This tunnel helps to minimize the risk of leakage when the stomach is distended or the tube is removed.[4]

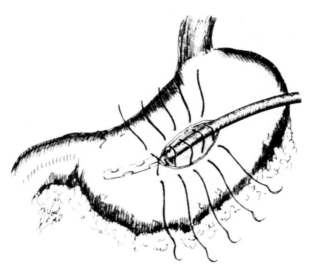

Fig. 5-3. Witzel temporary gastrostomy. Sutures placed for seromuscular tunnel. (From Rombeau JL, et al: Feeding by Tube Enterostomy (Enteral and Tube Feeding). Philadelphia, WB Saunders, 1984, p 278. With permission.)

Janeway Gastrostomy

The Janeway gastrostomy is preferred when the need for permanent tube feeding is anticipated. A gastric tube is created and brought through the abdominal wall to form a permanent stoma.[4] The gastric tube for the Janeway procedure may be constructed with the use of the stapler as described by Moss (Fig. 5-4).[5] The operative time is considerably reduced with use of the stapler. Once the tube has been created, a Foley catheter is inserted. The gastric tube is brought through the abdominal wall and a mucocutaneous stoma is created. The balloon on the catheter is inflated and the catheter attached to gravity drainage for 48–72 hours. If the stoma appears adequately perfused, feedings can be started when the gastric output is less than 300 ml/day.[4] On the eighth to tenth postoperative day the catheter can be removed from the gastric tube and reinserted for enteral feedings.

Percutaneous Gastrostomy

Gauderer et al. described a percutaneous endoscopic technique for placement of gastrostomy without laparotomy.[6] This technique involves endoscopic insufflation of the stomach followed by percutaneous puncture of the stomach with a 16-gauge Medicut catheter (Aloe Medical, St. Louis, MO). A No. 2 silk suture is passed through the catheter and into the stomach. The suture is snared and brought out through the mouth by way of the endoscope. The end of a specially prepared 16-Fr Pezzer catheter is drawn into the end of a second

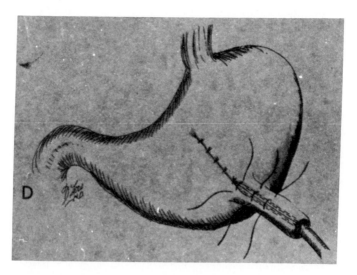

Fig. 5-4.   Janeway stapled gastrostomy. Creation of full thickness tunnel with stapler. (From Rombeau JL, et al: Feeding by Tube Enterostomy (Enteral and Tube Feeding). Philadelphia, WB Saunders, 1984, p 280. With permission.)

16-gauge Medicut catheter and attached in turn to the previously placed silk suture. The Pezzer catheter is lubricated and pulled retrograde through the patient's mouth, esophagus, and across the gastric and abdominal walls. A crossbar of heavy rubber tubing on the gastric side discourages extrusion of the catheter, and a second crossbar aids in anchoring the catheter to the abdominal wall. This type of gastrostomy may be performed under local anesthesia in most patients.

Possible Complications of Gastrostomy Tubes

Potential complications of gastrostomy include bleeding, peritonitis from leakage of gastric contents or feeding formula into the peritoneal cavity, tube dislodgement, skin erosion at the tube exit site, and wound infections that may lead to dehiscence and evisceration and possible bowel obstruction from migration of the feeding tube. Complications rates as high as 10–35 percent have been reported with gastrostomies.[7] This high complication rate may be attributed in part to the poor nutritional status and multiple medical problems of these patients. Wound healing and infection are frequent problems in these nutritionally depleted patients. Pulmonary complications are high because a great number of these patients are immobile.

A Foley catheter is readily available and can be used briefly for intragastric feedings, but it is not the ideal enteral feeding tube. The balloon can be damaged by gastric secretions and the diameter can change with time as gas passes across the balloon membrane. The balloon can also act as a stimulus to gastric peristalsis. The catheter tip may be carried along to the pylorus causing complete obstruction of the gastric outlet. Preferable tubes for gastrostomy feedings include the Malicot or mushroom catheters and the Pezzer catheter.

Nursing Care

Nursing care of the gastrostomy patient is an important aspect in the prevention and early detection of complications.[8] Immediately after surgery, a pressure dressing is applied to minimize swelling and bleeding. The stoma site and sutures are cleaned daily. Precautions with dressing changes initially are taken as with dressing a surgical wound. The dressing consists of a split 4×4 gauze sponge taped securely around the edges. The stoma is observed for redness, swelling, necrosis, or purulent drainage.

Leakage of gastric contents around the tube and onto the skin surface can lead to serious complications. Gastric secretions can cause rapid skin breakdown. The dressing should be checked each 8 hours for gastric drainage. Even if a small amount is present, cleaning of the stoma site and a fresh dressing are required.

The nurse can help prevent gastric leakage by securing the gastric tube to prevent migration. Without properly securing the tube, there is risk of the tube migrating into the stomach with peristalsis. If the tube moves only a few inches,

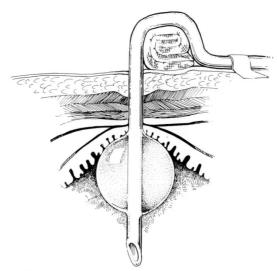

Fig. 5-5. Rolled gauze placed in this manner will provide adequate tension on the catheter to decrease risk of gastric contents leaking out on skin surface. (From DelRio D, et al: Handbook of Enteral Nutrition: A Practical Guide to Tube Feeding. El Segundo, CA: Medical Specifics Publishing, 1982, p 129. With permission.)

the mushroom tip or the balloon migrates away from the wall, breaking the seal, and thus allowing gastric contents to leak out onto the skin surface.[8] If the usual methods of taping do not prevent tube migration, an alternative should be used (Figs. 5-5 and 5-6).

Another complication associated with tube migration is possible esophageal or pyloric sphincter obstruction. If a patient begins to vomit immediately after a gastrostomy feeding, the feeding should be discontinued and location of the tube should be verified.

The position of the tube should be assessed frequently by a reference point on the tube that is made immediately following placement. Whenever the tube has moved a few inches, it should gently be pulled back and retaped.

Jejunostomy

Feeding into the jejunum has several advantages over intragastric feedings. Intrajejunal feeding virtually eliminates the problems of gastric overload, reflux, vomiting, and aspiration associated with gastric feedings. Feeding into the jejunum is not affected by the many mechanical and inflammatory processes in the upper GI tract that may limit gastric emptying. Intrajejunal feeding may be

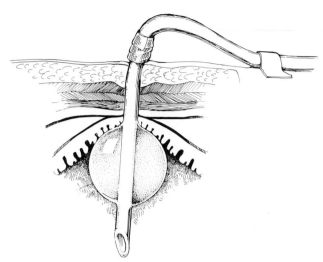

Fig. 5-6. This method is particularly helpful in children. Will hold catheter in proper place to prevent leakage of gastric contents. (Modified from DelRio D, et al: Handbook of Enteral Nutrition: A Practical Guide to Tube Feeding. El Segundo, CA: Medical Specifics Publishing, 1982, p 129. With permission.)

used for both temporary and long-term feeding whenever small bowel motility and absorptive capacity are adequate and in spite of disease states and conditions that may alter gastric, biliary, or pancreatic function.

There are two basic types of jejunostomies used for feeding: a *subserosal tunnel* similar to the Witzel gastrostomy and a *needle catheter* jejunostomy.

Witzel Jejunostomy

The Witzel jejunostomy is performed by choosing a loop of the jejunum 16 cm distal to the ligament of Treitz in order to allow easy attachment to the anterior abdominal wall.[4] A small puncture is made on the antemesenteric border, and a 16-Fr catheter is introduced 8 inches distally. A pursestring suture is inserted around the tube to fix it in place and the proximal 4–6 cm of tube are buried in a seromuscular tunnel. The catheter is brought out through the abdominal wall and the jejunum is sutured to the anterior parietal peritoneum (Fig. 5-7).

Originally a 12–16 mm rubber tube was used, but this technique had frequent complications that included leakage around the jejunostomy tube, obstruction of the bowel by the tube, and difficulty maintaining the position of the tube.[9]

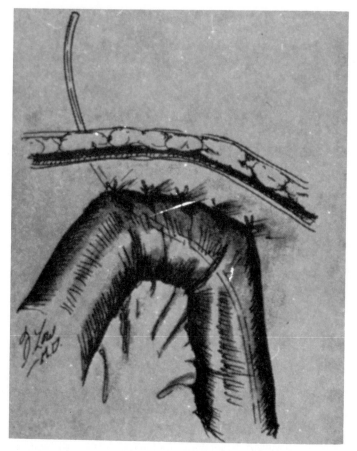

Fig. 5-7. Witzel jejunostomy. (From Rombeau JL, et al: Feeding by Tube Enterostomy (Enteral and Tube Feeding). Philadelphia, WB Saunders, 1984, p 282. With permission.)

Needle Catheter Jejunostomy

A modification of the Witzel jejunostomy has been advocated and termed the *needle catheter jejunostomy* (NCJ) or sometimes referred to as *feeding catheter jejunostomy* (FCJ). Usher first used polyethylene rather than rubber for the jejunostomy catheter in 1951.[10] The technique was later updated by Delaney et al. who used a commercially available catheter marketed for central venous cannulation for creating a FCJ.[11] Delaney et al. described the technique of NCJ for postoperative administration of fluids and defined formula diets.[12] A modification of this technique was later described and utilized by Page et al.[13] for adults and Andrassy et al.[14] for children.

The technique involves inserting a needle through a subserosal tunnel and entering the lumen of the bowel. A polyvinyl or silastic catheter is passed into the lumen of the bowel distally for approximately 15 cm. The needle is removed from the tunnel and pulled off the proximal end of the catheter. A pursestring suture is placed around the entry site of the jejunum and secured to create a snug fit around the catheter. The suture is tied around the catheter without occluding the lumen. The needle is passed percutaneously through the abdominal wall, and the catheter is passed out through the needle. The jejunum is attached to the parietal peritoneum at the exit site of the catheter with several sutures. A blunt-ended needle is placed in the proximal end of the catheter, and the catheter is secured to the skin edge with nonabsorbable sutures. Commercial kits are now available that contain all supplies needed to perform this procedure (Fig. 5-8).[15]

The NCJ can be used for short- or long-term nutritional support with a complication rate of less than 2 percent as shown by Page.[16] A long-term jejunal catheter, however has been developed by Kaminski that applies the fixation principles of the Hickman-Broviac catheter to jejunostomy.[17] The technique of placing this long-term jejunostomy tube utilizes the same principles as the Witzel technique. A specially designed silicone catheter with 2 sets of wings and a

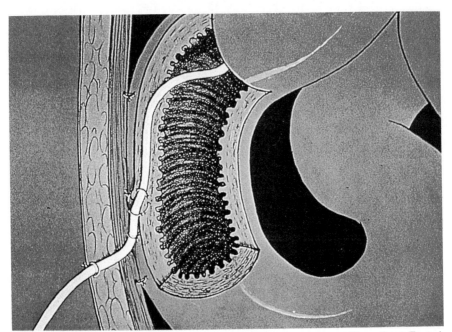

Fig. 5-8.   Schematic representation of needle catheter jejunostomy. (From Scott T, et al: Nutrition benefits of early postoperative jejunal feedings. Surg Rounds 6:26–32, 1983. With permission.)

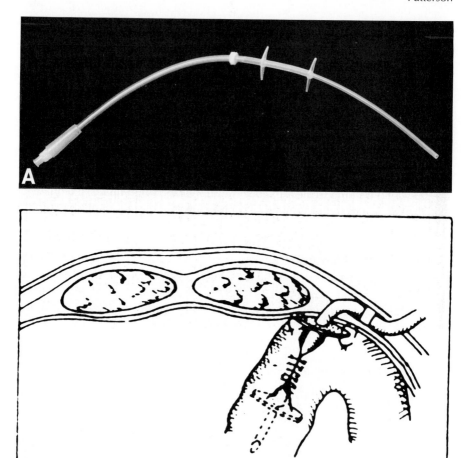

Fig. 5-9. (A) K-Tube. (B) Schematic representation of tube placement.

Dacron® cuff is inserted at the time of the laparotomy. The distal set of wings is placed within the lumen of the jejunum to temporarily secure the catheter while the Witzel tunnel is created. The proximal set of wings serves to attach the catheter to the bowel wall and the bowel wall to the abdominal wall at the catheter exit site. The catheter is brought out through a separate incision and the exit tunnel is constructed so that the Dacron® cuff lies within the subcutaneous tissues. The wings and Dacron® cuff serve to anchor the catheter securely for long-term nutritional support (Fig. 5-9). An operation is necessary to remove the catheter.

Another variation of the NCJ has been described by Cobb et al. for long-term jejunal nutritional support.[18] The catheter is permanently fixed to the abdominal wall in a fashion similar to the catheters used for home total

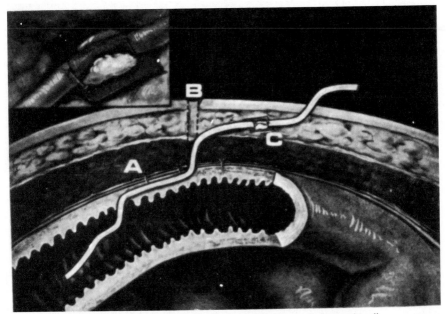

Fig. 5-10. (A) 5 cm serosal tunnel; (B) direct abdominal wall exit for short term placement; (C) subcutaneous fixation for long term placement. (From Cobb LM, et al: Early postoperative nutritional support using the serosal tunnel jejunostomy. JPEN 5:397–401, 1981. With permission.)

parenteral nutrition programs. A pledget of high density polypropylene mesh is secured to the catheter using a nonabsorbable monofilament suture and a small amount of medical grade silastic glue. The catheter is tunneled subcutaneously so that this mesh remains under the skin to fix it in position (Fig. 5-10). The tube can be removed by cutdown under local anesthesia.

Advantages of NCJ

The seromuscular tunnel prevents reflux of the feeding formula and ensures rapid closure of the catheter tract when it is withdrawn. Attachment of the jejunum to the abdominal wall avoids dislodgement of the catheter from the otherwise peristaltic jejunum and thus avoids the infusion of diet into the peritoneal cavity.

Patients who are candidates for NCJ include those undergoing major surgical procedures of the esophagus, stomach, duodenum, pancreas, or hepatobiliary system, particularly when the patient is malnourished preoperatively or a long period of nutritional deprivation is anticipated postoperatively.

Multiple trauma victims who undergo laparotomy are also candidates for jejunal feeding.

Contraindications to the insertion of the NCJ include local and systemic factors.[16] Local contraindications are Crohn's disease of the small intestine (potential for enterocutaneous fistula), extensive adhesions, and radiation enteritis. Systemic contraindications are ascites (risk of contamination and infection of ascitic fluid), profound immunosuppression (risk of necrotizing fasciitis), and coagulopathy (risk of bowel wall hematoma and obstruction).

Potential complications include: (1) dislodgement of the catheter, which may result in intraperitoneal infusion of feeding formula, peritonitis, or external loss of the catheter; (2) small bowel obstruction; (3) occlusion of the catheter; and (4) inflammation or infection at the catheter exit site.

Nursing Care

Following the surgical procedure, the jejunostomy feeding catheter is injected with opaque contrast solution, and the position of the catheter is verified by x-ray. Early postoperative feedings may be initiated within 24–48 hours postoperatively. If a feeding formula is not being infused, the catheter should be flushed with 10 ml of sterile water or saline every 8 hours to maintain the patency of the catheter. Serous drainage may be present in the immediate postoperative period; therefore daily dressing changes are done using the following procedure.[19]

1. Clean exit site with hydrogen peroxide and sterile cotton tip applicators.
2. Wipe with povidone-iodine swab. Repeat this step twice.
3. Allow povidone-iodine to dry. Pat dry with sterile gauze if needed.
4. Dress with gauze dressing daily the first 3–5 days.
5. For routine dressings after the initial 3–5 days, use a clear occlusive dressing. Change ever 5–7 days. If drainage is present or dressing not intact, clean and reapply new dressing.

To prevent kinking of the catheter, a small coil is made and taped securely (Fig. 5-11). Daily observations of the exit site are recorded. Any redness, drainage, or possible tube dislodgement is reported to the physician.

Care should be taken to avoid dislodgement of the catheter. Steps are taken at the time of the surgical procedure to anchor the catheter securely, but instructions to the patient to avoid tugging at the catheter when ambulating or turning are helpful.

Gastrostomy–Jejunal Tube

Rombeau and colleagues have recently described their experience with gastrostomy-jejunal feeding tube.[20] This type of feeding method provides the option of feeding via either the stomach or jejunum, permits proximal gastric decompression to avoid the possibility of aspiration while feeding into the

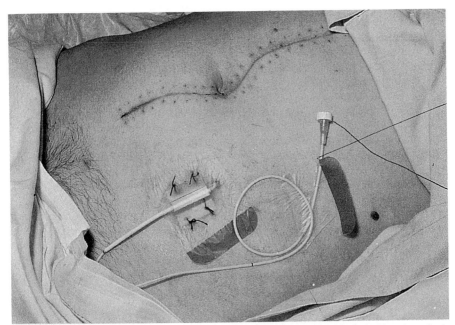

Fig. 5-11. Catheter is secured to abdominal wall with sheath and dressed with a clear occlusive dressing. (From Scott T, et al: Nutritional benefits of early postoperative jejunal feedings. Surg Rounds 6:26–32, 1983. With permission.)

jejunum, and provides a means whereby a feeding jejunostomy tube may be placed with the patient under local anesthesia. Added benefits of the gastrostomy-jejunal feeding tube are that crushed medication may be given through the tube and the tube is easily replaced.

The double lumen gastrostomy-jejunal tube is made of silicone and consists of a 24-Fr gastric tube with a 9.6-Fr jejunal tube within the wall of the gastric tube (Fig. 5-12). The jejunal tube is 20 inches long and is of sufficient length to ensure positioning of the tip beyond the ligament of Trietz. A 10 g mercury weight is present on the tip of the jejunal tube. A guidewire may be inserted during fluoroscopy to aid in proper placement of the jejunal tube.

A standard Stamm gastrostomy technique is used to place the gastrostomy-jejunal tube. The jejunal tube is passed through the stomach across the pylorus and positioned in the jejunum. The jejunal tube allows for infusion of both elemental formulas as well as those with a higher viscosity (e.g., polymeric diets).

Insertion of a gastrostomy-jejunal tube is indicated in patients expected to require long-term tube feeding or those who are at high risk for aspiration, or as an adjunct to gastrectomy or esophagectomy when gastric decompression or jejunal feeding is desired.

Complications associated with gastrostomy tube insertion can occur with use of the gastrostomy-jejunal tube. The incidence of aspiration and gastric

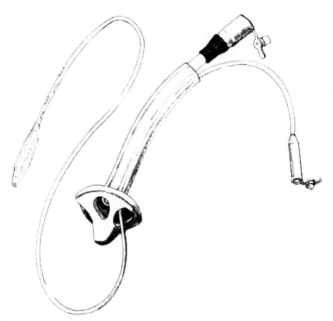

Fig. 5-12. Gastrostomy-jejunal tube. (From Rombeau JL, et al: Experience with a new gastrostomy-jejunal feeding tube. Surgery 93(4):574–578, 1983. With permission.)

leakage should be less if the ports are monitored to prevent excessive gastric filling. Complications associated with jejunostomy feeding tubes and catheters are also potential complications of the jejunal tube.

Nursing Care

The gastric and jejunal ports should be marked clearly to prevent possible confusion and inappropriate management of each tube. The following guidelines described by DelRio and colleagues should be helpful in providing nursing care to the patient with a gastrostomy-jejunal tube.[8]

1. Immediately following placement of the gastrostomy-jejunal tube, the gastrostomy tube should be attached to gravity drainage and the jejunal tube irrigated with water to maintain patency.
2. Dress the exit site in the same manner as a standard gastrostomy.
3. All medication should be instilled in the gastric port. Instillation into the jejunal tube may result in occlusion.
4. When a feeding formula is given into the jejunum, a continuous drip method is preferable. Infusion pumps will ensure a constant flow and bolus feeding can be avoided.

NONOPERATIVE ACCESS

Nasoenteral intubation is the simplest and most widely used route for nonoperative access to the GI tract. Until recently, the only available feeding tubes were large, rigid rubber or plastic tubing that were poorly tolerated by the patient. The size of the tube rendered the gastroesophageal junction incompetent, thus predisposing the patient to gastric reflux and aspiration. The large size of these tubes as well as their composition promoted ulceration of the nasal, pharyngeal, esophageal, and gastric mucosa and occasionally caused significant bleeding.

In 1952, Fallis and Barron introduced the use of a fine, weighted polyethylene catheter for nasoenteral feeding.[21] This technique increased patient comfort, and the combination of the weighted catheter and GI motility permitted the intubation of the jejunum for feeding purposes. This technique was not widely accepted at that time since there were no suitable liquid nutrients to be infused through the small caliber feeding catheter. This catheter serves as a prototype for a variety of commercially available fine, nasoenteral feeding catheters.

Nasoenteric Tubes

The soft, small-bore polyurethane and silicone tubes are being used with increasing frequency. Most of these tubes are 5–8-Fr in size, 36–43 inches in length, and manufactured with attached weights to assist in both introducing the catheter into the GI tract and maintaining it in the desired location (Fig. 5-13). These tubes have several advantages over the large-bore, stiff nasoenteric tubes. Oropharyngeal and esophageal irritation on intubation is minimized with the silicone or polyurethane tube. Use of the smaller sized tube may decrease the risk of aspiration since there is less compromise of the lower esophageal sphincter and thus decreased reflux of gastric contents. In addition, the patient's ability to swallow is usually not impaired by the small, softer tube.[22] The weighted tip allows for placement of the feeding tube past the pylorus into the duodenum or jejunum. The majority of the nasoenteral feeding catheters are accompanied by a stylet to facilitate catheter placement and in some instances to allow manipulation of the catheter under fluoroscopy. Most of the catheters are radiopaque. Table 5-1 lists some of the various nasoenteric tubes available.

Placement of Nasoenteric Tubes

Patient Preparation

First, explain the procedure to the patient and allow the patient to feel the tube. Remove stylet, if one is in place, to demonstrate the flexibility of the tube. Inform the patient that the procedure is not painful, but uncomfortable. Establish a signal by which the patient can stop you if needed.

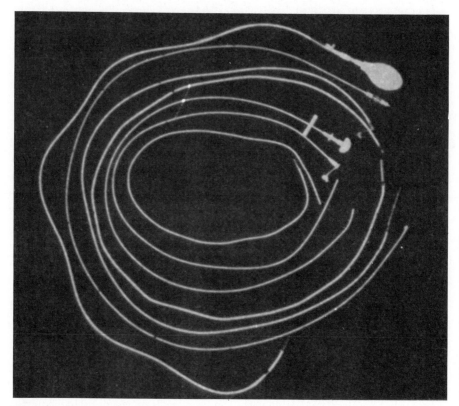

Fig. 5-13. Wide selection of commercially available nasogastric and nasoenteric feeding tubes. (From Silk DBA: Nutritional Support in Hospital Practice. Boston, MA: Blackwell Scientific Publications, 1983, p 89. With permission.)

Next, assemble needed equipment. Allowing the patient to drink water from a straw facilitates passage of the tube. An emesis basin should be on hand.

Determine length of tube to be inserted for nasogastric feedings. Mark the tube to provide a baseline for daily monitoring for tube position. Measuring the total distance from nose to ear to xiphoid (Fig. 5-14) will provide an estimate of the distance from the nose to the stomach in 98 percent of patients.[23] For tubes that are placed into the duodenum or jejunum, add 20–30 cm.

Have the patient in a sitting position if alert. A pillow behind the head will give additional support. If the patient is comatose, place in a semi-Fowlers position if clinical condition permits.

Determine the most patent nostril by direct visualization. Lubricate the tip of the feeding tube with a water-soluble lubricant or activate the lubricant according to the manufacturer's directions.

Table 5-1
New Developments in Enteral Feeding Techniques

	French gauge	Length (inches)	Feature	Use
Dobbhoff tube	8	43	Insertion catheter included; 7 g mercury or tungsten tip; larger bore	Long-term nasogastric
Keofeed	5, 7.5, 9.6	43	Insertion catheter included	Long-term nasogastric
Duo-Tube	5, 6, 8	40	Insertion bulb device	Long-term nasogastric
Enter-Al tube			Can be inserted without stylet	Long-term nasogastric
Entriflex	8	36 or 43	Hydrophilic inner coating; insertion catheter included; 3 g mercury or tungsten tip; larger bore	Long-term nasogastric
Vivonex tungsten tip	8	45	Does not need stylet for placement	Long-term nasogastric
Moss tube	18	44	Placed during surgery	Short-term postsurgery
Needle-catheter jejunostomy kit	5	41	Everything needed for placement included	Short/long-term postsurgery
K-Tube	8	15	Dacron cuff for anchoring to abdominal wall	Long-term jejunostomy feeding

Feeding Tube Placement

Insert the tube gently along the floor of the nostril. A common mistake is to force the feeding tube which may cause kinking and discomfort. Instruct the patient, if alert and cooperative, to sip water through a straw when the tip of the tube is felt in the back of the throat. The glottis protects the trachea when swallowing and the peristaltic action will actually "pull" the tube down the esophagus. Have the patient continue to swallow until the desired length of tube

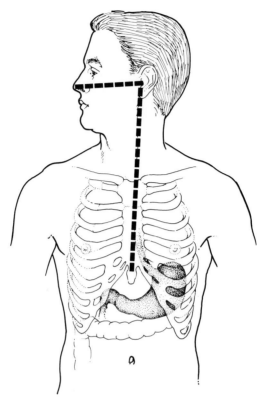

Fig. 5-14. Measuring total distance from nose to ear to xiphoid with approximate distance from nose to stomach.

has been passed. If the patient is comatose or uncooperative, pass the tube as described along the floor of the nostril. Check for position of the tube in the back of the throat with a tongue blade. Flex the patient's head toward the chest. This will close off the glottis to prevent the tube from entering the trachea. Gently advance the tube until the desired length has been placed.

Next, determine the position of the feeding tube tip. Aspirating through many of the small-bore, soft tubes to check for gastric placement is almost impossible since the tube has a tendency to collapse. Injecting air may be one way of checking gastric placement, but bubbling sounds may be transmitted from the chest to the upper abdomen, leading to the false impression that the stomach has successfully been catheterized. The only definitive method is via x-ray confirmation of the feeding tube. Proper placement will prevent inadvertent administration of diet into the tracheobronchial tree. If the catheter position is unacceptable, it must be adjusted and/or reinserted. When using catheters with side holes at the tip and a stylet present for insertion, it is important to make

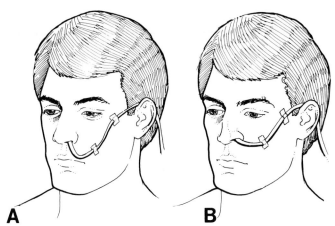

Fig. 5-15. (A) Correct taping method. (B) Improper taping method on right. Nares being pulled, increasing the risk for necrosis.

all adjustments prior to removing the stylet. One should never attempt reinsertion of the stylet in this type of feeding tube since possible exit of the stylet through one of the side holes may lead to perforation of the GI tract, especially the esophagus.

Once the feeding tube is in the proper place, the feeding tube should be taped securely. Figure 5-15 illustrates recommended techniques for taping. The feeding catheter should not be pulling on the nares. Pressures against the nares may cause excoriation and sloughing of tissue.

Duodenal or Jejunal Intubation

Transnasal intubation of the proximal small bowel is somewhat more difficult to achieve than access to the stomach. In the ambulatory patient, the feeding tube will spontaneously pass into the small intestine about half of the time if sufficient feeding tube is placed in the stomach. In the bedridden patient, this rarely occurs since the weighted tip tube rests in the dependent portion of the stomach and remains there. In some instances, successful cannulation of the proximal small bowel may be done under fluoroscopy with the use of a rigid stylet to manipulate the feeding tube through the pylorus.

Nursing Care

Monitoring the position of the feeding tube daily is important. A mark may be placed on the tube after proper placement and observed daily to ascertain that the tube has not been inadvertently displaced. The nares should also be inspected daily for any redness or sloughing. Cleaning the nares with cotton tip applicators and hydrogen peroxide is recommended. Petroleum jelly around the tube at the nares site may increase patient comfort. New tape should be applied when it becomes soiled or wet. Irrigation of the small-bore feeding tube should be done every 8 hours to maintain patency of tube, even if a continuous drip feeding if being delivered.

REFERENCES

1. Reyster HP, Noone RB, Graham WP III, et al: Cervical pharyngostomy for feeding after maxillfacial surgery. Am J Surg 116:610–614, 1968
2. Ware L, Garrett WS Jr, Pickrell K: Cervical esophagostomy: A simplified technique. Ann Surg 165:142–144, 1967
3. Olivencia JA, Beraudi RS: Temporary tube gastrostomy: A five year study. J Iowa Med Soc 67:362–366, 1977
4. Rombeau JL, Barot LR, David WL, et al: Feeding by Tube Enterostomy (Enteral and Tube Feeding). Philadelphia, WB Saunders, 1984
5. Moss G: A simple technique for permanent gastrostomy. Surgery 71:369–379, 1972
6. Gauderer MWL, Ponsky JL, Izant RF Jr: Gastrostomy without laparotomy: A percutaneous endocropic technique. J Pediatr Surg 15:872–875, 1980
7. Engel S: Gastrostomy. Surg Clin N Am 49:1289–1295, 1969
8. DelRio D, Williams K, Esvelt BM: Handbook of Enteral Nutrition: A Practical Guide to Tube Feeding. El Segundo, CA: Medical Specifics Publishing, 1982
9. Ryan JA, Page CP: Intrajejunal feeding: Development and current status. JPEN 8(2):187–198, 1984
10. Usher RC: Use of polyethylene catheter for jejunostomy feeding. Am J Surg 82: 408–510, 1951
11. Delaney HM, Garvey JW: Jejunostomy by a needle catheter technique. Surgery 73: 786–790, 1973
12. Delaney HM, Carnevale N, Garvey JW: Postoperative nutritional support using needle catheter jejunostomy. Ann Surg 186:165–170, 1977
13. Page CP, Carlton PK, Andrassy RJ, et al: Safe, cost effective postoperative nutrition. Am J Surg 138:527, 1978
14. Andrassy RJ, Woolley MM: Defined formula diet for pediatric surgical patient. Compr Therapy 15:48–53, 1979
15. Scott T, Patterson RS, Andrassy RJ: Nutritional benefits of early postoperative jejunal feeding. Surg Rounds 6:26–32, 1983
16. Page CP: Needle catheter jejunostomy. Contemp Surg 19:29–47, 1981
17. Kaminski MV: A new catheter for home enteral hyperalimintation. JPEN 4:604, 1980
18. Cobb LM, Carthill AM, Gilsdorf RB: Early postoperative nutritional support using the serosal tunnel jejunostomy. JPEN 5:397–401, 1981
19. Patterson RS, Andrassy RJ: Needle catheter jejunostomy. Am J Nurs 83:1325–1326, 1983
20. Rombeau JL, Twomey PL, McLean GK, et al: Experience with a new gastrostomy-jejunal feeding tube. Surgery 93(4):574–578, 1983

21. Fallis LS, Barron J: Gastric and jejunal alimentation with fine polyethylene tubes. AMA Arch Surg 65:373–381, 1952
22. Matarese LE: Enteral alimentation: Equipment: Part III. Nutri Support Serv 2(2):48–49, 1982
23. Hanson RL: Predictive criteria of nasogastric tube insertion for tube feeding. JPEN 3:160–163, 1979

Marcia A. Ryder

6

Parenteral Nutrition Delivery Systems

P arenteral nutrition is a complex form of therapy designed to provide daily nutritional requirements by the intravenous route. Therapeutic success is dependent on appropriate nutrient prescription, sterile compounding, catheterization technique, dressing management, and continuous patient monitoring. Management of venous access and the delivery system is the most difficult aspect of total parenteral nutrition (TPN) both in the hospital and in the home. This chapter is devoted to the discussion of central venous access, issues in management, and related complications of parenteral nutrition.

CENTRAL VENOUS ACCESS

Central venous access is required for infusion of hypertonic solutions. Parenteral nutrition solutions may have an osmolality 3–5 times greater than normal serum osmolality. High blood flow and rapid dilution in the central venous system reduces the risk of phlebitis, venous thrombosis, and sclerosing of vein walls. Access to the superior or inferior vena cava may be accomplished through any tributary that is sufficient in size to accommodate a catheter. The idea of inserting a catheter into the right heart was first introduced by Forssmann of Germany in the early 1900s for administration of emergency drugs and avoidance of the hazards of percutaneous intracardiac injections. Cubital, femoral, and external jugular veins were commonly used in the earlier days of central venous access. In 1952, however, Aubaniac introduced the infraclavicular approach to catheterization, and in 1966 the internal jugular approach was performed by Hermosura, Vanages, and Dickey.[1] These techniques with some variations are currently in use for catheterization in TPN. Unfortunately, the

NUTRITIONAL SUPPORT IN NURSING
ISBN 0-8089-1889-3

procedures for accessing the central venous system are not without potential risk of serious complications, a result of the immediate proximity of multiple anatomic structures to the access vessels. Thus the physician performing the procedure should have a thorough knowledge of the vascular anatomy and adjacent structures.

Anatomy

Subclavian Veins

The subclavian vein extends from the outer border of the first rib to the sternal head of the clavicle and arches behind the clavicle over the first rib to the insertion of the scalene muscle (Fig. 6-1). The vein rests in a depression on the first rib and the pleura. It reaches its most cephalad position in its arch over the rib, medial to the midpoint of the clavicle. At the medial border of the scalene muscle, the subclavian joins the internal jugular to form the innominate vein. Anteriorly it relates to the costoclavicular ligament, the pectoralis and subclavius muscles, and the clavicle that covers the entire course of the vein. Posteriorly it relates to the brachial plexus, the subclavian artery, and the anterior scalenus muscle. As it crosses the rib, the muscle separates the vein from the subclavian artery. Superiorly it relates to the suprascapular and transverse cervical branches

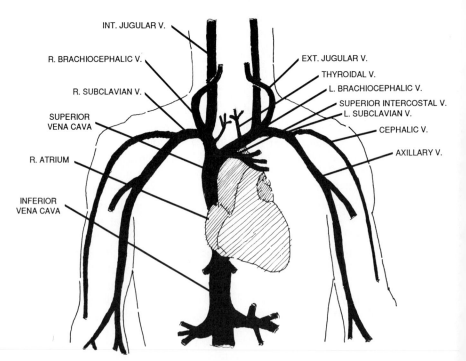

Fig. 6-1. Anatomy of the central venous system.

of the thyrocervical trunk. The thoracic duct enters the internal jugular vein near its junction with the subclavian vein. The right subclavian vein receives the right lymphatic duct in a similar location. The right innominate vein (2.5 cm in diameter) and the left innominate vein (6 cm in diameter) join to form the superior vena cava.

Internal Jugular Veins

The internal jugular veins are alternatives to the subclavian approach. These veins join the subclavian vein medial to the insertion of the anterior scalenus muscle on the first rib. The vein runs downward and lateral to the internal and common carotid arteries. The right internal jugular is larger than the left and is more distant from the artery.

External Jugular Veins

The external jugular veins lie in the superficial fascia beginning just behind the angle of the mandible. They descend obliquely across the sternocleidomastoid muscle, perforate the deep fascia just above the clavicle, and drain into the subclavian vein.

Peripheral Veins

The basilic vein originates from the medial side of the metacarpal network. It passes proximally along the medial side of the arm and joins with the antecubital vein in the antecubital space.

The cephalic vein rises from the lateral side of the arm. It passes proximally along the lateral side and empties into the axillary vein at the beginning of the subclavian vein.

The axillary vein is a continuation of the basilic vein. It passes obliquely across the axilla toward the middle third of the clavicle and becomes the subclavian vein at the lateral border of the first rib.

Femoral Veins

The femoral veins is formed by the posterior popliteal, saphenous, and lateral circumflex femoral veins. It empties into the internal iliac vein to the common iliac vein and on to form the inferior vena cava.

The advantages and disadvantages of the use of each of these vessels for venous access are described in Table 6-1.

Vein Selection

Vein selection should be given careful consideration. The patient's clinical situation and anatomic factors, as well as the experience and skill of the physician, should be taken into account when selecting the vessel to be cannulated. Femoral and peripheral access have not been widely accepted for prolonged venous access due to infection and thrombosis. Recent reports,

Table 6-1
Selection of a Central Vein for Venous Access

Vein	Advantages	Disadvantages
Subclavian	Large caliber vein (2.5 cm) with high flow rate Easily accessible in a fixed position Configuration of the chest wall allows for optimal dressing management, Patient mobility, and Patient comfort Accommodates catheter without occluding the vein	Blind technique—increased risk of insertion complications Difficult to puncture in hypovolemic state
Internal jugular	Vein may distend as much as 2.5 cm Easily accessible Decreased risk of pneumothorax	Increased risk of arterial puncture or lacerations Increased risk of infection due to difficulty in maintenance of sterile dressing Continuous motion of catheter with movement of the head Patient discomfort Enlargement and diameter vary considerably with respiration
External jugular	Easily accessible Easily visualized Decreased risk of pneumothorax or arterial puncture	Small caliber vessel—increased risk of thrombophlebitis Increased risk of infection due to difficulty in maintenance of sterile dressings Difficult insertion due to tortuous path of catheter Continuous motion of catheter with movement of head Patient discomfort
Peripheral veins Brachial	Eliminates complications of subclavian and jugular vein insertions Easier to maintain sterile dressings	Increased risk of thrombophlebitis
Cephalic Axillary		Difficulty threading catheter past the axillary junction Advancement of catheter with arm movements increasing risk of perforation and vessel trauma
Femoral	Large caliber vessel with high flow rate Eliminates complications of subclavian and jugular vein insertions	High risk of infection Insertion site contaminated Difficulty maintaining sterile dressing Risk of inferior vena cava, hepatic vein, thrombosis, and renal vein and/or thromboembolic complications

however, have shown high success rates for axillary vein catheterization[2] and for a new type of catheter, the *half-way catheter*, in the basilic or cephalic veins.[3]

Nonetheless, the subclavian vein is the preferred vessel, and the jugular vein the alternative. Infraclavicular and supraclavicular approaches have little difference in success or complication rate in spite of a higher rate of malposition with the infraclavicular approach.[4,5]

The left subclavian vein is sometimes preferred over the right because the pathway of the catheter to the superior vena cava is more direct and the apex of the lung is lower on the left side. Padberg et al.[6] identified a higher thrombosis rate in the left subclavian vein and recommended the right side for catheterization despite a higher incidence of malposition from a right insertion. The risk of accident with the subclavian route is increased for patients with neck and shoulder generative joint disease, obesity, cachexia, chest wall deformities, scoliosis, and high anxiety. Patients with chronic severe pulmonary disease are also at excessive risk for pulmonary complications due to their overinflated tense lungs and diminished pulmonary reserve.[7]

Internal jugular vein catheterizations are widely reported to have lower complication rates than the subclavian veins,[8,9] yet two more recent studies have shown higher complication rates with the internal jugular approach[7,10] in adults as well as children.[11] The right internal jugular is sometimes preferred over the left since it is shorter in length and is the most direct route to the superior vena cava. Internal jugular access should be avoided in patients with endotracheal tubes and tracheostomies because of contamination with secretions. Long-term internal jugular access is less desirable because of increased incidence of thrombosis in these smaller veins.

Complication and success rates are also related to the experience of the physician. The success rates of inexperienced physicians may be equal to or less than those of experienced physicians, but higher complication rates are more likely to be produced with less experienced operators.[10,12]

Catheter Materials

Prior to 1945, only ureteric catheters or soft rubber tubes were available for central venous catheterizations. In 1945, Meyers[13] and Zimmerman[14] utilized polyethylene cannulae for intravenous feeding in children. Polyethylene materials proved to be highly thrombogenic and led to the use of other materials such as polyvinyl chloride and Teflon; however, these also proved to be thrombogenic. Currently, silicone rubber and polyurethane catheters are the most frequently used.

Material composition of catheters is important because of its potential for platelet affinity, thrombophlebitis, bacterial colonization, and ease of insertion. Further discussion of this topic may be found under Postinsertion Complications of Catheter Septicemia and Thrombosis.

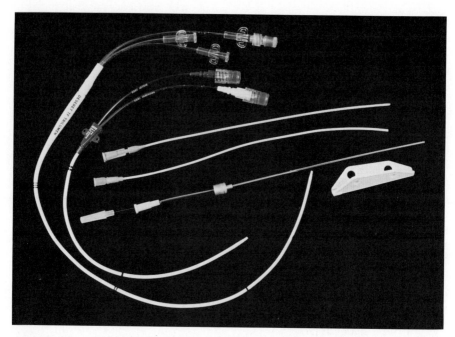

Fig. 6-2. Examples of percutaneous catheters (top to bottom): Triple lumen catheter, Deseret (Sandy, UT); double lumen catheter, Arrow-Howes (Reading, PA); single lumen hydromer-coated catheter, U.S. Viggo (Tampa, FL); single lumen silastic catheter, Travenol (Deerfield, IL); single lumen polyvinylchloride catheter with internal wire, needle, and needle guard, Deseret (Sandy, UT).

Catheter Designs

Catheters are categorized by the method of insertion, that is, they are inserted by needle venipuncture and threaded percutaneously or inserted by surgical implantation. Examples of each type of catheter are pictured in Figures 6-2 and 6-3.

Percutaneous Catheters

The single lumen catheter is constructed of a single piece of tubing with a plastic hub. The multilumen catheter is a single catheter with two or three noncommunicating internal lumens. Each lumen exits the catheter at intervals of 2.2 cm, which allows for simultaneous administration of incompatible mixtures. Unused lumens can be heparinized for intermittent use. Tips of these catheters are beveled for ease of insertion but may increase the risk of perforation.

Indwelling and Implanted Catheters

Indwelling and implanted Silastic catheters are inserted into the vein by percutaneous venipuncture or surgical cutdown. An additional portion of the catheter is tunneled into the subcutaneous space. It is exited through the skin at

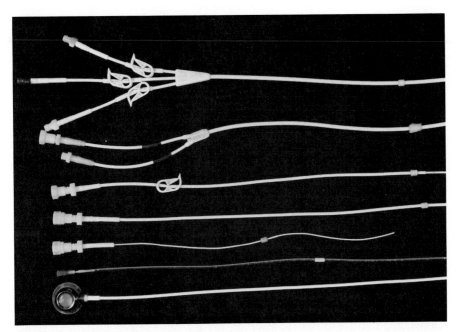

Fig. 6-3. Examples of indwelling and implanted catheters (top to bottom): Triple lumen catheter, Davol (Cranston, RI); double lumen catheter, Cook (Bloomington, IN); Broviac® catheter, Davol (Cranston, RI); Hickman® catheter, Davol (Cranston, RI); infant Broviac® catheter, Davol (Cranston, RI); Groshong® catheter (protective sleeve not shown), Cath Tech (Salt Lake City, UT); implanted port, Davol (Cranston, RI).

a convenient location for easy visualization by the patient to perform self-care. Fibrotic tissue growth around an adhered Dacron® cuff located in the subcutaneous tract acts as a barrier to prevent migration of bacteria through the tunnel and into the bloodstream. In addition, the ingrown cuff anchors the catheter to prevent dislodgement. These catheters can be heparinized for intermittent use and provide access for blood sampling. The external portion of the catheter is repairable if damaged or severed. The Hickman® catheter is a modification of the Broviac® catheter that was first used in 1970 as an "artificial gut" for TPN.[15] The Hickman has a larger lumen, 1.6 mm in diameter compared with 1.0 mm in the Broviac. Davol Company (Cranston, RI, original manufacturer of the Hickman and Broviac catheter) and others now produce multilumen Silastic indwelling catheters. The indwelling catheter has become widely accepted for long-term venous access and for self-administration of intravenous infusions in the home. Recently, another type of indwelling Silastic catheter has been introduced. The Groshong C.V. catheter (Cath-Tech., Salt Lake City, UT) incorporates a two-way valve adjacent to a closed rounded tip. This valve or slit opens to allow for both infusion and blood aspiration, but when the catheter is not in use, the valve closes and remains closed under normal central venous pressure conditions. This reduces the potential for air entry and backflow of blood into the catheter. As a result, clamping is not required and the catheter can be maintained with normal saline instillation.[16] Studies are currently underway to establish the efficacy of this design.

Implanted intravenous or intra-arterial devices differ from indwelling devices in that they are totally implanted under the skin. The device consists of two parts: (1) the Silastic catheter and (2) a metal or plastic chamber with a thick silicone rubber disc (Fig. 6-4). Access to the septum requires puncture of the skin with a non-coring needle. This type of device requires minimal routine care and maintenance. The obvious advantage of no external apparatus is particularly feasible in noncompliant patients and inviting for cosmetic reasons. Usage is more appropriate for intermittent access rather than daily skin puncture and securing the needle for nocturnal infusions.

Catheter Insertion

Prior to central venous catheter insertion, a physical and nutritional assessment should be completed to establish the indications for parenteral alimentation and appropriate insertion site for cannulation. Catheter insertion into the central veins is a surgical procedure that requires operative consent. The

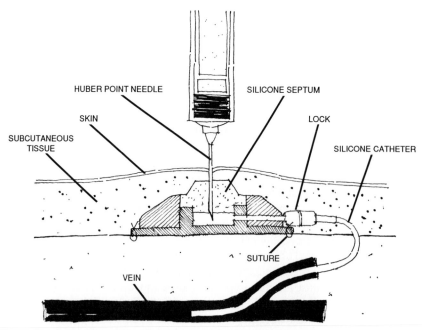

Fig. 6-4.   Cross section of an implanted port.

physician should discuss with the patient the necessity for parenteral nutrition, expected outcome of the therapy, and the risks associated with the catheterization procedure and administration of parenteral nutrition.

Percutaneous Catheters

Preoperative Preparation

Preoperative teaching by the nurse is an essential component to the success and safety of the operation. Patients should clearly understand the aspects of the procedure requiring their cooperation. The nurse should explain positioning, expectation of pain control, and maintenance of sterility. Demonstration of the catheter and explanation of its position in the body is also helpful. For patients who are highly anxious or combative, sedation is required, since these states greatly increase the risk of complication. Catheter insertion may be done in a patient's room with the following precautions:

1. Environment should be free of contaminating materials;
2. Curtains should be drawn between patients and doors should be closed;
3. Family and visitors should be restricted from the room;
4. The number of persons in attendance should be minimized;
5. Strict attention should be paid to infection control precautions or isolation techniques as indicated.

Patients with platelet counts of less than $100,000$ mm^3 may require infusion of blood products to prevent bleeding complications. Hydration status should be evaluated and corrected for adequate venous dilatation.

Positive end expiratory pressure (PEEP) in mechanically ventilated patients should not be greater than 5 cm at the time of venipuncture because of the increased risk of pneumothorax. If the PEEP cannot be reduced during insertion, sites other than the subclavian should be considered.

Before initiating the procedure or opening sterile equipment, bowel and bladder elimination needs should be tended to, necessary pain medications administered, and patients on ventilatory support suctioned. With subclavian venipunctures, a moderate sized towel roll should be placed between the scapulae under the upper thoracic spine. When supine, this allows the shoulders to drop back toward the bed to reduce the angle of the needle upon insertion. The greater the angle of the syringe on advancement of the needle, the greater the risk of pneumothorax.

All equipment should be assembled and prepared for use before the actual procedure is started. Many catheter manufacturers assemble catheters in kits with accompanying items for catheter insertion. In most cases, still additional items remain to be collected. Custom-kit manufacturers build kits to design specifications matching institutional policies and procedures. This type of kit containing all necessary items can be cost effective and time efficient, as well as increase compliance to procedures. Suggested components are listed in Table 6-2.

Contamination of a catheter inserted through inadequately prepared skin is one etiologic factor in catheter-related septicemia. Generally, shaving should be avoided since skin nicks and abrasions are potential sites for infection. The perineal area and heavy hair growth of the chest, arm, or neck of males, however, may be contaminating as well as painful on tape removal, and should

Table 6-2
Sterile Central Venous Catheter Insertion Tray

Nonsterile preoperative preparation	2	surgical masks
	1	moisture proof underpad
	1	triple swabsticks containing 70% isopropyl/10% acetone
	1	pair latex gloves
	1	iodophor detergent scrub sponge (available iodine .75%)
	1	absorbent towel
Sterile insertion items	1	sterile gown
	1	1 oz. packet containing povidone-iodine topical solution U.S.P. 10% (available iodine 1%)
	1	lollipop sponge stick
	1	fenestrated drape
	1	30 ml ampule 1% lidocaine HCL, injection
	1	25 ga × 5/8 inch needle
	2	22 ga × 1½ inch needles
	2	20 ga × 1½ inch filter needles
	2	12 cc syringes nonluer-lok
	1	10 ml ampule sodium chloride for injection
	6	4 inch × 4 inch gauze sponges
	1	hemostat
	1	scissors
	1	needle holder
	1	3-0 nylon suture with curved needle
	1	luer-lok extension tubing
Sterile dressing material	1	1 oz. packet hydrogen peroxide topical solution U.S.P. 3%
	1	povidone-iodine ointment U.S.P. 10% (available iodine 1%)
	2	2 in. × 2 in. gauze sponges
	1	swabstick with skin protectant
	1	roll rayon tape

be shaved or clipped with care. The skin preparation begins with cleansing of the skin with alcohol-acetone or alcohol alone. These defatting agents mechanically and chemically remove oils, dirt, secretions, and so on. This is followed with a 2-minute povidone-iodine detergent scrub that is patted dry on completion.

Following an application of povidone-iodine solution, a liberal amount of Xylocaine is injected for local anesthesia. If excessive amounts are used, the anatomy may be distorted. The clinician should bear in mind that the actual venipuncture is made approximately 3–4 inches away from the site of skin puncture so that the entire pathway of the needle is anesthetized.

The initial intravenous (IV) solution should be isotonic so that in the event the catheter is malpositioned, a hypertonic solution is not infused into lung tissue or smaller vessels.

All procedures for central venous access require surgical asepsis. The operating surgeon should wear a mask and gloves. A sterile gown is recommended to prevent inadvertent contamination of the sterile field and lengthy guidewires.

Catheter Insertion

One method of catheter insertion is the "through-the-needle" technique. This procedure is accomplished as follows:

1. The venipuncture is made;
2. The syringe is removed from the needle;
3. The catheter is threaded through the needle;
4. The catheter hub is tightened into the needle hub and the needle withdrawn from the skin;
5. The guidewire is removed from the catheter;
5. The IV tubing is connected and infusion started;
7. The needle guard is snapped into place over the needle.

The remaining needle and needle guard are at times cumbersome to manage, especially with jugular insertions.

More recent catheter designs, including the multilumen catheters, have replaced this method with an "over-the-wire" technique. This technique, originally described by Seldinger,[17] reduces mechanical problems of catheter care and is performed as follows:

1. Venipuncture is made;
2. The syringe is removed from the needle;
3. A spring guidewire is inserted through the needle;
4. The needle is removed;
5. The catheter is threaded over the guidewire;
6. The guidewire is withdrawn from the catheter;
7. The IV tubing is connected and infusion started.

The thin wire permits a smaller gauge needle for venipuncture instead of the larger bore needle that is required for passage of a catheter.

As previously stated, the subclavian and jugular veins are the preferred vessels for central venous access in parenteral nutrition. Figure 6-5 illustrates four insertion techniques for catheterization of these vessels.

The ideal position of the catheter tip is at the junction of the superior vena cava and the right atrium. Measurement of the distance from the site of insertion following the path of the subclavian or the internal jugular vein to the third intercostal space will determine the length of catheter to be inserted. Left subclavian insertions require more length than the right, and the same applies for the jugular veins.

Proper suturing of the catheter is an important aspect of the insertion procedure. A loose suture should be placed through the skin directly at the insertion site and knotted. The suture is then placed around the catheter and tied securely. Colonization of the skin tract may occur if the catheter is sutured at a distance away from the insertion site, allowing the contaminated portion of the catheter to slip in and out through the skin. Additional suturing is usually not required. Wings or suture tabs are not recommended because (1) they cannot be lifted to adequately cleanse the skin underneath during dressing change; (2) they require two suture sites that increase potential for irritation and infection; and (3) if the catheter is not secured tightly to the wing device, the catheter may inadvertently slip out, resulting in malposition or loss of the catheter.

Catheterization of the central venous system is not without serious risk. The complications of catheter insertion are described later. Because a majority of these can be detected on radiograph, it is essential that a postinsertion chest x-ray be taken before beginning parenteral nutrition solutions. The x-ray may reveal catheter malposition or injury to adjacent structures.

During catheter insertion, catheter tip location can be assessed by free flow of venous blood in the syringe or by lowering the IV solution below the level of the heart and observing for free flashback of blood in the tubing. These methods may be deceiving, however, since the flashback of venous blood may originate from a branch vessel or hematoma and may not be apparent on x-ray. A 250–500 cc infusion of isotonic solution prior to the x-ray is suggested so that a hydrothorax may be detected and corrected before initiating the hypertonic solutions.

Catheter Exchange

Catheter exchange is accomplished in the same manner as the "over-the-wire" technique. Patient preparation is the same as the original insertion. The guidewire is inserted into the existing catheter, followed by removal of the catheter with the guidewire remaining in place. The new catheter is then threaded over the wire through the insertion site. Finally, the guidewire is removed, leaving the new catheter in position. This method of catheter exchange can be performed with minimal risk to the patient. [18–21]

Indications for catheter exchange may include:

- Evaluation of suspected catheter-related septicemia,
- Redirection of a malpositioned catheter,
- Exchange of one type of catheter for another type,
- Mechanical problems with the existing catheter, or
- Initiation of parenteral nutrition.

The ability to exchange the catheter becomes a distinct advantage over removal and reinsertion of a new catheter by venipuncture. It also allows for uninterrupted administration of parenteral nutrition solutions. There is evidence that catheter-related sepsis can be eliminated with catheter exchange[21] if the skin tract is not infected. [18]

The most serious but rare (0.1–0.2 percent) complication associated with this procedure is pulmonary embolism.[21] This is related to dislodgement of venous thrombus or stripping of the fibrin sheath on catheter removal. Another potentially serious occurrence may be cardiac arrhythmia. This occurs as a result of stimulation or irritation of the myocardium by a guidewire that has been advanced into the atria or more notably the ventricle. Consequently, the heart rate and rhythm must be monitored during passage of the wire. In most cases the arrhythmias can be corrected by retraction of the wire; if not, emergent administration of antiarrhythmic drugs may be necessary.

Indwelling and Implanted Catheters

Home parenteral nutrition patients (HTPN) require venous access by means of an indwelling or implanted catheter. Percutaneous catheters are not recommended for home use since the risk of complication, complexity of care, and patient education time are increased. Candidacy for HTPN is ideally determined by the nutrition support team and the patient after careful assessment of these issues. Appropriateness for catheterization must be evaluated as well as the need for TPN therapy.

Assessment issues include the following:

1. Acceptance by the patient and family of the patient's need for HTPN therapy;
2. Intellectual capabilities of the patient and/or family;
3. Motivation by the patient and/or family to learn;
4. Family support;
5. Physical limitations of the patient affecting ability to perform catheter care and infusion procedures;
6. Type of catheter needed (i.e., single lumen, multilumen, implanted port).

Careful consideration should be given in determining the type of catheter to

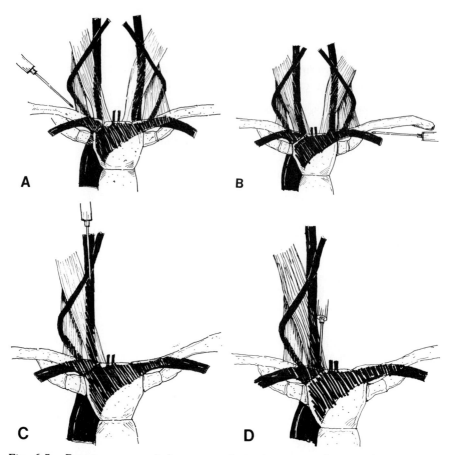

Fig. 6-5. Percutaneous central venous catheter insertion techniques. Insertion site: **Subclavian**. The patient is positioned with rolled towel between scapulae (longitudinally, arms at side, head turned away from side of insertion, head flat in bed, in the Trendelenburg position (15–20° tilt). If the guidewire method is used, the head should be turned toward the side of insertion while threading the wire to avoid entry into jugular vein. Procedure: (A) Supraclavicular approach: The physician stands at the head of the bed. The anterior scalenus muscle is palpated at the tubercle on the first rib at the posterior border of the sternocleidomastoid. The needle is passed over the tubercle to the costoclavicular space. The vein is entered 1 to 1.5 cm under the skin. The syringe is detached and catheter is advanced according to method of insertion. (B) Infraclavicular approach: The physician stands at the side of the bed. The skin is punctured 1 cm below the clavicle at the junction of the medial one-third and lateral two-thirds of the clavicle where it curves posteriorly. The needle is passed below the clavicle and advanced horizontally toward the suprasternal notch. When blood is freely aspirated, the syringe is detached and the catheter is advanced according to the method of insertion. Insertion site: **internal jugular**. The patient is positioned with a folded towel or small pillows under shoulder (transversely), arms at side, head turned 10–15° away from insertion site, Trendelenburg position (15–20° tilt). Procedure: (C) High anterior approach: The physician is at the head of the bed. The carotid artery is palpated at the medial border of the sternocleidomastoid and lower border of the thyroid cartilage. The puncture site is 4

be placed. Additional lumens increase potential for infection and time and equipment needed to care for them. In the case of the implanted device, the patient needs to understand that skin puncture is required for access. This may not be tolerable despite the advantage of no external catheter. These issues are often complex and may require a considerable amount of time to address. Nevertheless, careful weighing of the issues will affect the outcome. In most cases, the nutrition support nurse is the most appropriate person to make these assessments.

Preoperative Preparation

Preoperative teaching should be instituted as soon as the decision for catheter placement is made. The patient must have a clear understanding of the expectations and requirements of home care including catheter care, equipment and supplies, hours of solution administration, and home followup. Demonstration of the catheter and explanation of catheter insertion are also important. One of the major factors in the success of HTPN is the psychosocial component.[22] The patient and family usually have many questions and concerns. Sufficient time should be allowed for discussion, reassurance, and emotional support (see Chapters 9 and 10).

Both implanted and indwelling catheters are inserted in the operating room or a treatment room with the availability of emergency equipment, fluoroscopy, and/or x-ray. Adult patients typically receive preoperative sedation and local anesthesia. If the central veins have been used extensively because of prior critical illness, a preoperative venogram may be indicated to assess vascular patency. With the use of light anesthesia, many patients remember the operative experience. This makes preoperative explanation of the insertion procedure of significant importance. An unpleasant experience during catheter insertion may have a negative impact on acceptance of the catheter and the postoperative teaching program.

Methods of Insertion

The veins most commonly selected for catheter placement are the cephalic vein at the deltopectoral groove and the subclavian and the internal jugular vein.

⟨————————————————————————————————

cm below the angle of the mandible, 5 cm above the clavicle, and 1 cm inside the lateral border of the sternocleidomastoid. The needle is inserted under the sternomastoid aiming at the junction of the middle and inner thirds of the clavicle with a 30–45° posterior angle with the skin. When blood is freely aspirated, the syringe is detached and the catheter inserted according to the method of insertion. (D) Supraclavicular junctional approach: The physician stands at the head of the bed. The puncture site is 3 cm above the clavicle at the lateral border of the sternocleidomastoid. The needle is advanced toward the suprasternal notch with the needle at a 30° angle with the skin. When blood is freely aspirated, the syringe is lowered to the direction of the vein. The syringe is detached and the catheter advanced according to the method of insertion.

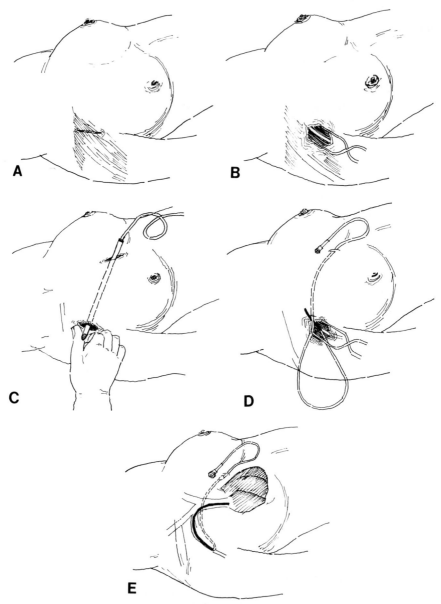

Fig. 6-6. Insertion techniques for indwelling Silastic catheters. Cutdown technique: Patient is positioned supine with head turned to contralateral side: (A) Local anesthetic is injected over the cutdown site and along the skin tunnel. A cutdown is performed over the vessel selected and the vein is isolated. The cephalic vein is isolated in the deltopectoral groove: the internal jugular vein is isolated at the posterior border of the sternocleidomastoid muscle in its midportion. (B) A skin tunnel is made by blunt dissection of the subcutaneous tissue with a long forcep or trocar. The instrument is

If subclavian and jugular or superior vena cava thrombosis has occurred, the saphenous or femoral vein can be accessed. The inferior epigastric and iliac vein have also been reported for use.[23] If both upper and lower venous systems are occluded, direct right atrial catheterization via thoracotomy may be indicated.[24]

The two methods of insertion are the cutdown and the percutaneous method, illustrated in Figure 6-6. Either technique can be used to insert both the indwelling and implanted catheters. The Groshong catheter with the closed tip requires tunneling of the catheter after it has been inserted into the vein. The catheter is pulled through the tunnel in the opposite direction of the Hickman catheter, from the insertion site to the exit site. A connector similar to a blunt needle adapter is inserted into the catheter and is supported with a protective sleeve (Fig. 6-7).

The implanted venous access port requires a subcutaneous pocket for implantation of the disc. The selected vein is accessed by the percutaneous

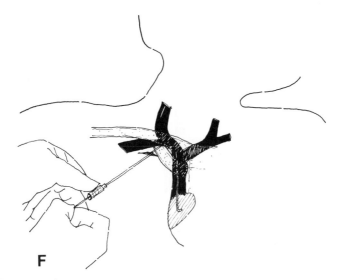

F

Fig. 6-6 continued
brought out through the skin by a small incision at the preselected point. (C) The catheter tip is grasped and pulled through the tunnel, positioning the Dacron cuff 1-2 cm above the exit site of the catheter. The catheter is cut to the proper length after measuring the distance from the insertion site to junction of the superior vena cava and the right atrium. (D) The catheter is heparinized and inserted through a venotomy in the vein. (E) Fluoroscopy confirms proper positioning. The cutdown site is sutured and a retaining suture is placed at the exit site. Percutaneous technique: Patient is positioned the same as for subclavian or jugular percutaneous insertion. Procedure: (F) Local anesthetic is injected over the insertion site and along the skin tunnel. Venipuncture is made with a 18-gauge needle. A springwire guide is advanced into the vessel. The 18-gauge needle is withdrawn with the wire in place.

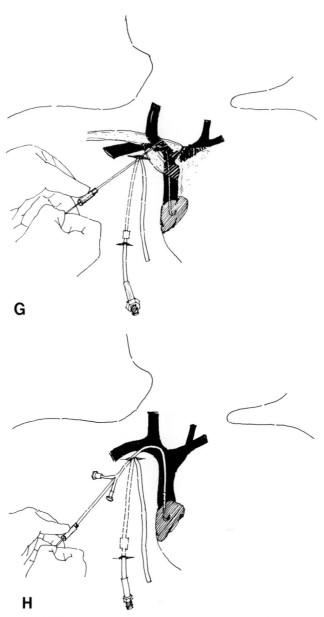

G

H

Fig. 6-6 Continued (G) A skin tunnel is made by blunt dissection of the subcutaneous tissue with a long forcep or trocar beginning at the point of exit of the wire. The instrument is brought out through the skin by small incision at the preselected point. The catheter tip is grasped and pulled through the tunnel-positioning the Dacron cuff 1–2 cm above the exit site of the catheter. The catheter is cut to the proper length after measuring the distance from the insertion site to the junction of the superior vena cava and right atrium. (H) A vessel dilator and peel-away introducer sheath is threaded over the wire and into the vessel. The wire is removed and blood return confirmed with blood aspiration through the dilator. The dilator is removed and the tip of the catheter is advanced through the peel-away sheath into place.

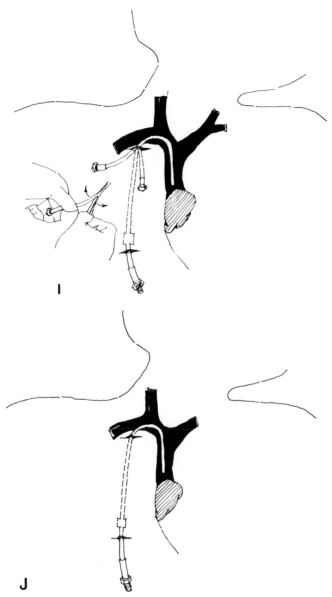

Fig. 6-6 continued (I) Verification of catheter and tip location should be confirmed by fluoroscopy, x-ray, and blood aspiration through the catheter. The handles of the peel-away sheath are grasped and pulled outward and upward at the same time until the sheath is completely peeled away from the catheter. advanced through the peel-away sheath into place. (I) Verification of catheter and tip location should be confirmed by fluoroscopy, x-ray, and blood aspiration through the catheter. The handles of the peel-away sheath are grasped and pulled outward and upward at the same time until the sheath is completely peeled away from the catheter. (J) The insertion site is sutured or steristripped and a retaining suture placed at the exit site.

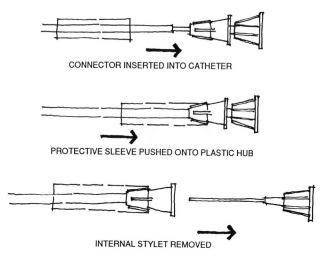

CONNECTOR INSERTED INTO CATHETER

PROTECTIVE SLEEVE PUSHED ONTO PLASTIC HUB

INTERNAL STYLET REMOVED

Fig. 6-7. Tunneling of the Groshong catheter after insertion into the vein.

method and the wire left in place. The skin over the third or fourth rib lateral to the sternum is anesthetized, and a subcutaneous pocket that will accommodate the portal is constructed in a cephalad direction. The trocar is then directed subcutaneously to the venipuncture site, the catheter pulled through the tunnel, and the distal end attached to the disc. The disc is then sutured to the fascia. The peel-away sheath and dilator are passed over the wire and the catheter introduced as illustrated in the percutaneous method in Figure 6-6. The subcutaneous pocket is then closed in layers leaving only an incision (Fig. 6-8).

ISSUES IN THE MANAGEMENT OF INFUSION SYSTEMS

Despite the multitude of mishaps that can occur during the insertion of central venous catheters, the majority of complications are related to administration of the solutions and care of the infusion system.[19] Many questions related to these topics remain unanswered, and further research is needed.

Several reports have demonstrated that the intervention of a nutrition support nurse and/or nutrition support team has significantly reduced infection rates and/or length of hospital stay in patients receiving specialized nutrition support.[25–31] Meticulous care by highly trained, motivated individuals can affect morbidity, mortality, and health care costs that are associated with bacteremias, septicemias, and multiple catheter placements.

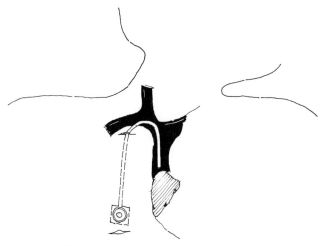

Fig. 6-8. Placement of an implanted port in a subcutaneous pocket.

Dressing Management

Percutaneous Catheters

Migration of bacteria from the skin surface along the subcutaneous tract of the catheter to the bloodstream has been considered a major factor in the pathogenesis of catheter sepsis. Percutaneous catheters are inserted through the skin directly into the vessel. This affords a relatively short distance for microorganisms to gain access to the blood. Consequently, initial and repeated sterilization of the skin is necessary to prevent colonization of the skin and tract.

Prior to 1978, the most common procedure for dressing changes were alcohol/acetone cleansing, povidone-iodine prep, povidone-iodine ointment, and gauze and tape on a Monday-Wednesday-Friday schedule.[32,33] In 1977, Thomas reported the use of a transparent polyurethane dressing for central venous catheters.[34] Since then, several studies have indicated that transparent dressings may be as effective a dressing material as the standard gauze and tape and perhaps more cost and time efficient.[32–39] It is important to note that in all of these studies the skin prep was usually the same (i.e., alcohol/acetone and povidone-iodine application). Povidone-iodine ointment was also used in all of these studies except one. The use of povidone-iodine ointment in reduction of catheter sepsis remains questionable despite the type of dressing material; however, it is recommended for use over antibiotic ointments in central venous access because of its antifungal properties.[40]

Table 6-3
Sterile CVP/TPN Dressing Change Kit

Nonsterile Items	1	polybacked waterproof towel
	1	face mask
Extension Tube Change	1	Povidone iodine Prep Pad
	1	sterile luer-lok extension tubing
Sterile Dressing Change Items	1	CSR overwrap
	1	pair sterile gloves
	4	alcohol/acetone swabsticks
	3	povidone iodine swabsticks
	1	povidone iodine ointment
	1	pkg. 2 × 2 inch gauze sponges
	1	protective dressing swabstick
	1	roll or pack of tape or transparent dressing

A prepackaged sterilized kit is recommended for sterile dressing changes. These kits may also be custom designed. They contain all sterile components, increase compliance to a standard procedure, and are cost and time efficient. A list of suggested components is found in Table 6-3. The kit described also includes items for extension tube change. Most dressing change protocols incorporate the catheter hub and tubing junction under the dressing. This junction, as all connection points, are potential portals of entry for bacteria and should be cleansed with povidone iodine prior to disconnection. The waterproof towel is placed on the bed for collection of the soiled dressing and components discarded after their use. Four alcohol/acetone swabsticks are included: 3 for cleansing the skin and 1 for cleansing the catheter itself. Cliniguard protective dressing (Clinipad Corp., Guilford, CT) is recommended for protection of skin integrity and healing of irritated skin. Tincture of benzoin will increase adherence of the dressing, but is a skin irritant and may further damage broken skin.

The frequency of dressing change is dependent on the following: type of dressing material used; activity of the patient; presence of contaminating drainage, secretions, or excessive perspiration; condition of the catheter site; and integrity of the old dressing on inspection. Schwartz-Fulton et al. reported the average dressing life for gauze and tape dressings to be 2.1–2.4 days,[32] and Powell et al.[39] reported 2.1 days. Average dressing life for transparent dressings varied from 5 days as reported by Powell et al.[39] to as long as 16.2 days as reported by Curtas and Grant.[35] The key issue is a dry, sterile, intact dressing. The patient must be assessed daily for potential catheter sepsis and the dressing evaluated frequently for necessity of change. Some patients may require daily changes while others can be maintained by the standard frequency of dressing change.

Indwelling Catheters

Implantation and ingrowth of the Dacron cuff on indwelling Silastic catheters provide a barrier against migration of bacteria through the skin tunnel to the blood. The space from the cuff to the exit site of the catheter, however, remains a potential site for local infection. Consequently, a dressing should be used over the exit site. The presence of the ingrown cuff permits use of a clean technique in dressing management. The same skin preparation, dressing materials, and frequency of change used with percutaneous catheters are recommended for indwelling catheters. The use of clean technique versus sterile technique and the reduction of time and cost of procedures makes this catheter more appropriate for home use.

Again, kits are useful. In many cases bulk supplies are difficult to manage in the home. The simpler the equipment and procedure, the higher the compliance rate and lower the complication rate. Certainly the tremendous cost of the treatment of catheter infection or sepsis far exceeds the minimal cost of a dressing change kit. An insert contained in the kit with directions for the procedure is valuable for teaching purposes and provides written instruction for the patient for home care.

Catheter Irrigation

Adult sized catheters generally do not require heparin irrigation with continuous infusions. The purpose of heparin instillation is to maintain patency of the catheter for intermittent use. This is particularly useful for implanted and indwelling catheters and for a lumen(s) of a multilumen catheter that is no longer needed. Single lumen percutaneous catheters could also be capped and irrigated for intermittent use, but this carries the risk of loss of the catheter should total occlusion occur.

Heparin is the drug of choice for maintaining catheter patency. Procedures for the care of the Groshong catheter specify normal saline for catheter irrigation.[16]

Recommendations for the volume and dosage of heparin vary widely. The volume required to replace the existing volume is dependent on the internal diameter and length of the catheter. An infant Broviac catheter in a neonate may contain as little as .2 ml compared to 1 ml in an adult Hickman, while the middle lumen of a 20-cm triple lumen percutaneous catheter holds .25 ml. Catheter volume after implantation is determined simply by aspirating through the heparin-filled catheter and measuring the volume in the syringe at the first appearance of blood. Enough volume should be used to accomplish a thorough mechanical flush and instill new heparin at the same time. The dosage of heparin should be of sufficient strength to prevent clotting of the catheter. The goal is to heparinize the catheter, not the patient. Suggested volumes and dosages are listed in Table 6-4.

Table 6-4
Heparinization of Central Venous Catheters

Catheter Type	Dosage	Volume
Indwelling/Implanted Catheters		
Infant (neonate)	10 units/ml	.5–1 ml
Infant/pediatric	100 units/ml	1–2 ml
Adult	100–1000 units/ml	3–5 ml
All leukemics	100 units/ml	
Percutaneous Catheters		
Multilumen		
Middle port	100 units/ml	1 ml
Proximal port	100 units/ml	1 ml

All catheters must be flushed and capped on discontinuation of an infusion. Most HTPN patients infuse their solutions at night over 12 hours, so the catheter is subsequently flushed daily. Frequency of flushing catheters not routinely used is again highly variable among protocols, from daily to weekly to monthly. Further studies are needed in this area.

Catheter Occlusions

Occlusion should occur relatively infrequently with proper management of catheters. The advent of effective fibrinolytic agents to restore catheter patency has prevented removal of thrombosed catheters.

Low-dose urokinase is effective in restoring patency of catheters occluded by fibrin clots.[41–44] It is not effective for clearance of obstructed catheters by substances other than blood products such as drug precipitates. Urokinase is an enzyme (protein) produced by the kidney and found in the urine. It acts on the endogenous fibrinolytic system by conversion of plasminogen to the enzyme plasmin that breaks down fibrin clots to fibrinogen. Urokinase has a half-life of 11–23 minutes and is eliminated primarily by hepatic metabolism. The small 5000 unit dose required does not affect serum fibrinolytic activity or coagulation assays. There have been no adverse reactions reported as a result of using low-dose urokinase for catheter clearance. Theoretical problems include bleeding, skin rash, fever, and allergic reactions such as bronchospasm.

Streptokinase is a nonenzymatic protein isolated from group C beta-hemolytic streptococci (half-life of 10–18 minutes). Hurtubise et al.[44] found that dilute solutions of streptokinase or urokinase were as equally efficacious as thrombolytic agents in central venous catheters. No adverse reactions could be attributed to either drug. Streptokinase is antigenic, however, and allergic responses including anaphylaxis may occur, especially if the catheter has been ruptured and the drug is injected into the subcutaneous tissue.

Initial treatment of catheter occlusion is aspiration of the clot with a syringe. Connecting a syringe of normal saline and gently alternating flush and aspiration of the catheter often "massages" the clot loose, especially if it is small. If this is not successful, urokinase is indicated. Sterile technique is essential with all catheter manipulations. No more than actual catheter fill should be instilled. A percutaneous catheter holds from .15 to .6 ml and implanted catheters from .2 to 1.2 ml depending on internal diameters in length. Excessive pressure on injection should be avoided to prevent rupture of the catheter or expulsion of the clot into the circulation. The drug should be allowed to remain in the catheter for at least 5 minutes. Repeat aspiration attempts can be made every 5 minutes if the catheter is not cleared on the first attempt. If the catheter is not opened within 30 minutes, the catheter may be capped and aspirated again at 60 minutes. A second injection of drug may be necessary.[45] When patency is restored, aspiration of 3–5 ml of blood assures removal of all drug and clot residual.

Filtration

In 1979 the National Coordinating Committee on Large Volume Parenterals (NCCLVP) recommended to multiple organizations including the American Medical Association, the American Nurses Association, the Center for Disease Control (CDC), the Joint Commission on Accreditation of Hospital (JCAH), Food and Drug Administration (FDA), and so on, that patients receiving hyperalimentation should have inline IV filtration. This filter should be both particulate and microbe retentive.[46] Filtration is an inexpensive, simplified method of preventing very hazardous and expensive complications. Several issues must be taken into account if filtration is not utilized.

Sepsis

The majority of microorganisms that survive and proliferate in simple intravenous solutions are gram-negative bacteria. TPN solutions primarily support the growth of fungi. Bacterial or fungal contamination of intravenous sources may occur at any time during manufacture, admixture, and administration of the solutions. Inadvertent contamination may result in bacterial levels of 10^8 organisms.[47] Immune deficient patients (neonates, burn patients, transplant patients, malnourished and critically ill patients) are at an increased risk for infection that may lead to substantial morbidity and mortality. A .22 μm filter will block the passage of virtually all bacteria and fungus.[48] Positive cultures of inline filter membranes have been reported in the range of 2.8–42.9 percent. If the trapped contaminants are gram-negative bacteria, endotoxins may be released. Endotoxins are phosphoglycolipid complexes derived from the walls of gram-negative bacteria. Endotoxin leakage is of interest because of the predictable rise in body temperature. This is associated with circulating interleukin-1, which is a peptide that mediates most responses to infections and to inflammatory and immunologic disease.[47] In addition to fever, septic shock may occur. The fever may be treated by removal of the catheter, increased or additional antibiotics, additional laboratory monitoring, or invasive clinical testing for the source of fever. All of these are very expensive treatment modalities. The Posidyne (PALL) 96 half-filter has been shown to be bacterial and endotoxin retentive up to 144 hours.[49] It has also been favorably tested for pyrogen retention following antibiotic administration through the filter.[50] The ability to retain the filter inline for 96 hours not only severely reduces the cost of filters and tubing, but also prevents daily manipulations of the line. If endotoxin retentive filters are not used and antibiotics are administered through the filter, filter tubing changes are recommended every 24 hours,[48] especially if antibiotics are administered through the filter.[51]

Infusion of Particulate Matter

Despite technological advances, IV solutions contain considerable amounts of particulate matter. Both the size and number of particles may increase by as much as 25-fold when medications are added to the solution.[52] Particulate matter may include unreconstituted medications, fragments from glass vials, syringes, needles, and rubber seals, or cotton fibers from alcohol swabs. Infusion of particulates may have adverse effects. Particulate matter may initiate a foreign body inflammatory response that may result in granuloma formation.[53] In a study by Rapp and Bivins,[54] patients receiving unfiltered parenteral solutions tended to have significantly higher white blood cell (WBC) counts than those receiving infusions in which a final filter was used. Increased WBCs may be due to reactive infusion particulates lodging in the pulmonary vascular bed eliciting an inflammatory response. In addition, occlusion of the capillary bed may inhibit oxygenation and normal metabolism and cause cellular damage and tissue death.[55]

Air Embolism or Hemorrhage

Air embolism is a potentially lethal complication related to the use of central venous catheters (see Postinsertion Complications). The use of an air-eliminating, position-insensitive, luer-locking filter at the catheter hub can virtually eliminate the potential for introduction of air in the administration tubing or as a result of disconnection. This is of particular concern not only in hospitalized patients, but also in the home when disconnection during nocturnal infusions may go undetected. In addition, hemorrhage from the catheter cannot occur since the size of a red blood cell is much larger than .22 μm and prevents blood from passing through the membrane.

Despite the small increase in cost, a bacteria- and endotoxin-retentive, air-eliminating filter will result in a net savings because of the reduction of filter and tubing changes, fewer complications, and the expensive treatment of those complications when they occur.

COMPLICATIONS RELATED TO THE ADMINISTRATION OF PARENTERAL NUTRITION

Complications related to central venous catheters can be major or minor in consequence. Major complications are events requiring further invasive treatment while minor complications do not require further intervention.

Complications of Catheter Insertion

The increased potential for complications of central venous catheter insertion occurs as the result of the immediate proximity of multiple anatomic structures to the central vasculature (Fig. 6-9). For example, the subclavian artery is immediately posterior to the subclavian vein, the brachial plexus is superior, and the pleura and lung are inferior. The carotid artery is laterally adherent to the internal jugular vein. The superior aspect of the pleura and lung are adjacent to the inferior and distal portion of the internal jugular vein. The thoracic duct on the left and numerous lymphatic channels surround the subclavian veins bilaterally. Complications of catheter insertion along with catheter sepsis, air embolism, and perforation constitute the most life-threatening complications associated with TPN therapy.

Pneumothorax

A pneumothorax is caused by inadvertent entrance into the pleural cavity and/or laceration of the lung. Clinical manifestations depend on the size and type of pneumothorax, but typical symptoms include pain, dyspnea, and hypoxia.

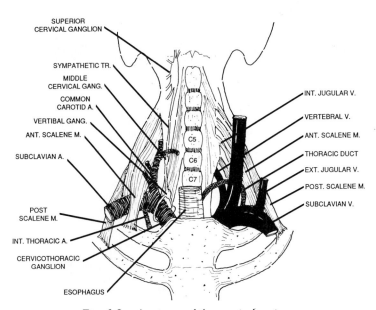

Fig. 6-9. Anatomy of the cervical region.

During catheter insertion, a needle puncture of the lung causes inspired air to escape from the surface of the injured lung into the pleural space. Placement of a chest tube is often required. A tension pneumothorax is an emergent problem (Fig. 6-10). This is most likely to occur in patients on mechanical ventilation, especially those with high inspiratory pressures. This increased airway pressure forces gas through the defect into the pleural space under high pressure. The heart shifts away from the side of the defect resulting in reduction of venous return and rapid clinical deterioration with cyanosis, venous distention, hypotension, reduction of cardiac output, and death. Immediate insertion of a large-bore needle or chest tube is required to avoid death.

Delayed pneumothorax is a relatively unrecognized complication.[56,57] It is caused by a slow pleural leak often associated with a difficult insertion procedure. Repeat postinsertion x-rays should be considered in the following situations:

1.   Difficult insertions requiring multiple attempts,
2.   Suspicion of pleural injury associated with aspiration of air during insertion or subcutaneous emphysema with normal postinsertion chest x-ray,
3.   The presence of another major complication,
4.   Patient complaints of persistent pleuritic pain or back pain after insertion,

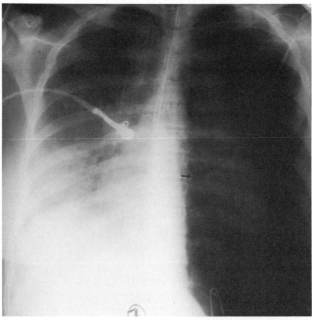

Fig. 6-10.   Tension pneumothorax after TPN catheter insertion. Note the shift of the heart to the right.

5. Preoperatively after previous difficult insertion of a central venous line, and
6. Postoperatively when a subclavian catheter is inserted intraoperatively.

Hemothorax

Arterial trauma by the inserting needle is the usual cause of injury to the vein whether cannulated or not. The blood collects in the pleural space either as free fluid or a subpleural collection at the apex of the chest. Extensive dissection may occur in the chest wall and extrapleural space without demonstration of intrapleural blood. Malposition into a pleural space that contains blood may lead to erroneous impressions that the catheter is in the vascular space when blood return with syringe aspiration or lowering the bag is achieved. A large hematoma in the neck may cause respiratory distress due to deviation of the trachea. Immediate bleeding is usually stopped by a compressive hematoma, but delayed bleeding, arteriovenous fistula formation, or the development of a false aneurysm is not uncommon following arterial trauma. Chest tube drainage may be necessary and in some cases thoracotomy is required for repair. Malposition of the catheter into the pleural space or injury to pulmonary vessels may lead to potentially lethal results.[58,59] Coagulopathies should be corrected before venipuncture.

Arterial Cannulation

Central venous catheters may inadvertently be placed into the central arterial vasculature rather than the venous system. Hypotension or hypoxemia may mask detection by pulsatile or bright red blood return (Fig. 6-11). Diagnosis is made by observation of the course of the catheter on x-ray. TPN solutions should never be infused intra-arterially. Clotting factors may need to be administered prior to catheter removal.

Hydrothorax or Hydromediastinum

The occurrence of hydrothorax or hydromediastinum results from perforation of the vein by the catheter or introducer on insertion, or by delayed perforation due to erosion of the catheter through the vein wall (Figs. 6-12 and 6-13). A catheter that has entered the vein but subsequently exited the vein into the mediastinum or pleural space may not be apparent on x-ray. Clinical manifestations vary according to the volume and rate of extravasation. Signs and symptoms may be manifested as general deterioration of condition, low-grade fever, slight dyspnea, or chest pain. Signs and symptoms become progressively worse as the hydrothorax increases. Hypoxia, respiratory distress, sepsis, and cardiovascular collapse may result if untreated. Delayed bilateral hydrothorax may occur from a hydromediastinum due to fluid shifting across the mesothelium of the parietal pleurae. Injection of contrast medium into the catheter is useful in diagnosis. Treatment involves removal of the catheter and drainage of the hydrothorax. Caution should be used with left subclavian and left internal

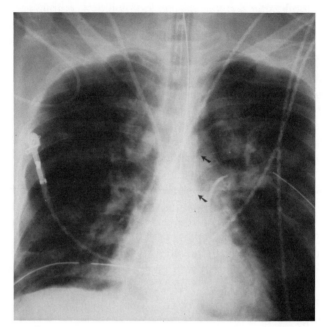

Fig. 6-11. Arterial cannulation of a TPN catheter with the tip in the aorta. The insertion was complicated by a pneumothorax. Hypoxemia and hypotension prevented detection by pulsatile blood flow and coloration of the blood.

jugular insertions when inserting the catheter into the superior vena cava toward the right atrial junction so that the catheter runs parallel to the superior vena cava. Catheter tips may perforate the vein if the tip rests on the opposite wall of the superior vena cava after making the turn downward. The use of softer, more flexible catheters will reduce the risk of these complications.

Catheter Embolism

Catheter embolism occurs as a result of improper technique by shearing off a portion of the catheter while withdrawing the catheter through the inserting needle (Fig. 6-14). Rupture of Silastic catheters may occur with use of excessive pressure while attempting to dislodge an occluded catheter. These transected fragments lead to embolization of the right atrium, right ventricle, pulmonary artery, or lung. Arrhythmias may be precipitated. Thrombus formation around this segment may occur, providing a nidus for infection. Removal of the fragment is accomplished by snaring the fragment under fluoroscopy with a hooked guidewire system, stone basket, wire loop technique, or endoscopic forceps. If this is not successful, thoracotomy may be required. Use of the

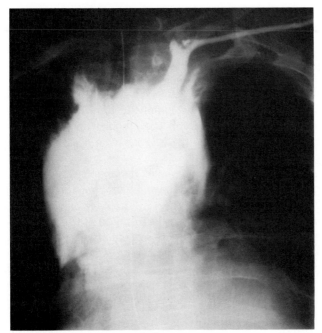

Fig. 6-12. Perforation of the superior vena cava by an introducer sheath. Injection of contrast material demonstrates extravasation into the mediastinal space.

"over-the-wire" rather than "through-the-needle" technique of catheter insertion will eliminate this complication.

Air Embolism

Air embolism is the most lethal complication of catheter insertion but fortunately its occurrence is rare. Negative intrathoracic pressure is transmitted to the portion of the central venous system leading to the heart. Subsequently, air embolism may occur when an opening from the outside of the body is made to one of these veins. This is more likely to occur on deep inspiration when the patient is in an upright position, dehydrated, or hypovolemic.[60,61] This complication can be avoided during catheter insertion by: (1) rehydration of dehydrated or hypovolemic patients; (2) placing the patient in the Trendelenburg position; (3) use of small-bore needles for venipuncture; and (4) placing a finger over the needle hub or catheter hub with disconnections and removal of the wire (see Postinsertion Complications, Air Embolism).

Nerve Injury

Both the brachial plexus and phrenic nerve are in close proximity to the central veins. The phrenic nerve can be damaged in both internal jugular and subclavian insertions by the needle or a malpositioned catheter.

Numbness and tingling sensations in the arm may be experienced for minutes to hours, or permanent weakness may occur. Paralysis of the hemi-diaphragm can result from phrenic nerve damage.

Lymphatic Injury

Lymphatic injury, lymphatic fistula, or chylothorax may be experienced with puncture or laceration of the lymphatic trunks or thoracic duct. These lymphatic vessels are in proximity to both jugular and subclavian veins. The thoracic duct empties into the left subclavian vein at its junction with the left internal jugular vein.

Clinical manifestations of lymphatic damage include: (1) aspiration of lymphatic fluid on insertion; (2) drainage of lymphatic fluid from the catheter insertion site, which may be excessive; or (3) drainage of lymph into the thoracic cavity. Drainage may not be seen from the insertion site if a chest tube is in place.

Differential diagnosis is made by evaluation of the drainage fluid for lymphocyte count and/or triglyceride level. The triglyceride level is of no value, however, if the patient does not have fat intake via the gastrointestinal tract.

Removal of the catheter is necessary for closure of the fistula. Transthoracic surgical ligation and repair may be necessary for continued leakage not resolved by catheter removal.[9]

Tracheal Puncture

Puncture of the trachea can occur with internal jugular vein insertions using the posterior approach. When the inserting needle is directed too medial and the skin is entered too caudal, puncture of the larynx or trachea may result. If the patient is intubated, puncture of the inflated cuff is possible, requiring emergency reintubation. Leakage of air may lead to subcutaneous emphysema, pneumo-mediastinum, or air trapping between the chest wall and the pleura.[62]

Catheter Malposition

Catheter malposition has been reported to occur in 1–33 percent of attempts.[63] It is generally accepted that catheter placement requires radiographic confirmation of position.

Erroneous positions may include subclavian insertion with the catheter ascending into the jugular vein and vice versa, or the catheter may cross the thorax to the contralateral subclavian vein. The right subclavian vein is mostly associated with catheter malposition.

Small tributaries of the central veins might be cannulated accidentally. These vessels include the left internal mammary vein, inferior thyroidal veins, superior intercostal veins, or pericardiophrenic vein—all branches of the left brachiocephalic vein—or the right internal mammary and azygous veins, which branch from the superior vena cava. Malposition to these tributaries appears to be more common via the left brachiocephalic than the right because of its longer, more oblique course and more frequent branches.

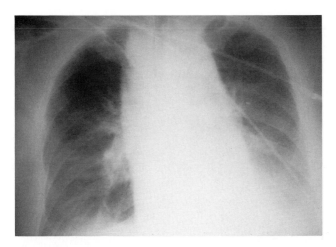

Fig. 6-13. Erosion of a TPN catheter that was malpositioned in a tributary vein resulting in a hydromediastinum.

Various complaints by the patient may indicate aberrant positioning. Misplacement into the jugular vein may be exhibited as pain in the neck or ear; the internal mammary vein causes sharp anterior chest pain; and the innominate vein creates pain in the ipsilateral shoulder blade. The primary dangers of aberrant central venous catheters are inaccurate venous pressure measurements, thrombophlebitis, perforation, ectopic infusions of toxic solutions, and catheter knotting.[64] Catheters advanced into the heart remain in constant motion because of the muscular action. This, along with torque forces applied along the length of the catheter, may lead to perforation of the right atrium or ventricle with resultant pericardial tamponade (see Postinsertion Complications, Pericardial Tamponade). Another aberrant route of a catheter that is advanced beyond the superior vena cava is through the heart into the inferior vena cava. This may cause laceration or thrombosis of the hepatic vein and/or inferior vena cava.

Migration of catheters at some time after the initial insertion may occur more often than once thought. Vazquez and Brodski[65] report an overall rate in silicone catheters of 5.31 percent. They attribute the problem to a function of physical forces acting on the soft, flexible silicone catheter in a high flow venous system rather than to placement technique. Recognition and repositioning of the catheter is important since infusion of hypertonic solutions into veins of smaller caliber may result in phlebitis and venous thrombosis (Fig. 6-15). Knotted or coiled catheters may traumatize the vein and are more likely to break and embolize or perforate the vein wall.

Malpositioned catheters may spontaneously reposition themselves, but if

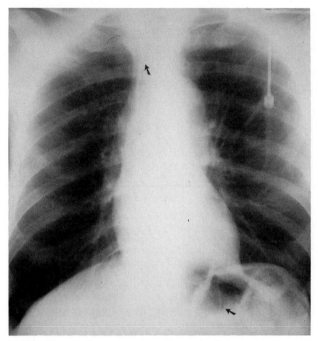

Fig. 6-14. Catheter segment sheared off during catheterization utilizing the "through-the-needle" technique. Note the
catheter fragment in the left lower lobe.

not, repositioning may be accomplished by the use of a guidewire under
fluoroscopy.[66]

Careful evaluation of postinsertion and subsequent x-rays, particularly in
home patients, is warranted. Administration of an isotonic fluid bolus prior to the
postinsertion x-ray may be of benefit by showing a detectable fluid level if the
catheter is in the pleural space.

POSTINSERTION COMPLICATIONS

Catheter-Related Septicemia

Incidence

Plastic catheters for intravenous infusions were introduced in 1945, but the
first reports of infections related to intravascular devices did not appear until
1963.[67] The subject was barely mentioned at the first International Conference
on Nosocomial Infections held in 1970.[68] An estimated 50,000 cannula-related

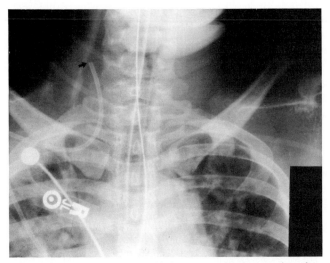

Fig. 6-15. Migration of a Hickman® catheter months after catheter insertion. Thrombosis of the internal jugular vein was found on autopsy.

septicemias in 20 million infusion recipients occur each year in the United States. On the average, 20–40 percent of patients in whom a nosocomial bacteremia is acquired do not survive.[69] In addition, these nosocomial bacteremias portend 14–19 days of additional hospitalization and $3600 to $4390 in excess hospital costs. The character of the blood pathogen does not appear to greatly influence mortality except for two organisms, *Pseudomonas aeruginosa* and *Candida*. Case fatality rates in septicemia caused by these organisms exceed 60 percent in most centers.[70] In addition to bacteremic complication, local infection of the insertion site results in morbidity and prolonged hospital stay. Such local infections, although usually less severe, presumably occur much more commonly than bacteremias.[71]

Risk Factors

Multiple risk factors are related to catheter-acquired infections. Patient-related risk factors include:

1. Age. Susceptibility is increased in the elderly and the neonate.[72,73]
2. Severity of the underlying illness. Mortality is highest in patients with fatal underlying disease because of a diminished host defense mechanism.
3. Presence of local infection. Hematogenous microbiologic seeding ranges from 5.8–19.5 percent.[73]
4. Antibiotic therapy. May lead to bacterial resistance or fungal overgrowth.

5. Abdominal surgery. Increases risk of disseminated candidiasis.[74,75]
6. Malnutrition.
7. Corticosteroid or other immunosuppressive therapy.
8. Other invasive vascular devices.
9. Loss of skin integrity in burned patients.[76]
10. Malignancies.
11. Drug addiction.
12. Acquired immunodeficiency syndrome (AIDS).

Other risk factors are hospital-related and include:

1. Catheter material. Silastic catheters and hydromer-coated catheters may be less thrombogenic,[77] reducing fibrin sleeve formation and subsequent nidus for infection. Catheter materials have varying affinities for adherence of slime-producing organisms.[78–81]
2. Type of catheter (single lumen, multilumen, pulmonary artery, Hickman, etc.). Infection rates are generally higher in Swan-Ganz and multilumen catheters and should be utilized for TPN administration with caution.[19,82–85]
3. Location of insertion. Pinilla reported infection rates to be 20 percent in the antecubital vein, 12 percent in the internal jugular, 7 percent in the subclavian vein, and 29 percent with pulmonary artery catheters at the internal jugular site compared with 7 percent in the subclavian veins.[86]
4. Duration of catheterization. Numerous reports have reported that phlebitis and septicemia increase with duration of catheterization.
5. Method of insertion (percutaneous vs. cutdown). Catheters placed by the percutaneous method have lower colonization rates than with cutdown insertions.[87]
6. Technical aspects of catheter insertion. Skill of the surgeon, adequate skin preparation, emergent vs. elective insertion.
7. Dressing management. Dressing material, technique employed, frequency of change, skin preparation, use of antibiotic vs. antiseptic ointments.
8. Handwashing technique.
9. In-use contamination.
10. Proximity of tracheostomy or wounds.
11. Composition of the infusate.
12. Sterility of the infusate.
13. Presence of sideports, manometers, stopcocks, etc.
14. Presence of nutrition teams with strict protocols for care.

Pathogenesis

Any intravenous system or device for vascular access is a direct link between the environment with its multitude of organisms and the patient's bloodstream. Pathogens may be introduced into the vascular system by:

1. Contamination during catheter insertion.

2. Migration of bacteria along the subcutaneous tract.
3. Contaminated parenteral solutions.
4. Nonsterile manipulation or contamination of any of the components of the infusion system.
5. Hematogenous "seeding" of the intravascular segment during periods of bacteremia or fungemia.

Catheterization of the central venous system is an invasive procedure that requires surgical asepsis. Preoperative skin preparation, sterile draping, and aseptic technique are required. The site at which the catheter penetrates the skin and the subcutaneous tract is presumably one of the more important routes of bacterial and fungal access. The theory of migration of bacteria as an etiologic factor of catheter sepsis is based on the strong association between organisms present on the skin surrounding the catheter wound and organisms recovered from the catheter tip and blood in septicemia. The most common organisms isolated from catheter tips are ubiquitous on the skin of hospitalized patients and hands of personnel. The number of passes with the insertion needle has also been shown to correlate with catheter sepsis.[88]

Contamination of parenteral solutions occurs at a rate of 3–38 percent.[72,89–93] Since growth of microorganisms is different with different organisms and solutions, pathogenesis is reflected by the etiologic factors. Several studies have demonstrated that Candida proliferates well in TPN solutions[90,94–99] and in lipid emulsions.[100–104] Exuberant growth of Candida is supported in TPN solutions utilizing casein hydrolysates compared with synthetic amino acids.[105,106]

Organisms may be introduced into the infusion system by nonsterile manipulations while adding medications to the bag or bottle, injecting medication into the tubing, using devices in the line, changing administration tubings, withdrawing blood samples, declotting occluded lumens, or with influx of unfiltered air and through hairline cracks in bottles.[89,91,107–115] When additives are made on the patient wards, in-use contamination of infusion fluid may exceed 30 percent.[114] High contamination levels have been found with the use of stopcocks:[115,116] 55 percent of side ports were shown to be contaminated,[117] and a 22 percent contamination rate was documented with CVP measurements.[118] Stiges-Serra et al.[119–121] and Linares et al.[122] in a series of studies found that contamination of the catheter hub was the most common portal of entry for bacteria causing catheter-related sepsis, particularly Staphylococcus epidermidis. Two other studies demonstrated that breaks in aseptic technique when manipulating central lines[123] or solution leaking at the catheter hub[124] resulted in Staphylococcus epidermidis septicemia.

Hematogenous seeding of the catheter has been well documented[73,125–132] as a cause of secondary catheter sepsis and can occur when a distant foci is a primary source of sepsis or transient bacteremia.

Catheter sepsis is a result of bacterial and/or fungal attachment and proliferation in the fibrin sheath[133] surrounding the catheter. Good correlation of catheter sepsis and thrombus formation has been demonstrated,[134] and microscopic examinations have revealed organisms deep within the thrombus.[81,135,136] Scanning electron microscopy demonstrates that intravenous cannulae in situ become coated with a cellular fibrinous matrix that appears to accumulate with time. Clusters of bacteria could be seen within this matrix.

Catheter colonization can also occur without fibrin sheath formation by (1) adherence of hydrophobic bacteria (*Staph. aureus, Serratia marcescens, Klebsiella pneumoniae*) to liquid hydrocarbons in the catheter material[138] and (2) attachment of coagulase negative staphylococci by lodgement in surface irregularities, slime layer production, or by "foot processes" that project from the bacterial cell wall to the catheter surface in single or multiple linear configurations.[139] *Pseudomonas aeruginosa* also produce slime or exopolysaccharides that allow for attachment. This glycocalyx or matrix material protects the organisms from antibiotic penetration. These findings have been observed in both plastic[81,137–139] and Silastic catheters.[140]

Detection

Because of the multitude of variables involved in the pathogenesis of catheter sepsis, determination of its origin is exceptionally difficult. Many researchers designate multiple determinates in the definition of catheter-related septicemia, but most define it as a positive growth of organisms on the catheter tip with concordant organism growth in the blood. Diagnosis of central venous catheter sepsis may be evaluated on three levels: clinical, qualitative bacteriologic, and semiquantitative or quantitative bacteriologic.[141]

Clinical diagnosis relies on defervescence of fever and/or chills following removal or exchange of the catheter. Unless the catheter is no longer needed, this method is disadvantageous since a high percentage (75–85 percent) of catheters are falsely removed[6,25,132,141,142] and new venipuncture is required.

The qualitative approach depends on identification of microorganisms on the catheter tip with the same organisms in the blood. Broth cultures of the catheter tip demonstrate the presence of microorganisms but not the quantity. Colonization, therefore, cannot be differentiated from infection. Peripheral blood cultures are reported to have the predictive positive value of 36–38 percent.[143,144] The addition of blood cultured from catheter aspiration increases this value to only 46 percent.

The third method, semiquantitative or quantitative bacteriologic, allows for differentiation between colonization and infection. The semiquantitative method described by Maki et al.[145] is accomplished by sterilely rolling the subcutaneous and/or tip segment of the removed catheter on the surface of a blood agar plate (Fig. 6-16). Fifteen or more colony-forming units are defined as an infection. The quantitative method[146,147] is performed by inserting a needle to the proximal end of the extracted segment, immersing it into 2–10 ml of trypticase soy broth, and flushing 3 times. The broth is then diluted and streaked on blood agar.

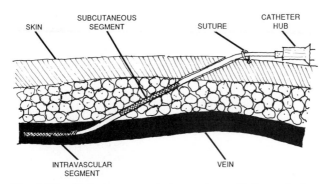

Fig. 6-16. Catheter segments for semi-quantitative culturing.

Infection is defined as the presence of 1000 or more colony-forming units. The quantitative method may also be used for blood culturing. Raucher et al.[147] described higher colony counts of blood drawn from the catheter than peripheral blood with this method. He also concluded that inability to withdraw blood through the catheter may be a sign of increased susceptibility to catheter infection. Cooper and Hopkins[148] identified a rapid, inexpensive method of culturing the catheter by gram staining and examining the catheter in oil immersion fields under the microscope.

Treatment

Options in the management of catheter sepsis include removal of the catheter, which usually controls the infection, or exchange of the catheter over a guidewire. Removal of the catheter may be a major disadvantage in the critically ill when lack of venous access and exaggerated risks due to respiratory failure and clotting disorders exist. Recent evidence indicates that prompt exchange of the catheter over a guidewire can eradicate sepsis and significantly reduce the risk of new catheter insertion.[18-21] Appropriate culturing of the catheter can be accomplished and additional therapy determined if needed. Intravenous low-dose heparin administration has been advocated for prevention of sepsis[149-151] despite conflicting reports that it will not affect fibrin sleeve formation.[152,153] Antibiotic prophylaxis at the time of catheter insertion does not appear to reduce the incidence of TPN-related sepsis.[154] Antibiotic therapy may be indicated with persistent positive blood cultures. *Candida* infections are of major concern because once the organism is within the intravascular compartment, it may disseminate to virtually any organ (kidney, brain, eye, bone, skin, heart, lungs, spleen, liver, or skeletal muscle). Diagnosis of disseminated candidiasis is difficult and has a mortality rate of 50 percent.[155] Amphotericin B is the therapeutic agent of choice, and more recent data indicate that treatment should be aggressive following catheter removal.[135,155-157] Focal infections may also occur from dissemination of bacteria as well as yeasts (Fig. 6-17).

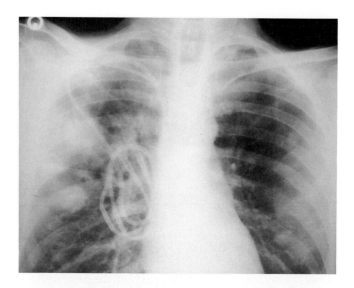

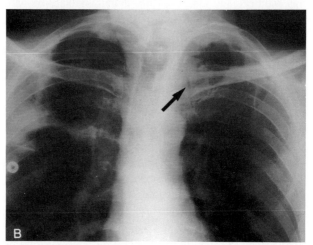

Fig. 6-17. *Staph. aureus* pneumonia and osteomyelitis of the left clavicular head secondary to indwelling catheter tunnel infection and catheter septicemia. (A) The catheter was removed, antibiotic therapy instituted, and surgical removal of the clavicular head performed. (arrow) (B)

Venous Thrombosis

Originally it was postulated that thrombosis would not exist as a complication of central venous catheterization because of the high flow rate and large caliber of the central veins. This has been disproven, however, and 3 types of clot formation have been identified: fibrin sleeve formation, mural thrombosis, and occlusive thrombosis. A review of a published series by Lindblad[158]

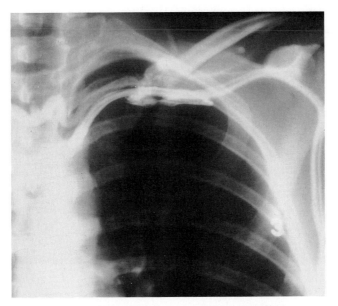

Fig. 6-18. Indwelling catheter tip improperly positioned in the subclavian vein. This venogram demonstrates thrombosis and fibrin sheath formation resulting in retrograde flow within the sheath to collateral circulation. The patient presented with left shoulder and back pain.

indicates that fibrin sleeve formation exists in 80 percent of patients investigated, and mural or occlusive thrombosis in 19 percent. More recent prospective studies have reported catheter-related thrombosis of the subclavian vein and the superior vena cava in 20–40 percent of all patients.[159–161]

The fibrin sleeve tends to originate at the point of venipuncture and from there propagates downward to the tip encasing the catheter. The fibrin formation can also develop on the tip or in sections along the catheter at points of contact with the vein wall. Fibrin sleeve formation may result in continued deposition of platelets and fibrin if other predisposing factors of thrombosis are present (Figs. 6-18 and 6-19).

The first step in the coagulation cascade is the deposition and adherence of platelets. The platelet has been likened to a sponge and is said to carry many of the coagulation factors absorbed on its surface and additional platelet factors within its body. Once the platelets adhere, they contract and become depleted of their intracellular granules, forming a release reaction that in turn results in further aggregation of platelets and formation of a platelet plug. Fibrin is then laid down and a coagulum of red and white cells resect as the thrombus takes form.[77]

Platelet adherence varies with catheter materials. A 1985 study by Borow and Crowley[77] compared thrombogenicity of several catheter materials including silicone, polyvinylchloride, polyurethane, and hydromer-coated polyure-

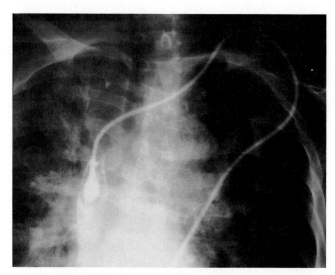

Fig. 6-19. This venogram identifies a large fibrin clot at the tip of an indwelling catheter in the superior vena cava. Flow in the SVC is severely reduced. The patient presented with right ear and neck pain.

thane. A wide range of thrombogenicity was noted, with the most thrombogenic being polyurethane and the least thrombogenic the hydromer-coated polyurethane. The next least thrombogenic catheter was silicone. In the Wolfe et al.[19] study of TPN complications, the hydromer-coated catheter was used for 2 years with no incidence of clinical thrombosis. A 1984 study by Linder et al.[162] found that the incidence of clinical thrombophlebitis and platelet adherence was higher in the silicone catheter than the polyurethane. It should be noted that in this study both catheters were of equal stiffness. They, as well as others,[159,163–166] have found a correlation between stiffness and thrombus formation: the stiffer the catheter, the higher the risk of thrombus formation. The soft, flexible catheters satisfy the "flotation principle" and avoid traumatic contact with the vein endothelium.

Thrombus formation may occur within 24 hours of insertion.[167] Duration of catheterization appears to increase thrombosis rates. This seems reasonable since the layers of the sleeve may continue to be laid down over a period of time until total occlusion occurs.[167–169]

Patients needing central venous access often have activated coagulation systems because of trauma or severe disease. This promotes the development of clot formation. A study by Imperial et al.[170] suggests that antithrombin III deficiency is prevalent among patients requiring TPN and that patients with malignancy, inflammatory bowel disease, and septicemia with concomitant antithrombin III deficiency are at high risk for developing catheter thrombosis.

Other factors affecting thrombus formation may include misplacement of the catheter in small tributaries of the central veins, infusion of hyperosmolar solutions into the subclavian vein, jugular vein, or vessels of smaller diameter, hypersensitivity reactions,[171,164] and repeated cannulations (Fig. 6-20).

Attempts to reduce thrombus formation have been made by heparin-coating the catheter. This has not proven to be effective. The coating process increases the stiffness of the catheter, which in turn increases pressure damage to the vein wall.[163,168] The addition of low dose heparin (1–2 IU/ml) to the infusion fluids has been found by some to reduce the incidence of fibrin sleeve formation,[169] thrombophlebitis, and catheter-associated sepsis,[172,173] whereas with others it has not been beneficial.[167,174] Studies where higher doses of heparin were administered have had better results with reduction of the occurrence of catheter-associated thrombosis.[160,170,175]

Fibrin sleeve formation usually goes undetected unless the entire catheter becomes encased and retrograde flow of infusing solutions drains out through the catheter insertion site. The clot at the tip of the catheter may allow infusion but no blood return on aspiration due to the "ball valve" effect of the clot suspended from the catheter tip. Other clues of thrombus formation may be increased resistance on flushing of the catheter, discomfort on flushing, and frequent triggering of the pump occlusion alarm. Clinical manifestations of total occlusion include edema of the neck, shoulder, and/or arm of the catheterized side, and possibly observable collateral circulation on the chest wall. Many occlusions go undetected clinically, but are discovered when attempts to recannulize the vein are unsuccessful or on autopsy.

One possible consequence of fibrin sleeve or thrombus formation is catheter sepsis since the clot provides a growth medium for microorganisms and may extend and suppurate.[176,177] Others include propagation of the clot with caval occlusion, inability to cannulate the vein for future access, chronic venous insufficiency, thrombotic valvular vegetation, catheter malfunction, and pulmonary embolism. A prospective study by Jeejeebhoy et al.[178] and Ahmed and Payne[179] found pulmonary emboli in 5 percent of patients receiving TPN. Ryan et al.[25] in their study of 200 patients found that 8 of 34 patients who died were noted at autopsy to have thrombosis of the superior vena cava and 3 had pulmonary emboli. These emboli may occur as a result of stripping of the clot on catheter removal or dislodgement of the clot by a guidewire. This can occur while the catheter is in place as well as days to weeks after catheter removal.

Usual treatment of thrombosis is removal of the catheter and heparin therapy. Heparin administration after a clot has been established is primarily done to prevent further propagation but may be ineffective in this regard.[180–182] Dissolving clots with thrombolytic therapy of either streptokinase or urokinase offers a noninvasive option for resolution of clot with minimal risk of bleeding.[183–186] Thrombolytic agents are effective in patients with relatively fresh clot, but less effective in organized thrombus.[187]

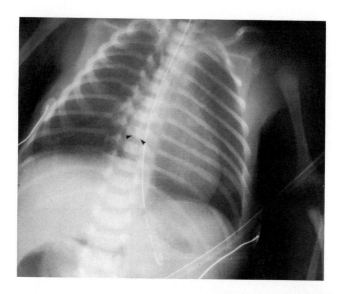

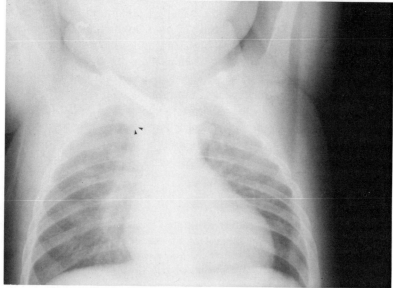

Fig. 6-20. (A) An infant Broviac® catheter inserted for TPN into the right internal jugular vein and exited behind the ear. The tip was placed into the right atrium. (B) Several months later the mother complained of frequent triggering of the pump occlusion alarm and resistance on catheter irrigation. The catheter had migrated out of the vein into the subcutaneous tissue behind the ear. Peripheral blood cultures were positive.

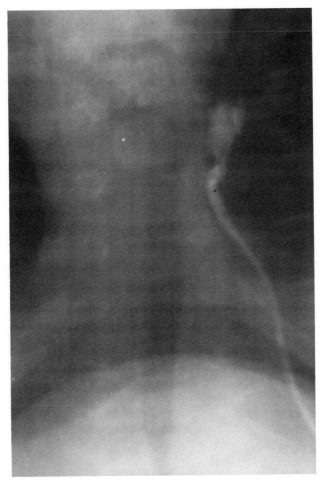

Figure 6-20 continued (C) A large fibrin clot had developed on the tip of the catheter. The catheter was removed and antibiotic therapy instituted.

Air Embolism

The complication of air embolism is possible (1) during catheter insertion (*see* Complications of Catheter Insertion); (2) as a result of a crack in the catheter hub; (3) with disconnection of catheter connections; (4) with run-drys of intravenous solutions; (5) with rupture of a silicone catheter,[188] or (6) after removal of the catheter. The precipitating factor is the development of a negative pressure gradient between the intrathoracic end of the catheter and the end open to the atmosphere. This potential is increased in dehydration, hypovolemia, and with the patient in an upright position.

A review of 24 patients by Kashuk and Penn[60] indicates that the mortality rate of air embolism in these patients was 50 percent. Among the survivors, 5 (42 percent) had neurologic damage.

Determination of the route of entry of bubbles into the arterial system is difficult, but the gas must pass either through an anatomic shunt (propatent foramen ovale) or through the pulmonary capillaries themselves. A patent foramen ovale is present in 20–25 percent of the population.[189] Usually it is clinically unimportant since higher left atrial pressures keep the foramen ovale closed. It does become significant when the pressures of the right atrium exceed those of the left, allowing air to pass from the venous to the arterial circulation. The primary function of the lungs is gas exchange. Its secondary function is that of a blood filter effective in trapping thrombi, platelet aggregates, and various emboli. Air in the right side of the heart churned into bubbles smaller than 10 μm can traverse the pulmonary vasculature. Although the lungs are normally superb bubble filters, certain conditions may facilitate the passage of venous bubbles through the pulmonary vasculature and into the arterial system. These include certain pharmacologic agents, namely aminophylline, oxygen toxicity, excessive volumes of gas,[190] intermittent positive pressure ventilation, and PEEP.[189] Arterial air is a serious threat if blood flow to vital organs is obstructed by air bubbles, especially the brain and heart. In humans the average lethal rate of injection has been calculated to be between 70–150 ml/sec.[61] As little as 100 ml of air forced rapidly into the venous system can be fatal[191,192] and 20 ml may be enough to harm a critically ill patient.[193] A 14-gauge needle with an internal diameter of .072 inches can transmit 100 ml of air per second. The time required to instill 200 ml of air is approximately 5 times greater through a catheter 25 cm long than through a 5-cm needle of the same bore.[61]

Early recognition and diagnosis is imperative since death can occur within minutes. The pathologic effects of venous air embolism depend on the site and rate of administration as well as body position when the emboli reach the heart. Characteristic symptoms include sudden cardiovascular collapse, increased venous pressure with concomitant drop in blood pressure, tachycardia, hypoxia, neurologic defects, and a loud "churning" or "mill wheel" murmur over the precordium which is caused by frothing of air bubbles at the pulmonic valve. Local hypoxia with pulmonary hypertension may predispose a fluid leak and pulmonary edema. Cardiac arrest and death occur due to obstruction of the pulmonary arterial outflow tract by air bubbles; consequently, reestablishment of an adequate cardiac output is of paramount importance. The patient should immediately be placed into a left lateral steep Trendelenburg position to decrease the amount of air entering the outflow tract of the right ventricle. Air may be aspirated through a catheter advanced into the heart or through a Swan-Ganz catheter while it is withdrawn from the pulmonary artery to the superior vena cava.[194] Percutaneous aspiration using a large spinal needle may also be attempted. External or internal cardiac massage is necessary if cardiac arrest occurs.

Air embolism can also occur along the subcutaneous track after removal of a central venous catheter.[60] The entrance site should be covered with an air occlusive dressing and left in place for 24 hours.

Air embolism is best treated prophylactically. Integrity of the system is of prime importance. Luer-lok connections and air-eliminating filters are strongly recommended since high morbidity and mortality rates are associated with this complication.

Cardiac Tamponade/Perforation of the Great Veins

Despite its rare occurrence, cardiac tamponade is the most lethal complication of central vein catheterization with a mortality rate between 78–95 percent.[195–197] A late diagnosis of the problem is the reason for the high mortality rate.

Several factors affect the potential for the occurrence of perforation and subsequent tamponade. These are catheter material, site of catheter insertion, and position of the catheter tip. Most cases of perforation occur with stiff catheters constructed of polyethylene or similar materials. There are recent reports, however, of tamponade with Silastic,[198–200] polyurethane,[200] and multilumen catheters.[199,201] Beveled or tapered tips facilitate tissue penetration, especially with the multilumen catheter. Catheters inserted into the basilic or cephalic vein can advance up to 10 cm in a proximal direction with abduction of the arm, rotation of the torso, or flexion of the elbow. Advancement of jugular or subclavian catheters is only 1–3 cm with neck or shoulder movement.

Probably the most important factor is the location of the tip. The length of the catheter should be measured during insertion so that the tip will lie at the right border of the manubrium, midway between the angle of Louis and right sternoclavicular joint. The tip of the catheter should be parallel to the wall of the vein and proximal to the pericardial shadow. If the catheter is positioned in the atrium or ventricle, perforation may occur rapidly, especially with a beveled tip. Cardiac or caval wall lesions may be gradual, with initial thrombus formation and adherence of the tip to the endocardium or vein wall. Horizontal orientation of the left brachiocephalic vein and its 90° angle with the superior vena cava may result in positioning of the catheter tip against the right lateral vein wall on left side insertions if the catheter is not advanced far enough. The constant motion of the cardiac and respiratory cycles creates endothelial injury, mural thrombi, and possible erosion and perforation.

Tamponade can occur within hours of insertion or days or weeks later. Clinical symptoms include retrosternal or epigastric pain, shortness of breath, venous engorgement of the face and neck, restlessness and confusion, hypotension, paradoxical pulse, muffled heart sounds with mediastinal widening, pleural effusions, or cardiac arrest. Cardiac tamponade is immediately treatable by discontinuation of the infusion, aspiration through the catheter, and/or performing pericardiocentesis. Treatment must be rapid and aggressive.

SUMMARY

The plethora of reports of catheter complications clearly indicate that even though complication rates may be and have been reduced, they are not totally eliminated. Since most of these increase morbidity and mortality, quality assurance mechanisms are necessary for identification of the complications and their rate of occurrence. This should form the basis for investigation and correction and instigate appropriate changes in policies and procedures.

ACKNOWLEDGMENT

The author wishes to express her gratitude to Steven Ryder for his support and for production of the illustrations.

REFERENCES

1. Kalso E: A short history of central venous catheterization. Acta Anaesth Scand 81(suppl):7–10, 1985
2. Gouin F, Martin C, Saux P: Central venous and pulmonary artery catheterizations via the axillary vein. Acta Anaesth Scand 81(suppl):27–29, 1985
3. Linder LE, Wojciechowski J, Zachrisson BF, et al: "Half-way" venous catheters. IV. Clinical experience and thrombogenicity. Acta Anaesth Scand 81(suppl):40–46, 1985
4. Sterner S, Plummer D, Clinton J, et al: A comparison of the supraclavicular approach and the infraclavicular approach for subclavian vein catheterization. Ann Emerg Med 15:421–424, 1986
5. Ross A, Anderson J, Walls A: Central venous catheterization. Ann R Coll Surg Engl 62:454–458, 1980
6. Padberg FT, Ruggiero J, Blackburn G, et al: Central venous catheterization for parenteral nutrition. Ann Surg 193:264–270, 1981
7. Kaiser WC, Koornick AR, Smith N, et al: Choice of route for central venous cannulation: Subclavian or internal jugular vein? A prospective randomized study. J Surg Onc 17:345–354, 1981
8. Jernigan WR, Gardner WC, Mahr MM, et al: Use of the internal jugular vein for placement of central venous catheter. Surg Gynecol Obstet 130:520–524, 1970
9. Khalil KG, Parker FB Jr, Mukherjee N, et al: Thoracic duct injury: A complication of jugular vein catheterization. JAMA 221:908–909, 1972
10. Bo-Linn G, Anderson D, Anderson K, et al: Percutaneous central venous catheterization performed by medical house officers: A prospective study. Cathet Cardiovasc Diagn 8:23–29, 1982
11. Pybus A, Poole J, Crawford M, et al: Subclavian venous catheterization in small children using the Seldinger technique. Anesthesia 37:451–453, 1982
12. Sznajder J, Zveibil F, Bitterman H: Central vein catheterization failure and complication rates by three percutaneous approaches. Arch Intern Med 146: 259–261, 1986
13. Meyers L: Intravenous catheterization. Am J Nurs 45:930–931, 1945
14. Zimmerman B: Intravenous tubing for parenteral therapy. Science 101:566–568, 1945

15. Brozenec S: Surgical implants: Medication and alimentation devices. AORN J 37(7):1353–1368, 1983
16. Technical Information Bulletin. Salt Lake City, UT, Catheter Technology Corporation, Aug 1, 1985
17. Seldinger S: Catheter replacement of the needle in percutaneous arteriography. Acta Radiol 39:368–376, 1953
18. Ryder M, Wolfe BM, Flynn N: Safety and efficacy of catheter exchange for replacement and/or evaluation of sepsis in central venous catheters. ASPEN Clinical Congress, Dallas, TX, February 1986
19. Wolfe BM, Ryder M, Nishikawa R, et al: Complications of parenteral nutrition. Am J Surg 152:93–99, 1986
20. Newsome H, Armstrong C, Mayhall G, et al: Mechanical complications from insertion of subclavian feeding catheters: Comparison of de novo percutaneous venipuncture to change of catheter over guidewire. JPEN 8(5):560–562, 1984
21. Bozzetti F, Terno G, Bonfanti G, et al: Prevention and treatment of central venous catheter sepsis by exchange via a guidewire: A prospective controlled trial. Ann Surg 198(1):48–52, 1983
22. Ryder M, Wolfe BM: Psychosocial limitations to home parenteral nutrition. Nutr Clin Prac 1(4):200–204, 1986
23. Maher J: A technique for the positioning of permanent central venous catheters in patients with thrombosis of the superior vena cava. Surg Gynecol Obstet 156:659–660, 1983
24. Oram-Smith JC, Mullen JL, Harken AH, et al: Direct right atrial catheterization for total parenteral nutrition. Surgery 83:274–276, 1978
25. Ryan JA, Abel RM, Abbott WM, et al: Catheter complications in total parenteral nutrition: A prospective study of two hundred consecutive patients. New Engl J Med 290:757–761, 1974
26. Nehme AE: Nutritional support of the hospitalized patient: The team concept. JAMA 243(19):1906–1908, 1980
27. Shildt RA, Slottman L, Rose M, et al: Organization of a nutrition support team at a medical center: One year's experience. Military Med 147:55–58, 1982
28. Keohane PP, Jones BJM, Attrill H, et al: Effect of catheter tunneling and a nutrition nurse on catheter sepsis during parenteral nutrition: A controlled trial. Lancet 2:1388–1390, 1983
29. Gilster SD: The impact of a team approach on catheter related infections. Nutr Supp Serv 5(4):22–24, 1985
30. Nelson D, Kien C, Mohr B, et al: Dressing changes by specialized personnel reduce infection rates in patients receiving central venous parenteral nutrition. JPEN 10(2):220–222, 1986
31. Faubion W, Wesley J, Khalidi N, et al: Total parenteral nutrition catheter sepsis: Impact of the team approach. JPEN 10(6):642–645, 1986
32. Schwartz-Fulton J, Colley R, Valanis B: Hyperalimentation dressing and skin flora. NITA 4:354–357, 1981
33. Copeland EM, MacFayden BV, Diudrick SJ: Prevention of microbial catheter contamination in patients receiving parenteral hyperalimentation. South Med J 67:303–306, 1974
34. Thomas MA: Opsite wound dressing for subclavian line care. JPEN 1:41A, 1977
35. Curtas S, Grant J: Evaluation of Opsite as a total parenteral nutrition dressing. NITA 4:414–415, 1981

36. Powell C, Regan C, Fabri P, et al: Evaluation of Opsite catheter dressings for parenteral nutrition: A prospective, randomized study. JPEN 6(1):43–46, 1982

37. Palidar P, Simonowitz D, Oreskovich M, et al: Use of Opsite as an occlusive dressing for total parenteral nutrition catheters. JPEN 6(2):150–151, 1982

38. Vasquez R, Jarrard M: Care of the central venous catheterization site: The use of a transparent polyurethane film. JPEN 8(2):181–186, 1984

39. Powell C, Traetow M, Fabri P: Opsite dressing study: A prospective randomized study evaluating Povidone iodine ointment and extension set changes with 7-day Opsite dressings applied to total parenteral nutrition subclavial sites. JPEN 9(3):443–446, 1985

40. Maki DG, Band J: Study of polyantibiotic and iodophor ointments in prevention of vascular catheter related infection. Abstract. Am J Med 70:739–744, 1981

41. Lawson M, Bottino J, Hurtubise M, et al: The use of urokinase to restore the patency of occluded central venous catheters. Am J IV Ther Clin Nutr 29–32, 1982

42. Delaplane D, Scott J, Riggs T, et al: Urokinase therapy for a catheter related right atrial thrombus. J Pediatr 100:149–151, 1982

43. Glynn M, Langer B, Jeejeebhoy K: Therapy for thrombotic occlusions of long-term intravenous alimentation catheters. JPEN 4:387–390, 1980

44. Hurtubise M, Bottino J, Lawson M, et al: Restoring patency of occluded central venous catheters. Arch Surg 115:212–213, 1980

45. Abbokinase®, Open-cath: Urokinase for catheter clearance. North Chicago, IL, Abbott Laboratories, July 1984

46. National Coordinating Committee on Large Volume Parenterals: Recommendations to pharmacists on solving problems with large volume parenterals. Am J Hosp Pharm 33:231, 1976

47. Baumgartner T, Schmidt G, Thakker K, et al: Bacterial endotoxin retention by inline intravenous filters. Am J Hosp Pharm 43:681, 1986

48. Holmes C, Kundsin R, Ausman R, et al: Potential hazards associated with microbial contamination of inline filters during intravenous therapy. J Clin Micro 12(6):725–731, 1980

49. Spielberg R, Martin J: Evaluation of the endotoxin/bacterial retention capabilities of IV filters during simulated extended infusions. Ref No. IV-1001, Aug 1985

50. Schmidt G, Baumgartner T, Thakker K, et al: Contaminated intravenous filters and their relative pyrogen retention after antibiotic administration. Presented at American Society for Nutrition Support Services Annual Meeting, Miami, FL, January 20, 1985

51. Rusmin S, DeLuca P: Effect of antibiotics and osmotic change on the release of endotoxin by bacterial remained on intravenous inline filters. Am J Hos Pharm 32:378–380, 1975

52. Harrigan C: Care and cost justification of final filtration. NITA 8:426–430, 1985

53. Rapp R, Bivins B: Cost effectiveness of inline filters in the era of DRG's. Infect Med 66, 1984

54. Rapp R, Bivins B: Particulate infusions: Local and systemic response? Clin Pharm 1:551–552, 1982

55. Jonas A: Potentially hazardous effects of introducing particulate matter into the vascular system of man and animals. Washington, DC: Proceedings of the FDA symposium on safety of large volume parenteral solutions, 1966

56. Sivak S: Late appearance of pneumothorax after subclavian venipuncture. Am J Med 80:323–324, 1986

57. Slezak F, Williams G: Delayed pneumothorax: A complication of subclavian vein catheterization. JPEN 8(5):571–574, 1984

58. Mattox K, Fisher R: Persistent hemothorax secondary to malposition of a subclavian venous catheter. J Trauma 17(5):387–388, 1977

59. Murray J, Allen P, Swan P: Isolated intrapulmonary hemorrhage anesthesia. 40:468–470, 1985

60. Kashuk JL, Penn I: Air embolism after central venous catheterization. Surg Gynecol Obstet 159:249–252, 1984

61. Ordway CB: Air embolism via CVP catheter without positive pressure. Ann Surg 179:479–481, 1973

62. Konichezky S, Saguib S, Soroker D: Tracheal puncture, a complication of percutaneous internal jugular vein cannulation. Anesthesia 38:572–574, 1983

63. Webb JG, Simmonds SD, Chan-Yan C: Central venous catheter malposition presenting as chest pain. Chest 89(2):309–311, 1986

64. Langston C: The aberrant central venous catheter and its complications. Diag Radiol 100:55–60, 1971

65. Vazquez RM, Brodski EG: Primary and secondary malposition of silicone central venous catheters. Acta Anaesth Scand 81(suppl):22–25, 1985

66. Schaefer CJ, Geelhoed GW: Redirection of misplaced central venous catheters. Arch Surg 115:789–791, 1980

67. Maki D: Preventing infection in intravenous therapy. Hosp Pract 11:95–104, 1976

68. Brachman PS, Eickhoff T (eds): Proceedings of the First International Conference on Nosocomial Infections (Center for Disease Control, August 3–6, 1970, Atlanta, GA). Chicago: Am Hosp Assoc 1–334, 1971

69. Maki DG: Sepsis arising from extrinsic contamination of the infusion and measures for control, in Phillips I, Meens P, D'Arcy P (eds): Microbiologic Hazards of Intravenous Therapy. Lancaster, England, MTP Press Ltd, 1978, pp 99–141

70. Maki DG: Epidemic nosocomial bacteremias, in Wenzel R (ed): Handbook on Hospital Acquired Infections. West Palm Beach, FL, CRC Press, Inc, 1981, pp 371–512

71. Henderson DK: Catheter acquired infection in total parenteral nutrition, in: Infection control during parenteral nutrition. ASPEN, 10th Clinical Congress, Dallas, TX, February 9, 1986:18–27

72. Bozzetti F, Terno G, Cameroni E, et al: Pathogenesis and predictability of central venous catheter sepsis. Surgery 9:383–389, 1982

73. Maki DG: Nosocomial bacteremia. Am J Med 70:719–732, 1981

74. Edwards J, Foos R, Montegomerie J, et al: Ocular manifestations of candida septicemia: Review of seventy-six cases of hematogenous candida endopathalmitis. Medicine 53:47–75, 1974

75. Seelig M: The role of antibiotics in the pathogenesis of candida infections. Am J Med 40:887–917, 1966

76. Maki DG: A semi-quantitative culture method for identification of catheter related infection in the burn patient. J Surg Res 22:513–520, 1977

77. Borow M, Crowley J: Evaluation of central venous catheter thrombosity. Acta Anesth Scand 81(suppl):59–64, 1985

78. Christensen G, Simpson W, Bisno A, et al: Adherence of slime producing strains of staphylococcus epidermidis to smooth surfaces. Infect Immun 37:318–326, 1982

79. Franson T, Sheth N, Rose H, et al: Scanning electron microscopy of bacteria adherent to intravascular catheters. J Clin Microbiol 20(3):500–505, 1984

80. Bayston R: A model of catheter colonization in vitro and its relationship to clinical catheter infections. J Infect 9:271–276, 1984

81. Cheesbrough JS, Elliott T, Finch R: A morphological study of bacterial colonization of intravenous cannulae. J Med Microbiol 19:149–157, 1985

82. Hoover P, DeSilva M: Sepsis related to multilumen intravascular catheters: A challenge for the infection control practitioner. Abstract, APIC, 12th Annual Ed. Conference, Cincinnati, OH, May 1985

83. Kelly C, Ligas J, Smith C: Sepsis due to triple lumen central venous catheters. Surg Gynecol Obstet 163(1):14–26, 1986

84. Pemberton L, Lyman B, Lander V, et al: Sepsis from triple vs. single lumen catheters during total parenteral nutrition in surgical or critically ill patients. Arch Surg 121:591–594, 1986

85. Pfeiffer J: Bacteremia outbreak linked to use of multilumen catheters. Hosp Inf Control 13:102–103, 1986

86. Pinilla J, Ross D, Martin T, et al: Study of the incidence of intravascular catheter infection and associated septicemia in critically ill patients. Crit Care Med 11(1):21–25, 1983

87. Samsoondar W, Freeman J, Coultish I: Colonization of intravascular catheters in the intensive care unit. Am J Surg 149:730–732, 1985

88. Sitzmann J, Townsend T, Siler M, et al: Septic and technical complications of central venous catheterization. A prospective study of 200 consecutive patients. Ann Surg 202(6):766–770, 1985

89. Arnold TR, Hepler CD: Bacterial contamination of intravenous fluids opened in unsterile air. Am J Hosp Pharm 28:614–619, 1971

90. Deeb EN, Natsios GA: Contamination of intravenous fluids by bacteria and fungi during preparations and administration. Am J Hosp Pharm 28:764–767, 1971

91. Miller WA, Smith GL, Latiolais CJ: A comparative evaluation of compounding costs and contamination rates of intravenous admixture systems. Drug Intell Clin Pharm 5:51–60, 1971

92. Wilmore DW, Dudrick SJ: An inline filter for intravenous solutions. Arch Surg 99:462–463, 1969

93. Duma RJ, Warner JF, Dalton HP: Septicemia from intravenous infusions. New Eng J Med 284:257–260, 1971

94. Boeckmann CR, Krill CE Jr: Bacterial and fungal infections complicating total parenteral alimentation in infants and in children. J Pediatr Surg 5:117–126, 1970

95. Brennan MF, O'Connell RC, Rosal JA, et al: The growth of Candida albicans in nutritive solutions given parenterally. Arch Surg 103:705–708, 1971

96. Freeman R, Lemire A, MacLean LD: Intravenous alimentation and septicemia. Surg Gynecol Obstet 135:708–712, 1972

97. Sanderson J, Deitsi M: Intravenous hyperalimentation without sepsis. Surg Gynecol Obstet 136:577–585, 1973

98. Shadomy S, Shadomy HJ: Growth of candida in casin hydrolysate solutions. New Eng J Med 286:612–613, 1972

99. Baggerman C: Microbial growth in infusion fluids. Pharmacy International 1:257–261, 1981

100. Maki DG: Growth properties of microorganisms in infusion fluid and methods of

detection, *in* Phillips I, Meers PD, D'Arcy PF (eds): Microbiologic Hazards of Intravenous Therapy. Lancaster, England, MTP Press Ltd, 1977, pp 13–47

101. Melly MA, Meng HC, Schaffner W: Microbial growth in lipid emulsions used in parenteral nutrition. Arch Surg 110:1479–1481, 1975

102. Deitel M, Kaminsky M, Fuksa M: Growth of common bacteria and candida albicans in 10 percent soybean oil emulsion. Can J Surg 18:531–535, 1975

103. Crocker KS, Noga R, Filibeck D, et al: Microbial growth comparisons of five commercial parenteral lipid emulsions. JPEN 8(4):391–395, 1984

104. Jarvis W, Highsmith A: Bacterial growth and endotoxin production in lipid emulsion. J Clin Microbiol 19(1):17–20, 1984

105. Gelbart SM, Reinhardt GF, Greenlee HB: Multiplication of nosocomial pathogens in intravenous feeding solutions. Appl Microbiol 26:874, 1973

106. Goldmann DA, Maki DG: Infection control in total parenteral nutrition. JAMA 223:1360–1364, 1973

107. Perceval AK: Contamination of parenteral solutions during administration. Med J Aust 2:954–956, 1966

108. Robertson MH: Fungi in fluids—a hazard of intravenous therapy. J Med Microbiol 3:99–102, 1970

109. Sack RA: Epidemic of gram-negative organism septicemia subsequent to elective operation. Am J Obstet Gynecol 107:394–399, 1970

110. Kundsin RB: Microbial hazards in the assembly of intravenous infusion, *in* Johnston IDA (ed): Advances in Parenteral Nutrition. Lancaster, England, MTP Press, Ltd, 1983, p 319

111. Syndman DR, Murray SA, Kornfeld SJ, et al: Total parenteral nutrition related infections, prospective epidemiologic study using semiquantitative methods. Am J Med 73:695–699, 1982

112. Schwartz-Fulton J, Valanis B: Sepsis related to intravenous and hyperalimentation catheters, a summary of recent research findings. NITA 4:248–255, 1981

113. Brismar B, Nyström B: Thrombophlebitis and septicemia—Complications related to intravascular devices and their prophylaxis. A review. Acta Chir Scand 530(suppl):73–77, 1986

114. Denyer SP, Blackburn JE, Worral AV, et al: In-use microbiological contamination of intravenous infusion fluids. J Pharmacol 227:419–425, 1981

115. McCarthur B, Hargiss C, Schoenknecht RD: Stopcock contamination in an ICU. Am J Nurs 75:96–97, 1975

116. Dryden GE, Brickler J: Stopcock contamination. Anesth Analg 58:141–142, 1979

117. Oberhammer EP: Contamination of injection ports on intravenous cannulae. Lancet 2:1027, 1980

118. Hoshal VL Jr: Intravenous catheters and infection. Surg Clin N Am 52:1407–1417, 1972

119. Sitges-Serra A, Puig P, Linares J, et al: Hub colonization as the initial step in an outbreak of catheter related sepsis due to coagulase negative staphylococci during parenteral nutrition. JPEN 8(6):668–672, 1984

120. Sitges-Serra A, Linares J, Garau J: Catheter sepsis: The clue is the hub. Surgery 97(3):355–357, 1985

121. Sitges-Serra A, Linares J, Perez J, et al: A randomized trial on the effect of tubing changes on hub contamination and catheter sepsis during parenteral nutrition. JPEN 9(3):322–325, 1985

122. Linares J, Sitges-Serra A, Garau J, et al: Pathogenesis of catheter sepsis: A prospective study with quantitative and semiquantitative cultures of catheter hub and segments. J Clin Microbiol 21(3):357–360, 1985

123. Forse RA, Dixon C, Bernard K, et al: Staphylococcus epidermidis: An important pathogen. Surgery 86:507–514, 1979

124. Deitel M, Krajden S, Saldanha CF, et al: An outbreak of staphylococcus epidermidis septicemia. JPEN 7:569–572, 1983

125. Colvin MP, Blogg CE, Savege TM: A safe long-term infusion technique? Lancet 2:317–320, 1972

126. Fleming RC, Witzke DJ, Beart RW Jr: Catheter related complications in patient receiving home parenteral nutrition. Ann Surg 192:593–599, 1980

127. Henzel JH, DeWeese MS: Morbid and mortal complications associated with prolonged central venous cannulation; awareness, recognition and prevention. Am J Surg 121:600–605, 1971

128. Jeejeebhoy KN, Langer B, Tsallas G, et al: Total parenteral nutrition at home: Studies in patients surviving four months to five years. Gastroenterology 71:943–954, 1976

129. Moncrief JA: Femoral catheters. Ann Surg 147:166–172, 1958

130. Mogensen JV, Fredericksen W, Jensen JK: Subclavian vein catheterization and infection: A bacteriologic study of 130 catheter insertions. Scand J Infect Dis 4:31–36, 1972

131. Bernard RW, Stahl WM, Chase RM Jr: Subclavian vein catheterization: A prospective study—II. Infectious complications. Ann Surg 173:191–200, 1971

132. Blackett RL, Bakran A, Bradley JA, et al: A prospective study of subclavian vein catheters used exclusively for the purpose of intravenous feeding. Br J Surg 65:393–395, 1978

133. Hoshal VL, Ause RG, Hoskins P: Fibrin sleeve formation on indwelling subclavian central venous catheters. Arch Surg 102:353–358, 1971

134. Stillman RM, Soliman F, Garcia L, et al: Etiology of catheter associated sepsis: Correlation with thrombogenicity. Arch Surg 112:1497–1499, 1977

135. Strindin W, Helgerson R, Maki DG: Candida septic thrombosis of the great central veins associated with central catheters. Ann Surg 202(5):653–658, 1985

136. Anderson AO, Yardley JH: Demonstration of candida in blood smears. N Engl J Med 286:108, 1972

137. Locci R, Peters G, Pulverer G: Microbial colonization of prosthetic devices. I. Microtopographical characteristics of intravenous catheters as detected by scanning electron microscopy. Zentralbl Bakteriol Mikrobiol Hyg [B] 173:285–292, 1981

138. Ashkenazi S, Weiss E, Drucker M: Bacterial adherence to intravenous catheters and needles and its influence by cannula type and bacterial hydrophobility. J Lab Clin Med 107(2):138–140, 1986

139. Franson T, Sheth N, Rose H, et al: Scanning electron microscopy of bacteria adherent to intravascular catheters. J Clin Microbiol 20(4):500–505, 1984

140. Bayston R: A model of catheter colonization in vitro and its relationship to clinical catheter infections. J Infect 9:271–276, 1984

141. Bjornson HS, Colley RN, Bower RH, et al: Association between microorganism growth of the catheter insertion site and colonization of the catheter in patients receiving total parenteral nutrition. Surgery 92:720–727, 1982

142. Sanders R, Sheldon G: Septic complications of total parenteral nutrition: A five year experience. Am J Surg 132:214–219, 1976
143. Bozzetti TG, Terno G, Bonfanti G, et al: Blood culture as a guide for the diagnosis of central venous catheter sepsis. JPEN 8:396–398, 1984
144. Bozzetti F: Central venous catheter sepsis. Surg Gynecol Obstet 161:293–301, 1985
145. Maki DG, Weise C, Sarafin HW: A semiquantitative culture method for identifying intravenous catheter related infection. New Eng J Med 296:1305–1309, 1977
146. Cleri DJ, Corrado ML, Seligman SJ: Quantitative culture of intravenous catheters and other intravascular inserts. J Infect Dis 141:781–786, 1980
147. Raucher H, Harris M, Hodes D: Quantitative blood culture in the evaluation of septicemia in children with broviac catheters. J Pediatr 104(1):29–33, 1984
148. Cooper G, Hopkins C: Rapid diagnosis of intravascular associated infection by direct gram staining of catheter segments. New Eng J Med 312(18):1142–1148, 1985
149. Tanner WA, Delaney PV, Hennessy TP: The influence of heparin on intravenous infusions: A prospective study. Br J Surg 67:311–312, 1980
150. Bailey MI: Reduction of catheter associated sepsis in parenteral nutrition using low-dose intravenous heparin. Br Med J 1:1671–1673, 1979
151. Tanner WA, Delaney TP, Hennessy TP: The influence of heparin intravenous infusions: A prospective study. Br J Surg 67:311–312, 1980
152. Ruggiero RP, Aisenstein TJ: Central catheter fibrin sleeve: Heparin effect. JPEN 7:270–273, 1983
153. Brismar B, Malmborg A: Prophylaxis against microbial colonization of venous catheters. J Hosp Infect 2:37–43, 1981
154. McKee R, Dunsmuir R, Whitby M, et al: Does antibiotic prophylaxis at the time of catheter insertion reduce the incidence of catheter related sepsis in intravenous nutrition? J Hosp Infect 6:419–425, 1985
155. Edwards J: Disseminated candidosis. Infect Dis Newsletter 4:81–84, 1985
156. Henderson D, Edwards J, Montgomerie J: Hematogenous candida endopthalmitis in patients receiving parenteral hyperalimentation fluids. J Infect Dis 143(5): 655–661, 1981
157. Montgomerie J, Edwards J: Association of infection due to candida albicans with intravenous hyperalimentation. J Infect Dis 137(2):197–201, 1978
158. Lindblad B: Thromboemboli complications and central venous catheters. Lancet 2:936–937, 1982
159. Brismar B, Hardstedt C, Jacobson S: Diagnosis of thrombosis by catheter phlebography after prolonged central venous catheterization. Ann Surg 194:779, 1981
160. Fabri PJ, Mirtallo JM, Ruberg RL, et al: Incidence and prevention of thrombosis of the subclavian vein during total parenteral nutrition. Surg Gynecol Obstet 155: 238, 1982
161. Lokich JL, Becker B: Subclavian vein thrombosis in patients treated with infusion chemotherapy for advanced malignancy. Cancer 52:1586, 1983
162. Linder LE, Curelaru I, Gustavsson B, et al: Material thrombogenicity in central venous catheterization: A comparison between soft, antebrachial catheters of silicone elastomer and polyurethane. JPEN 8(4):399–406, 1984

163. Hoar P, Stone G, Wicks A, et al: Thrombogenesis associated with Swan-Ganz catheters. Anesthesiology 48:445–447, 1978
164. Stephens WP, Lawler W: Thrombus formation and central venous catheters. Lancet 2:664–665, 1982
165. Ratcliffe PJ, Oliver DO: Massive thrombosis around subclavian cannulas used for haemodialysis. Lancet i:1472–1473, 1982
166. Welch GW, McKeel DW Jr, Silverstein P, et al: The role of catheter composition in the development of thrombophlebitis. Surg Gynecol Obstet 138:421–424, 1974
167. Hoshal VL, Ause RG, Hoskins PA, et al: Fibrin sleeve formation on indwelling subclavian central venous catheters. Arch Surg 102:253, 1971
168. Peters WR, Bush WH, McIntyre RD, et al: The development of fibrin sheath on indwelling venous catheters. Surg Gynecol Obstet 137:43–47, 1973
169. Ruggiero RP, Aisenstein TJ: Central catheter fibrin sleeve—heparin effect. JPEN 7(3):270–272, 1983
170. Imperial J, Bistrian BR, Bothe A, et al: Limitation of central vein thrombosis in total parenteral nutrition by continuous infusion of low-dose heparin. J Coll Nutr 2: 63–73, 1983
171. Freund H: Chemical phlebothrombosis. Arch Surg 116:1220–1221, 1981
172. Bailey MJ: Reduction of catheter associated sepsis in parenteral nutrition using low-dose intravenous heparin. Br Med J 1:1671–1673, 1979
173. Tanner WA, Delaney PV, Hennessy TP: The influence of heparin on intravenous infusions: A prospective study. Br J Surg 67:311–312, 1980
174. Bozzetti F, Scarpa D, Terno G, et al: Subclavian venous thrombosis due to indwelling catheters: A prospective study on 52 patients. JPEN 7(6):560–562, 1983
175. Brismar B, Hardstedt C, Jacobson S, et al: Reduction of catheter associated thrombosis in parenteral nutrition by intravenous heparin therapy. Arch Surg 117:1196–1199, 1982
176. Stein J, Pruitt B: Suppurative thrombophlebitis: A lethal iatrogenic disease. New Engl J Med 282:1452–1455, 1970
177. Munster A: Septic thrombophlebitis: A surgical disorder. JAMA 230(7):1010–1011, 1974
178. Jeejeebhoy KN, Langer B, Tsallas G, et al: Total parenteral nutrition at home: Studies in patient surviving four months to five years. Gastroenterology 71:943–953, 1976
179. Ahmed N, Payne RF: Thrombosis after central venous cannulation. Med J Aust 134:217–220, 1976
180. Chamorro H, Gopal R, Wholey MC: Superior vena cava syndrome: A complication of transvenous pacemaker implantation. Radiol 126:377–378, 1978
181. Dye LE, Sepoll PH, Russell R, et al: Deep venous thrombosis of the upper extremities associated with the use of the Swan-Ganz catheter. Chest 73:673–674, 1978
182. Ladefoged N, Stig T: Long term parenteral nutrition. Br Med J 2:262–266, 1978
183. Curnow A, Idowu J, Behrens E, et al: Urokinase therapy for silastic catheter induced intravascular thrombi in infants and children. Arch Surg 120:1237–1240, 1985

184. Kahn S, Goldstein J, Cope C: Low-dose streptokinase therapy for Swan-Ganz catheter indused thrombosis. Am Heart J 110(4):891–893, 1985
185. Smith N, Ravo B, Soroff H, et al: Successful fibrinolytic therapy for superior vena cava thrombosis secondary to long-term total parenteral nutrition. JPEN 9(1): 55–57, 1985
186. Rubenstein M, Creger W: Successful streptokinase therapy for catheter induced subclavian vein thrombosis. Arch Int Med 140:1370–1371, 1980
187. Rubin RN: Fibrinolysis and its current usage. Clin Ther 5:211, 1983
188. Haavik PE, Steen PA: Air embolism caused by rupture of a silicone central venous catheter. JPEN 8(5):579–580, 1984
189. Jacobsen WK, Briggs B, Mason L: Paradoxical air embolism associated with a central total parenteral nutrition catheter. Crit Care Med 11(5):388–389, 1983
190. Butler BV, Hills BA: Transpulmonary passage of venous air emboli. J Appl Physiol 59(2):543–547, 1985
191. Peters JL, Armstrong R: Air embolism occurring as a complication of central venous catheterization. Ann Surg 187:375–378, 1978
192. Munson ES, Paul WL, Perry JC, et al: Early detection of venous air embolism using Swan-Ganz catheter. Anesthesiology 42:223–226, 1975
193. James PM, Myers RT: Central venous monitoring, misinterpretation, abuses, indications and a new technique. Ann Surg 175:693–701, 1972
194. Marshall WK, Bedford RF: Use of a pulmonary artery catheter for detection and treatment of venous air embolism. Anesthesiology 52:131–134, 1980
195. Defalque RJ, Campbell C: Cardiac tamponade from central venous catheters. Anesthesiology 50:249, 1979
196. Eide J, Odelgaard E: Cardiac tamponade as a result of infusion therapy. A potentially amenable complication of central venous catheters. Acta Anesth Scand 27:181, 1983
197. Krog M, Berggren L, Brodin M, et al: Pericardial tamponade caused by central venous catheters. World J Surg 6:138, 1982
198. Harford FJ, Kleinsasser J: Fatal cardiac tamponade in a patient receiving total parenteral nutrition via a silastic central venous catheter. JPEN 8(4):443–446, 1984
199. Tocino I, Watanabe A: Impending catheter perforation of superior vena cava: Radiographic recognition. Am J Radiol 146:487–490, 1986
200. Suddleson EA: Cardiac tamponade: A complication of central venous hyperalimentation. JPEN 10(5):528–529, 1986
201. Maschke SP, Rogove HJ: Cardiac tamponade associated with a multilumen central venous catheter. Crit Care Med 12(7):611–613, 1984

Kathleen S. Crocker

7

Metabolic Monitoring During Nutritional Support Therapy

Routine laboratory monitoring and clinical assessment are required to ensure that nutritional support therapy is used in a safe and consistent manner. Although technical problems and infectious complications were encountered during the initial clinical use of nutritional support, metabolic complications were also described, which could result from the altering of metabolic events by parenteral and enteral nutrition therapy.

In 1972 Dudrick et al.[1] identified the metabolic complications associated with parenteral nutrition and suggested clinical approaches for their resolution and prevention. Ten years later, a study of 100 patients from a university hospital setting revealed that 63 percent of the patients who were parenterally fed developed at least one metabolic complication, while 29 percent of the patients developed more than one metabolic complication.[2]

Metabolic complications also have been reported during the use of enteral nutritional support. Azotemia as well as fluid and electrolyte imbalances such as hypernatremia and dehydration have been associated with the use of tube-feeding formulas that contain a high concentration of protein.[3–5] A 1981 study of 100 patients described the frequency of 11 metabolic complications that occurred during the use of tube-feeding formulas. At least 40 percent of the patients developed hyperkalemia while 29 percent developed at least one episode of hyperglycemia.[6]

The current availability of nutrient modules and disease-specific nutrients permits the clinical manipulation of metabolic events and further increases the possibility of metabolic complications during nutritional support therapy. The clinical (i.e., physical) assessment and monitoring of laboratory parameters are

NUTRITIONAL SUPPORT IN NURSING
ISBN 0-8089-1889-3

191

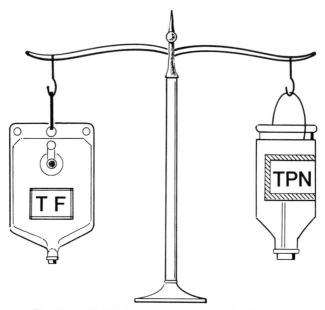

Fig. 7-1.   Metabolic complications can be the same.

the same regardless of whether parenteral or enteral nutrition is in use, as the metabolic complications that may occur are the same regardless of the route of delivery.

Nutrient administration should be considered in the same manner as medication administration. The nurse should understand the composition of each nutrient solution or formula administered to the patient, the expected metabolic response, and the potential complications of therapy. Such a knowledge base should enable the nurse to identify patients who are at risk for metabolic complications and to better monitor the patient's response to nutrient delivery. Finally, nursing guidelines should be established so that metabolic complications are either prevented or recognized and resolved by the appropriate member of the health care team.

NUTRIENT COMPOSITION

Enteral feedings via a nasogastric tube were first documented by the Egyptians in ancient times.[7] Attempts to deliver nutritional requirements via the parenteral route date back over 350 years. Parenteral nutritional support has been reviewed in detail by Cuthbertson[8] as well as in Chapter 1 of this text. Parenteral nutritional support as currently practiced had its origins in the 1930s when Elman demonstrated that lean body mass could be maintained using intravenous infusions of exogenous protein.[9]

Table 7-1
Variables of Nutrient Composition

Variable	Parenteral Solution	Enteral Formula
Derived source of nutrient	X	X
Intactness or complexity of nutrient	X	X
Nutrient bioavailability	X	X
Molecular form of each nutrient	X	X
Caloric density	X	X
Caloric distribution among macronutrients	X	X
pH of final composition	X	X
Osmolar effect of final composition	X	X
Digestibility		X
Viscosity		X
Residue		X
Palatability		X

Nutritional support solutions and formulas vary in composition. These variables are listed in Table 7-1. Despite the trend toward individualization of a solution's composition based on specific patient requirements, fixed or standardized formulations are still commonly used. For example, it is not uncommon to prescribe total parenteral nutrition (TPN) by liters, namely, 1 liter today, 2 liters tomorrow, and 3 liters on day three. Standard parenteral solutions of 25% dextrose and 4.25% amino acid/liter probably are used for the majority of hospitalized patients receiving TPN. Enteral formulas are supplied as ready-to-use liquids or dehydrated powders that require reconstitution. Ready-to-use enteral formulas are still the norm, although specific nutrient modules now allow manipulation of the composition of an enteral formula similar to that done with parenteral nutrition.[10]

The Macronutrients

Protein

Since the ultimate goal of nutritional support is nitrogen balance and preservation of lean body mass, the protein or nitrogen component of a parenteral solution or enteral formula is of major importance. During the 1930s Rose identified the essential amino acids and the ratios of each required for human protein synthesis.[11] Rose identified 8 essential amino acids: leucine, isoleucine, valine, phenylalanine, tryptophan, methionine, threonine, and lysine. Essential amino acids must be exogenously supplied because the body cannot produce them in sufficient quantities to meet anabolic needs. Cysteine and histidine have been found to be essential in infancy, while histidine and arginine have since been observed to be essential in chronic renal failure. The 9 nonessential amino acids—alanine, glutamine, tyrosine, aspartic acid, asparagine, glutamic acid, proline, serine, and glycine—can be produced endogenously as long as sufficient amounts of essential amino acids are present. Today's ability to manipulate the amino-acid structure of a solution, based on a desired organ response, is based on Rose's original study of renal failure patients.

Parenteral solutions. Historically the parenteral source of nitrogen was protein hydrolysates, which were derivatives of milk casein or beef blood fibrin. These formulations consisted of both di- and tripeptides as well as the D and L forms of free amino acids. The peptides required further degradation prior to their use in metabolic pathways. Although these initial solutions were inexpensive and proved clinically effective, their composition was basically fixed; that is, the proportions of the various amino acids and peptides could not be easily altered.

The manufacture of crystalline amino acids allowed the alteration of the proportion of each amino acid within a formulation.[12] Formulations of crystalline amino acids do not contain peptides. In contrast to the protein hydrolysates, crystalline amino acids are composed only of L-amino acids, the only amino-acid structure utilized by the human body.[13] When intravenous crystalline amino acids are used, nitrogen balance may be achieved using 0.5 g of protein equivalent per kg in the healthy adult, as compared with 0.8 g/kg when protein hydrolysates are used.[14]

As previously mentioned, the use of crystalline amino acids allows manipulation of the proportion and quantity of each amino acid within a parenteral formulation. This has resulted in the manufacture of solutions called *disease-specific* or *organ-specific*. Solutions containing only essential amino acids have been developed for patients in renal failure who are not being dialyzed,[15] while solutions containing high proportions of branched-chain amino acids are available for patients with hepatic encephalopathy.[16] The effect of amino-acid manipulation in septic or traumatized patients is the focus of current clinical investigation.[17]

Enteral formulas. A greater variety of protein sources are utilized for enteral formulas. Whole or intact protein is derived from eggs, milk, or meat. Protein isolates are derived from egg (lactalbumin), milk (casein), or soybean. Protein hydrolysates derived from casein, fish, meat, soy, or whey also contain mixed peptides. These large protein molecules must be digested into di- and tripeptides and amino acids before absorption across the gut lumen will occur. Defined peptides, namely, oligopeptides, di- and tripeptides, and L-crystalline amino acids, are absorbed as ingested and provide the nitrogen content of chemically defined or elemental formulas.[18]

Initially, protein absorption in the intestine was thought to occur only after macromolecular proteins were broken down into amino acids. Subsequent studies have shown that this is not the case. Di- and tripeptides are as easily and in some disease states more easily, absorbed than pure amino acids. The transport carrier system for di- and tripeptides seems to be independent of the transport carrier system for amino acids. This is particularly beneficial for patients with hereditary defects of amino-acid absorption (i.e., Hartnup disease, cystinuria). The affected amino acids of such diseases can be easily absorbed and transported when administered as oligopeptides instead of as crystalline amino acids.[19,20] This knowledge may be of benefit when dealing with the malnourished, hospitalized patient who has some degree of gastrointestinal (GI) dysfunction. For instance, when inflammatory disease alters the capacity of intestinal lumen absorption, there may be less damage to the oligopeptide transport system than to the amino-acid transport system. A more rapid and uniform absorption may occur if di- and tripeptides are used instead of crystalline amino acids.[18]

Carbohydrate

Parenteral solutions. Glucose is the most commonly used nonprotein source of energy in TPN solutions. Other carbohydrates such as fructose, xylitol, and sorbitol have been tried, but they too are eventually converted to glucose prior to their entry into metabolic pathways. Fructose not only is expensive but may cause a potentially fatal lactic acidosis, while xylitol is hepatotoxic.[21]

High concentrations of glucose are well-tolerated when infused via a central venous catheter. Daily intakes of 500–800 g/day can be achieved. A healthy adult can utilize 0.3–0.4 g of intravenous glucose per kg per hour.[22] As much as 1.2 g of intravenous glucose per kg have been administered without adverse reaction.[23] Glucose tolerance can be achieved in many patients when blood and urine glucose levels are closely monitored and exogenous insulin supplementation is provided as needed.

Enteral formulas. Carbohydrate is also the most common nonprotein source of energy used in commercially prepared enteral formulas. As much as 90 percent of an enteral formula may be carbohydrate. Only since the development of enteral nutrient modules can dependency on carbohydrate as the primary nonprotein source of energy be altered to any appreciable degree.

The type of carbohydrate used in the enteral formula will influence a patient's tolerance to the formula since carbohydrate molecules exert a strong osmotic effect. Large molecules of complex carbohydrates, called *polysaccharides*, such as starch, glycogen, and whole sugar, have a small influence on osmosis within the gut lumen. Simple sugars, called *monosaccharides*, such as glucose, fructose, and sucrose, greatly influence osmosis because of their small molecular size. In general, carbohydrates are hydrolyzed and absorbed directly at the brush border of the intestinal mucosa. Undigested simple sugar remaining in the intestinal lumen may enhance osmosis and cause an osmotic diarrhea.

Large molecular weight carbohydrates require the presence of pancreatic amylase for digestion and absorption. Smaller molecular weight carbohydrates, called *oligosaccharides*, are polymers of monosaccharides, consisting of 2–6 molecules of simple sugars. These do not require pancreatic amylase for digestion and absorption. Because absorption is not dependent on the presence of amylase, formulas containing oligosaccharides may be useful for patients with pancreatic insufficiency.[18]

Although the use of lactose increases the palatability of an enteral formula, most formulas are lactose-free. Many people are lactose-intolerant because of a deficiency of the enzyme lactase. Prior to absorption, lactose is broken down to the simple sugars, glucose and galactose. This does not occur unless sufficient amounts of lactase are present. Undigested lactose will exert an osmotic effect on the gut lumen causing diarrhea and other "dumping syndrome"-type symptoms.[24]

Sucrose has been used to enhance formula palatability but it too has limited usefulness because of its osmotic effect. Since large molecular weight starches are difficult to keep in suspension, smaller starch hydrolysates are used. These readily dissolve in water and influence osmosis to a lesser extent than the simple sugars.

Fat

The value of fat as a nutrient has been long recognized. As a nonprotein source of energy, fat has a high energy:weight ratio, yielding 9 kcal/g. Protein and carbohydrate yield only 4 kcal/g. Under certain metabolic conditions it is the preferred fuel utilized by the body. Fat is an essential nutrient, supplying the essential fatty acids needed to maintain the structural integrity of cellular membranes. Fatty acids also are necessary for the formation of prostaglandins.

Parenteral fat emulsions. An intravenous source of fat was first available in the 1920s.[12,25] Fat emulsions have a low osmotic pressure and can be administered peripherally without increased risk of thrombophlebitis. This led to an increased interest in their use as a source of energy for nutritional support since placement of a central venous catheter was not required for administration.

The initial use of fat emulsions in the United States met with little success. The cottonseed oil emulsion first available was not stable; the fat globules tended to coalesce, producing dangerously large particles within the body. Increased reports of fever, severe allergy-type symptoms, liver damage, and fat emboli caused the Federal Drug Administration to discontinue its use in 1954.[25] Further development of fat emulsions has been dependent on technical advances that allow mass manufacturing of a clinically safe emulsion. The components of the currently available fat emulsions mimic the particle size and biologic activity of naturally occurring chylomicrons and are safe for clinical use.

The fat emulsions best tolerated are those containing a base of either soybean or safflower oil. All contain the essential fatty acids—arachidonic, linoleic, and linolenic—but in different quantities. Arachidonic acid can be manufactured within the body if sufficient linoleic acid is supplied. The importance of linolenic acid remains somewhat unclear.[26] Both soybean and safflower oil contain a high percentage of linoleic acid, while soybean oil contains a higher percentage of linolenic acid. A source of linolenic acid is essential when fat emulsions are used in premature infants, who normally present with underdeveloped pathways for fat metabolism.[26]

All emulsions contain egg yolk phospholipids as the emulsifier. They also contain glycerol to increase the isotonicity of the product. Without the addition of glycerol, a fat emulsion is hypotonic. Fat emulsions currently are available as 10- and 20-percent emulsions, providing 1.1 and 2.0 kcal/ml, respectively.

A safflower oil-based fat emulsion was introduced into the United States during the 1970s. Its use initially met with some resistance, although the daily administration of a fat emulsion had characterized the European method of parenteral nutrition for many years. Used in small, intermittently delivered doses, fat emulsions initially were administered to treat essential fatty acid deficiencies in those patients chronically dependent on parenteral nutrition. The use of fat emulsions as a caloric source, providing 30–60 percent of daily nonprotein calories, is still a topic of controversy within the medical community, specifically, the value of fat as a sparer of protein. Conflicting studies promote or deny the ability of fat emulsions to enhance nitrogen balance when compared with the use of glucose as the sole energy source. This controversy in particular centers on the use of fat emulsions in the hypermetabolic patient, one originally thought not able to utilize fat as a fuel source.[27,28]

There is increasing evidence that the severe complications observed with the use of the cottonseed oil emulsions do not occur when soybean or safflower oil emulsions are used according to established guidelines. Since there are biologic differences among the currently available emulsions, it is important to guard against speaking of fat emulsions in general terms. The specific fat emulsion being used should be identified by name.

Enteral fat emulsions. The source of fat in most enteral formulas is long-chain triglycerides. These triglycerides are derived from corn-, sunflower-, soy-, or safflower-refined oils. The percentage of fat within the different formulas varies from less than 3 percent to as high as 50 percent. Unlike carbohydrate, fat is water-insoluble and does not affect osmotic pressure.

To digest and absorb long-chain triglycerides, pancreatic lipase and bile salts must be available. After hydrolysis, the long-chain triglycerides combine with proteins and phospholipids to form chylomicrons. These chylomicrons diffuse across the intestinal wall and enter the lymphatic circulation. Vessels of the lymphatic system drain into the thoracic duct, which in turn delivers lymph to the systemic circulation.

Of particular interest as an energy source are the medium-chain triglycerides. Because of a shorter chain length these particular triglycerides, under the influence of intestinal wall lipase, are absorbed passively across the intestinal brush border and are transported directly into the portal circulation. This process does not require the presence of pancreatic lipase or bile salts. Medium-chain triglycerides may be of value in those patients with pancreatic insufficiency or some degree of fat malabsorption.

Both long- and medium-chain triglycerides are metabolized to fatty acids and glycerol at the cellular level. Free fatty acids can be further metabolized to ketone bodies that may be utilized as a source of energy. Medium-chain triglycerides may be an effective source of fuel that can be utilized without the accompanying osmotic effect seen during the use of carbohydrate. The use of medium-chain triglycerides, however, does not satisfy the body's requirements for essential fatty acids. Essential fatty acid requirements must be met by other means if essential fatty acid deficiency is to be avoided.

The Micronutrients

Delivery of amino acids, carbohydrates, and fat will not result in anabolism and repletion of lean body mass unless electrolytes, vitamins, minerals, and trace elements are present in sufficient quantities. In addition, fluid requirements must be adequately assessed. Since fluid and electrolyte balance is affected by the use of carbohydrate- and protein-containing therapies, a discussion of fluid and electrolyte requirements is included in this section.

The requirements for micronutrients will differ depending on the route of administration. The daily requirements of specific micronutrients by administration route are listed in Table 7-2. The common sites of GI absorption of macro- and micronutrients are listed in Table 7-3. Use of the enteral route, unlike the parenteral route, must take into consideration the dietary form and bioavailability of each micronutrient, the absorptive capacity of the gut, and the recommended daily allowance. In the case of some micronutrients, for example, iron, intake may be high, but only a small percentage of what is ingested actually will be absorbed.

Guidelines for enteral micronutrient delivery are based on the Recommended Daily Allowances (RDA).[29] Guidelines for parenteral administration of trace elements are based on the recommendations of the American Medical Association.[30] These guidelines recommend the amount of micronutrients needed for maintenance, assuming that a deficiency does not exist. Additional supplementation must be provided when a deficiency does already exist. Wolman et al.,[31] for example, have recommended additional supplementation of zinc, the exact amount being dependent on daily fecal or fistula losses.

Table 7-2
Estimated Daily Maintenance Requirements of Selected Micronutrients

Micronutrient	Oral/Enteral	Parenteral
Sodium	50–150 mEq	1.4–2 mEq/kg or 50–250 mEq
Potassium	50–150 mEq	1.2–2.5 mEq/kg or 30–200 mEq
Chloride	—	50–250 mEq
Magnesium	300–350 mg	.35–.45 mEq/kg or 10–30 mEq
Calcium	800 mg	.2–.3 mEq/kg or 10–20 mEq
Phosphorus	800 mg	7–10 mmoles/1000 calories
Zinc	15 mg	4 mg
Copper	2–3 mg	22 μg
Chromium	—	20 μg
Manganese	2.5 mg	2.3 mg

Data From Recommended Daily Allowances. National Research Council, Food and Nutrition Board (ed 9). Washington DC, National Academy of Sciences, 1980, pp 137–165, p 178. Alpers DH, Clouse RE, Stenson WF: Manual of Nutritional Therapies. Boston, Little, Brown, 1983. Grant JP: Handbook of Total Parenteral Nutrition. Philadelphia, WB Saunders, 1980. With permission.

A complete review of micronutrients is beyond the scope of this chapter; however, those of particular concern will be emphasized. The reader is referred to Alpers et al.[32] for a detailed review of micronutrient requirements.

Fluid

The requirements for water are approximately 30 ml/kg/day or, on the average, 2–3 liter/day for an adult. A 1:1 ratio of ml:kcal also has been used to estimate daily fluid needs during nutritional support. Many patients who require nutritional support also require fluid restriction or aggressive fluid repletion.

Patients who have been ill prior to hospitalization may be severely dehydrated. Fluid and electrolyte balance often must be reestablished prior to the initiation or intensification of nutritional support. Other patients who have chronic liver or renal dysfunction may present with generalized anasarca due to their underlying disease and hypoalbuminemia. An aggressive refeeding schedule for these patients may result in fluid mobilization that may precipitate pulmonary edema and congestive heart failure.

Because calorically dense solutions of 2–3 cal/ml can be formulated, there is an increased potential for dehydration. Fluid balance must be closely monitored since free water administration has been restricted. Calorically dense solutions are of particular value when feeding the critically ill patient. Very often other fluid-intense therapies compete with the nutritional support solution for a share of the patient's daily fluid allotment. On more than one occasion in an intensive care setting, nutritional support has been discontinued or not even begun because of the need for severe fluid restriction.

Table 7-3
Gastrointestinal Sites of Macro- and Micronutrient Absorption

Duodenum	Jejunum	Entire Jejunum and Ileum	Ileum
Vitamin A	*Proximal*	Vitamin D	*Proximal*
Vitamin B12	Vitamin A	Vitamin E	Vitamin K
Iron	Vitamin B	Vitamin K	Disaccharides
Calcium	Folic Acid	Vitamin B1	*Distal*
Zinc	Iron	Vitamin B2	Vitamin B12
Glycerol	Zinc	Vitamin B3	Intrinsic Factor
Fatty Acid	Disaccharides	Vitamin B6	*Entire Length*
Monoglycerides	*Distal*	Iodine	Chloride
Amino Acids	Disaccharides	Calcium	Sodium
Monosaccharides	Dipeptides	Magnesium	
Disaccharides	*Entire Length*	Phosphorus	
	Folic Acid		
	Biotin		
	Copper		
	Zinc		
	Panthothenic Acid		
	Potassium		
	Ascorbic Acid		
	Glucose		
	Galactose		
	Glycerol		
	Fatty Acids		
	Monoglycerides		
	Amino Acids		

Electrolytes

Potassium is the most abundant intracellular ion, the vast majority of which is found within muscle cells.[33] The conversion from catabolism to anabolism requires potassium supplementation, since this ion is needed for glucose uptake, cellular glycogen synthesis, and protein synthesis. Provision of nutritional support without potassium supplementation will result in hypokalemia as extracellular potassium moves into the cell.

Serum levels of potassium are used to evaluate the adequacy of intake versus output. However, serum potassium is influenced by shifts in acid-base balance. Acidosis is accompanied by hyperkalemia. The transfer of hydrogen ions into the cell, with a temporary transfer of potassium ions into the extracellular fluid, is a normal compensatory mechanism. Urinary excretion of excess potassium will occur. Quick attempts at correcting the acidosis may result in a rebound hypokalemia.[33] For example, patients receiving ventilatory assistance may develop a respiratory acidosis that may be improved by adjusting the settings on the ventilator. If the acidosis is resolved in this manner, hypokalemia may occur unless frequent potassium blood levels are monitored and potassium supplementation provided accordingly.

Since potassium is primarily found in muscle, an increase in potassium uptake will reflect increased protein synthesis. Serial determination of total body potassium or balance studies based on 24-hour urine collections are often used to monitor the effectiveness of nutritional support. Grant suggested that serum potassium levels be maintained within a high normal range since a potassium:nitrogen ratio of 3.5:1 has been shown to be beneficial for optimal protein synthesis.[34]

Sodium is predominantly an extracellular ion. Of total body sodium, 80 percent is available for utilization. Serum sodium levels usually are not altered because of nutritional support therapy. Sodium supplementation may be required if sodium loss exists, as with increased GI output. Sodium restriction may be necessary when renal dysfunction or cardiac disease is present. The kidneys easily can reabsorb or excrete considerable amounts of sodium as needed. Consequently, if renal function is normal, a spot urine collection for sodium is an appropriate clinical marker of sodium homeostasis. A change in the serum sodium value usually indicates fluid overload or dehydration rather than an increase or decrease in the extracellular sodium content. For example, hypernatremia can be corrected by supplementing fluid intake, while hyponatremia can be corrected by restricting fluids.

Chloride is important in the maintenance of plasma tonicity, acid base regulation, and fluid volume. The concentration of chloride as well as the concentration of bicarbonate determines the osmotic pressure of extracellular fluid. Approximately 100 of the 300 mosm/liter are contributed by chloride. Because chloride is involved in so many metabolic events, a change in its concentration may not be a result of nutritional support therapy. A common reason for chloride loss is loss of gastric secretions. Loss of hydrochloric acid causes a hypochloremic alkalosis. Hyperchloremia may also be a feature of renal failure, as renal tubular acidosis causes excessive chloride reabsorption.[33]

Since the majority of calcium is present in bone, one would not expect changes in daily requirements during either protein breakdown or synthesis. Assessment of calcium status cannot be based solely on the observation of serum levels. Circulating calcium is bound to albumin; therefore, the presence of hypoalbunemia results in a falsely low serum calcium value. Measurement of ionized calcium is a more accurate parameter. Nomograms for correcting serum calcium values based on serum albumin or total protein are available.[34,36] Hypercalcemia is commonly seen in patients with bony metastases. Restriction of calcium and vitamin D may be required.

Bone pain and fractures have been reported in patients receiving long-term TPN therapy despite improvement in their nutritional status. The effects of continuously administering nutrients parenterally are largely unknown but appear to be associated with alterations of bone and mineral homeostasis. Hypercalciuria, hyperphosphatemia, low serum levels of 1,25-dihydroxy vitamin D and low levels of parathyroid hormone have been noted, but their cause remains unknown.[35]

Phosphorus is required for the maintenance of erythrocyte 2,3-diphosphoglycerate (2,3-DPG), which is needed to maintain a normal oxygen:hemoglobin ratio. Without it, a hemoglobin molecule will hold on to its oxygen and not release it to the cell. Hemolytic anemia and hemolysis may result. Phosphorus is also required for phagocytosis, bacterial killing, and calcium homeostasis.[37] The clinical implications of hypophosphatemia are of concern in a malnourished patient at risk for hypoxia or sepsis.

The most common cause of hypophosphotemia is the lack of supplementation during nutritional support. Parenteral solutions as well as enteral formulas inherently contain very little phosphorus. Since phosphorus enters the cell during glucose uptake, conversion to anabolism will increase the need for phosphorus supplementation. Phosphorus requirements also rise when exogenous insulin is used, again because of its relation to glucose utilization.[6] Hypophosphatemia during nutritional support has been implicated in the deaths of several patients.[38] Since phosphorus reabsorption and excretion are controlled by the kidneys, phosphorus intake is restricted when renal failure is present. Correction of renal failure without a concurrent increase in phosphorus supplementation may result in a rebound hypophosphatemia.

After potassium, magnesium is the next most abundant intracellular ion. Inside the cell, magnesium is bound to protein and is utilized in such activities as mitochondrial integrity and enzyme activation.[39] Serum magnesium levels accurately reflect body stores. Patients with excessive GI losses such as diarrhea and fistula drainage will require magnesium supplementation, while patients with renal failure will require restriction.

Trace Elements

The study of trace elements and their relation to nutritional support is still in its infancy. Trace element deficiencies during nutritional support therapy usually are a result of a lack of supplementation, as base solutions of carbohydrate, protein, and fat do not contain adequate quantities. The trace elements of concern during nutritional support are listed in Table 7-4.

Zinc deficiency is one of the most frequently reported trace element deficiencies associated with nutritional support. Zinc is a component of many enzymes and necessary for protein synthesis. A deficiency will present as a scaly, pustular rash around the nose and mouth that can spread over the entire body. Alopecia is also present. Over 90 percent of zinc excretion occurs via the GI tract. Excessive diarrheal losses can precipitate a deficiency state if associated with insufficient supplementation. As much as 15–30 mg/day may be required to maintain balance in patients with excessive diarrheal or fistula losses.[31] Clinical signs of zinc deficiency resolve in a matter of days once supplementation is implemented.

Chromium is important for normal glucose utilization. Its presence influences the sensitivity of peripheral tissues to the action of insulin.[34] Chromium deficiency with resultant glucose intolerance during prolonged TPN has been reported.[40]

Copper is a component of many enzymes such as ceruloplasmin. Copper status can be measured by copper or ceruloplasmin levels. A copper deficiency may present as an iron deficiency anemia. Copper is released into the circulation from hepatocytes and is excreted almost entirely in the bile. For patients with intra- or extrahepatic disturbances in biliary excretion, copper intake may require restriction.[41]

Selenium protects the cell from oxidant stress. It influences the fragility of red cells in the presence of an oxidizing agent. Several cases of selenium deficiency, some fatal, have been reported during prolonged TPN.[42] Irreversible cardiomyopathy has been well-documented in people living in agricultural areas with selenium-deficient soil, for example, Keshan disease in China. Clinically, selenium deficiency may present as limb pain during passive and active range of motion. This functional abnormality does reverse with selenium supplementation.

The body's store of iron can be measured by such tests as serum iron, total iron binding capacity, ferritin, and direct transferrin. Since iron is transported in plasma bound to transferrin, measurement of transferrin is a more accurate indicator of iron availability. Mathematical formulas based on body weight, hemoglobin concentration, and age are available for calculating total iron replacement.

Laboratory assays of trace element status are often expensive, difficult to obtain, and require a long turn-around time for results. Trace element-free needles, tubes, and containers are necessary because of the potential for environmental contamination. Serial trace element analysis of patients on chronic nutritional support and those at risk for deficiencies may be beneficial.

Vitamins

Vitamin requirements can be sufficiently provided via the parenteral or enteral route. Physiologic factors influencing the development of vitamin deficiencies may include exogenous supply, endogenous synthesis, function of enterohepatic circulation, storage capacity within various organs, increased utilization, or increased loss. Water-soluble vitamins are not stored by the body and must be administered daily. Healthy adults have large stores of fat-soluble vitamins, but those patients with chronic illnesses or malabsorption may have depleted their stores. The reader is referred to the review of Caldwell et al.[43] for an indepth discussion of this topic.

Table 7-4
Characteristics of Trace Elements

Trace Element	Function	Route of Excretion	Signs of Deficiency	Patients at Risk
Zinc	Growth & development Cell replication Component of metalloenzymes Protein synthesis Wound healing	Feces	Dermiitis (nasolabial folds, face, anogenital, heels, elbows, toes) Alopecia Anorexia Apathy, depression Taste changes	Cirrhotics Renal failure Inflammatory Bowel Disease Chronic Diarrhea Steroid Therapy Malnutrition Protein-losing syndromes
Copper	Formation of hemoglobin and red blood cells Iron metabolism Skeletal development	Hepatobiliary	Confusion Kinky hair Hair depigmentation Skin pallor Hypothermia Periorbital & pretibial edema Leukopenia, neutropenia, anemia Bone changes in infants	Chronic malnutrition Infants Biliary or intestinal fistula

Element	Function	Excretion	Deficiency Signs	Conditions
Chromium	Glucose utilization Insulin cofactor	Urine	Glucose intolerance Decreased respiratory quotient Weight loss Neurologic changes similar to peripheral neuropathy of diabetes	Prolonged NPO Glucose intolerance Elderly Increased insulin administration
Manganese	Enzyme systems (pyruvate carboxylase)	Bile	Not well documented Glucose intolerance Weight loss Retarded hair/nail growth Scaly dermititis Nausea and vomiting	
Selenium	Metallocofactor for glutathione peroxidase	Feces Urine	Cardiomyopathy Severe muscle pain and tenderness Changes in fingernails Increased liver function tests Increased red blood cells	Prolonged TPN

Summary

Manipulation of both macro- and micronutrients of both parenteral solutions and enteral formulas is possible. The individualization of a patient's particular nutrient requirements can be accomplished using fixed, standardized compounds, mixing additive modules to fixed solutions, compounding using individual nutrient modules exclusively, or by simple dilution of the solution or formula.

Initially, enteral formulas could be altered only by dilution. High levels of certain nutrients, sodium and potassium, for example, necessitated the discontinuance of enteral nutrition support in favor of parenteral nutrition support when the patient's condition required electrolyte restriction, as simple dilution resulted in a lower intake of calories and protein. In one study, as many as 42 percent of formula changes were occasioned by unacceptable electrolyte levels.[44] The use of enteral modular components has allowed the manipulation of enteral formulas in a manner similar to parenteral solutions.[10]

Those who prescribe and administer nutritional support should have access to a nutrient formulary. Each nutrient container should be labeled in detail. This label should state all contents, taking into consideration any nutrients inherent in the base solution as well as the final volume of the container. In particular, the electrolyte contents of nutritional support solutions and formulas should be acknowledged when serum electrolyte values are being evaluated. For example, as much as 80 mEq/liter of potassium can be found in frequently used enteral products. Several parenteral amino acid bases contain acetate and phosphorus. If this micronutrient intake is not considered unnecessary, supplementation of micronutrients may occur. This becomes a key for enteral formulas that may be repackaged in the dietary department prior to transport to the nursing unit. Particularly on enteral labels micronutrient content is not readily available.

The RDAs for vitamins and minerals are met when specific amounts of enteral formulas are used. A volume of 1.5–3 liters may be required to meet the RDA, depending on the enteral product in question. It may be necessary to supplement the patient with vitamins, minerals, and trace elements during the early stages of enteral feeding when diluted formulas are being used at low infusion rates. The manipulation of vitamins within parenteral solutions is also limited because multivitamin preparations are usually used. It may be difficult to omit just one particular vitamin from a solution. For example, if vitamin D is removed, a ready source of all other fat-soluble vitamins may not be available.

The use of nutritional support in the 1980s requires a high level of sophistication and understanding on the part of those prescribing, compounding, administering, and monitoring the use of this therapy. The nurse, who sees the patient on a daily basis, is a key member of the nutritional support team whose importance to patient care will only be enhanced by an increased knowledge of nutritional support theory.

Table 7-5
Metabolic Complications Commonly Associated with Nutrition Support

Macronutrients	Micronutrients
Carbohydrate: • Hyperglycemia • Hypoglycemia • Hyperglycemic, hyperosmolar, nonketotic dehydration • Fatty liver* • Hypercapnia* *Protein:* • Azotemia • Plasma amino acid imbalance *Fat:* • Poor plasma lipid clearance* • Hypertriglyceridemia* • Essential fatty acid deficiency*	*Fluid/electrolytes:* • Hyper/hypokalemia • Hyper/hyponatremia • Dehydration • Fluid overload • Hyper/hypomagnesemia • Hyper/hypophosphatemia • Acid-base imbalance* • Hyper/hypocalcemia *Trace Elements:* • Deficiencies: Zinc, Copper, Chromium,* Iron, Manganese,* Selenium* *Vitamins:* • Deficiency or toxicity • Altered clotting factors • Warfarin™ resistance†

*Only reported to occur during parenteral nutrition.
†Only reported to occur during enteral nutrition.

METABOLIC COMPLICATIONS

The metabolic complications frequently observed during administration of nutritional support therapy are listed in Table 7-5. Although each nutrient exerts a metabolic effect, only those most frequently seen are detailed in the following section. Further information on these complications is outlined in Table 7-6. Since many of the metabolic complications observed involve changes in the osmotic homeostasis of cellular compartments, a brief review of osmosis is presented.

Nutrient Composition and Osmosis

Cellular life normally occurs within a fixed osmolar range, 270–300 mosm/liter. Water moves across the semipermeable membrane of the cell from a dilute solution to a solution of higher concentration in order to maintain an iso-osmolar environment. This osmotic pull maintains fluid balance between the intracellular and extracellular compartments; changes in one compartment will automatically affect the other compartment. Plasma osmolality is maintained at the expense of all other fluid compartments. The majority of fluid derangements

Table 7-6
Metabolic Complications Related to Nutrition Support

Hyperglycemia	HHNC	Hypoglycemia	Hypercapnia	Hepatic Dysfunction (Fatty Liver)	Hypertri-glyceridemia
Causes: • Lack of monitoring of blood and urine sugar levels. • Lack of monitoring during initial refeeding. • Poor infusion control. • Inadequate exogenous insulin supplementation. • Lack of identification of patients at risk. • Development of infection or sepsis in a patient previously glucose-tolerant. *Prevention:* • Identification of patients at risk: those with sepsis, diabetes, hyper-metabolism, renal or pancreatic insuffi-ciency, elderly, those	*Symptoms:* • Hyperglycemia (blood glucose greater than 500 mg%/dl). • Glycosuria. • Serum osmolarity greater than 350 mOsm/l. • Clinical and labora-tory signs of dehydra-tion: negative fluid balance; weight loss; clouded sensorium, nausea, headache; thirst, poor skin turgor, sunken eye-balls; hypernatremia, azotemia, metabolic acidosis; late signs include hypotension, convulsions, coma. *Causes:* • Lack of identification of patients at risk. • Failure to respond to	*Symptoms:* • Posterior occipital headaches. • Tingling sensations of extremities and mouth. • Cold, clammy skin. • Thirst, dizziness, rapid pulse. • Blood sugar below 60 mg%/dl. *Causes:* • Abrupt cessation of TPN infusion. • Failure to reinsert clogged feeding tube and resume enteral nutrition delivery in patient who has re-ceived exogenous insulin. • Failure to monitor correction of recent glucose intolerance. • Overzealous	*Symptoms:* • Increased oxygen consumption. • Increased carbon dioxide production. • Measured respiratory quotient of 1.0 or greater. • Increased minute ventilation. *Causes:* • Use of high carbohy-drate nutrition solu-tions in ventilator-dependent patients. • Overestimation of nutritional requirements. *Prevention:* • Identify patients at risk (ventilator-dependent). • Monitor respiratory status during refeeding.	*Symptoms:* • Elevations in SGPT, SGOT, LDH, (less often) bilirubin. • Upper abdominal pain. • Jaundice. • Coma (late). *Causes:* • Excessive caloric intake. • Excessive reliance on glucose calories. • Inappropriate calorie:protein ratio. • Essential fatty acid deficiency. • Immature or inefficient hepatic metabolic pathways (neonates). • Toxicity of compo-nents within TPN solutions (sodium bisulfite, degraded	*Symptoms:* • Serum triglycer-ides greater than 200 mg/dl. • Appearance of milky (lipemic) serum during blood sampling. *Causes:* • Excessive delivery of intravenous fat emulsions. • Lack of monitor-ing of serum triglycerides. *Prevention:* • Obtain baseline serum triglyceride prior to first dose of intravenous fat emulsion. • Monitor serum triglyceride levels at least twice weekly during

receiving medications known to cause glucose intolerance, i.e., steroids.
- Clinical and laboratory monitoring: blood sugars, urine for sugar and acetone q6h, daily weights, intake and output records, calculation of fluid balance, check for clinical signs of dehydration.
- Continuous infusion control.
- Gradual increase of formula rates based on established patient tolerance.
- Use of short-acting insulin in adequate amounts to keep blood sugar below 150 mg%/dl.
- Provision of a percent of daily nonprotein calories as fat.

persistent hyperglycemia, increased serum osmolality, glycosuria, and fluid loss.
- Inadequate exogenous insulin supplementation.
- Inadequate replacement of fluid volume.
- Inconsistent infusion control.

Prevention:
- See comments under Hyperglycemia Prevention.

Treatment:
- Stop nutrition support therapy.
- Administer large amounts (initially 250 cc/hour) 0.45 normal saline with potassium 10–20 mEq/1.33.
- Administer exogenous insulin gradually (initially may require 10–20 units of regular insulin/hour).
- Monitor vital signs, intake and output hourly.

treatment of hyperglycemia.
- Lack of infusion control.

Prevention:
- Constant continuous infusion control.
- Treat glycosuria only if 2+ or greater.
- Discontinue TPN infusions by gradual tapering over a 4–12 hour period. If abrupt stoppage of TPN is necessary, hang 5–10% dextrose solution at 50 cc/hour or at previously ordered TPN rate.
- Have a liter of 10% dextrose available for emergencies, (i.e., breakage of TPN bottle, clotted central line, clogged feeding tube of patient on enteral nutrition receiving insulin).
- Monitor blood sugars of patients at risk.

- Provision of 30–60 percent of nonprotein calories as fat in nutrition regimens of ventilator-dependent patients.

tryptophan).
Prevention/Treatment:
- Monitoring of LFT.
- Accurate estimation of caloric requirements.
- Use of fat as a nonprotein calorie source.
- Maintain calorie:protein ratio at 150:1 or less.
- Avoid TPN if enteral feeding is possible.
- Cycle TPN.

therapy.
- Observe serum for a milky white appearance.
- Begin initial infusion of fat emulsion at rates lower than 60 cc/hour for the first 30 minutes.
- If hypertriglyceridemia is suspected, stop the infusion for at least four hours and measure serum triglycerides.
- Addition of heparin 1000 unit/liter of TPN may enhance plasma clearance of fat emulsion.

seen during nutritional support therapy affect the extracellular compartment. The osmotic balance between the gut and the vascular system is altered during enteral nutritional support, while the vascular system is directly affected when hypertonic nutrient solutions are infused intravenously.

Osmotic pressure is the ability of a fluid to hold water or to attract water to itself through a semipermeable membrane. Osmotic pressure is determined basically by the number of particles per unit of liquid. Particles that influence osmotic pressure include electrolytes, glucose, and the nonprotein nitrogen, urea.

The terms *osmolality* and *osmolarity* are often used interchangeably, but the distinction between the two should be understood. Osmolality is defined as the particle (solute) concentration per unit of water, expressed as mosm/kg of water. Osmolarity, on the other hand, refers to the number of particles per unit of solution and is expressed as mosm/liter of solution. Osmolarity takes into consideration solute plus solvent and is influenced by all particles present and the temperature of the solution. The difference between the two terms relates to a weight versus volume measure. In describing the characteristics of a solution (e.g., a parenteral or enteral nutritional solution), osmolarity is the more appropriate term. In describing the osmotic effect exerted by such a solution, osmolality is the more appropriate term because it refers to all particles influencing the osmotic pull per unit of water, as opposed to all particles influencing the osmotic pull per unit of serum. Serum osmolality describes the osmotic pressure of body fluid and is one of the most reliable parameters of fluid balance. Frequently, urine osmolality also is measured.

The number of particles in a given solution alters the osmotic pull—as the number of particles in a solution increases so does the osmolarity of that solution. Since a given volume of solvent can hold more small particles in solution than large particles, it follows that the smaller the particles in the solution, the greater the osmotic effect. For example, large complex carbohydrates and whole proteins have less of an osmotic effect than do simple sugars and amino acids. Fat does not contribute to osmosis because fat is an emulsion. Fat does not dissolve in water but rather is held in a suspension.

If the osmolarity of a particular nutritional support solution is not known, the nurse can estimate the osmotic effect by knowing the electrolyte content and the specific structure of the nutrients within the solution. For example, an enteral formula containing monosaccharides and amino acids would have more of an influence on osmosis than a formula containing oligosaccharides and di- and tripeptides, provided the electrolyte content of the two formulas was the same.

Hypotonic, isotonic, and *hypertonic* are terms used to compare the mosm/liter of a particular solution with that of plasma. Although plasma osmolality often is reported as part of a chemistry profile, plasma osmolality can be indirectly calculated if the blood urea nitrogen (BUN), sodium, and glucose levels are known by using the following equation.

$$\text{Serum osmolality} = 2(\text{Na}) + \frac{\text{BUN}}{3} + \frac{\text{BS}}{20}$$

A calculated osmolality is usually lower than a measured osmolality.[45]

The hypertonicity of a nutritional support solution will affect the selection of the route of administration. Hypertonic solutions administered intravenously via peripheral veins can result in a chemically created thrombophlebitis, a condition that is less frequent when administration of such solutions is via a large central vein. Hypertonic enteral formulas delivered jejunally can increase the potential for diarrhea. Because jejunal feedings bypass the stomach, the formula is not diluted by gastric secretions.

Carbohydrate-Related Complications

Hyperglycemia

As noted by Weinsier et al. and Vanlandingham et al., hyperglycemia is the most commonly observed metabolic complication regardless of the route of administration.[2,6] It is recommended that blood glucose level be maintained below 150 mg%/dl, a level difficult to maintain in the septic, diabetic, or hypermetabolic patient.

Hyperglycemia seen at the initiation of therapy may be caused by too rapid an infusion, the inability of the pancreas to increase the endogenous insulin supply on demand, or the lack of exogenous insulin supplementation. Patients with renal insufficiency may have a high renal threshold for glucose. Others may be receiving medications that alter the results of urine glucose testing. In these instances, assessment of glucose status should be based on blood glucose levels. The frequency of blood sugar monitoring is dependent on the instability of the patient's condition. Altering the formula or solution prescription to include more nonprotein calories like fat may resolve the glucose intolerance and decrease the need for exogenous insulin supplementation.

In a patient who previously was glucose-tolerant, the sudden presence of hyperglycemia may be predict impending infection or sepsis. Hyperglycemia and glycosuria have been shown to precede the clincal diagnosis of sepsis by 12–24 hours. Glycosuria may be observed before a rise in temperature or a rise in the white blood cell count.

Hyperosmolar, Hyperglycemic, Nonketonic Dehydration and Coma Syndrome

If hyperglycemia continues and is accompanied by glycosuria and diuresis, the syndrome of hyperosmolar, hyperglycemic, nonketonic dehydration and coma (HHNC) may develop. This syndrome is fatal in more than 40 percent of cases.[46] Development of HHNC during both parenteral and enteral nutrition has been reported.[47,48]

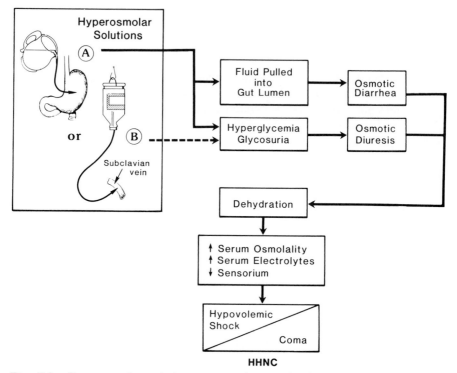

Fig. 7-2. Sequence of metabolic events resulting in development of hyperglycemic, hyperosmolar, nonketonic dehydration and coma (HHNC).

The sequence of events in the development of HHNC is illustrated in Figure 7-2, while its treatment is illustrated in Figure 7-3. When a hyperosmolar formula is introduced into the gut lumen in a haphazard fashion, or if the gut mucosa cannot assimilate the formula quickly, additional water will move into the gut lumen from the extracellular space. This is an attempt to neutralize the hypertonic effect of the formula and maintain an iso-osmolar environment.

The movement of water into the gut lumen occurs much faster than the transport of the nutrients out of the lumen, across the brush border of the gut mucosa, and onto the liver via portal circulation. The presence of this additional fluid within the gut lumen may be accompanied by patient complaints of fullness, nausea, or diarrhea, which are the clinical signs of formula intolerance. This is of particular concern when calorically dense, elemental diets are used.

Administration of the enteral formula by continuous infusion, beginning at dilute concentrations and/or slow rates of infusion will allow for gut adaptation. If diarrhea occurs, antidiarrheal agents such as tincture of opium or paregoric can be administered concurrently with the formula (Fig. 7-2).

Hyperglycemia will occur if enteral nutrient absorption proceeds, but,

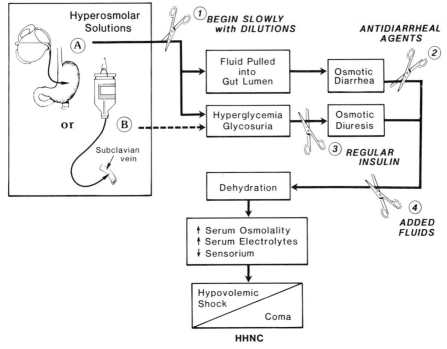

Fig. 7-3. Clinical intervention during HHNC.

because of a lack of endogenous insulin or a clinically created insulin resistance, glucose uptake by the cells is diminished. At this point, administration of either enteral formulas or parenteral solutions will alter metabolism in a similar way, contributing to the development of HHNC.

In the patient with adequate pancreatic beta-cell function, hyperglycemia will result in increased endogenous insulin release. In patients who were glucose-intolerant prior to nutritional support however, any additional insulin release will be meager, enough to prevent ketosis, but not enough to control the hyperglycemia. Hyperglycemia causes the cell to become dehydrated, which in turn suppresses the production of insulin. Unless exogenous insulin is supplied, the cycle of hyperglycemia, dehydration, and inadequate insulin production and release continues. Regular insulin should be used to maintain the blood glucose below 150 mg%/dl. If the hyperglycemia has persisted for any length of time, its correction should be gradual. If correction occurs too quickly, cerebral edema may develop as water from the blood (now rendered hypotonic in respect to the cerebral spinal fluid) moves into the cerebral spinal fluid.[34] Hyperglycemia will lead to glycosuria as the kidney attempts to excrete the increased solute load it has absorbed. Glucose is a very effective osmotic diuretic, even in the presence of adequate antidiuretic hormone.[48] Persistent glycosuria alters the normal osmotic gradient within the renal tubules, causing excretion of large volumes of urine (e.g., osmotic diuresis). If renal insufficiency already exists, the ability to concentrate the urine is one of the first functions to diminish, which also enhances diuresis. Persistent diuresis will lead to clinical signs of dehydration if fluid supplementation is not begun.

Initially during this cycle, the fluid loss is mainly water, but continued diuresis results in a loss of important electrolytes, primarily sodium and potassium. Total body sodium depletion and hypokalemia can result. These electrolyte losses eventually will be accompanied by changes in sensorium as fluid and electrolyte shifts involve the intracellular as well as the extracellular fluid compartments. Treatment should be aimed at replacement of sodium and water. At the same time, cautious use of insulin is suggested because sudden decreases in blood glucose, in the face of total body sodium deficits, may cause rapid fluid shifts within the central nervous system. This may result in edema, convulsions, coma, and death.[47]

Fluid supplementation is important. Simply increasing the infusion rate of the nutrient solution will only compound the dehydration. The use of isotonic saline and appropriate electrolyte replacement will repair these deficits and also prevent a shift of water back into the intracellular compartment, which would now be hypertonic because of dehydration.[47]

Hypoglycemia

Hypoglycemia most often is caused by abruptly stoping TPN, although endogenous insulin manufacture and release diminishes quickly when the supply of exogenous glucose is discontinued.[33] Clinical signs of hypoglycemia are commonly observed in patients who were receiving intermittent exogenous insulin supplementation. Abrupt disruption of glucose infusion as a result of catheter clotting, TPN bottle breakage, or infusion pump malfunction will decrease the availability of glucose during a time of peak insulin activity. Hypoglycemia can be prevented by slowly tapering the glucose infusion when therapy is being discontinued, although this tapering can be done in a matter of hours instead of the former practice of days. If a TPN solution must be quickly discontinued, the infusion of 5 or 10% dextrose in water usually provides sufficient glucose to prevent a rebound hypoglycemia.

Hypoglycemia is not a common concern when enteral nutrition support is used. If a patient is receiving intermittent injections of a long-acting insulin, however, a rebound hypoglycemia will occur if the enteral-formula infusion is stopped during peak insulin activity. This may occur if the feeding tube becomes dislodged or clogged and is not replaced. At special risk are those patients who frequently dislodge their feeding tubes. In the middle of the night the physician or nurse may elect to wait until morning to reinsert the feeding tube, especially if radiologic confirmation of the position of the tube tip is necessary. In this case, the night nurse should frequently check the patient for signs of hyperglycemia if the patient has received insulin but no alternative source of glucose has been provided. Tube-fed patients who need insulin supplementation should receive regular insulin on a frequent schedule. Use of long-acting insulin requires close coordination of enteral formula delivery and insulin administration with assurances that the feeding tube remains patent. The use of transitional feeding techniques presents a challenge when the patient is receiving exogenous insulin. Clinical assessment, plus accurate intake and output records and calorie counts, must be done daily.

Hypercapnia

Excessive production of carbon dioxide has been shown to occur in specific patients when nutritional support solutions contain a high concentration of glucose. Although published reports have involved the use of parenteral nutrition, the problem has been identified in those receiving enteral nutrition. Askanazi et al. have demonstrated that carbon dioxide production appropriately increased with a minimal increase in oxygen consumption in the nutritionally depleted, nonhypermetabolic patient who was fed a large glucose load. Carbon dioxide production also increased in the hypermetabolic patient, but this increase was accompanied by a large rise (70 percent) in minute ventilation, indicating a substantial increase in oxygen consumption.[49]

Increased carbon dioxide production is a critical factor in patients with marginal pulmonary function. The patient with chronic obstructive pulmonary disease, for example, is insensitive to rises in arterial carbon dioxide levels and would not be able to respond by excreting the additional carbon dioxide. Carbon dioxide retention would result. The increased oxygen consumption and increased carbon dioxide (e.g., the work of breathing) might precipitate respiratory distress, interfering with the patient's attempts at spontaneous respiration.[50] Respiratory failure precipitated by high carbohydrate loads during refeeding has been documented.[51] This sequence of events would be particularly harmful for the ventilator-dependent patient who is attempting to wean from the ventilator.

Composition of the nutritional support solution for pulmonary-compromised or ventilatory-dependent patients should be altered to provide 30–60 percent of the nonprotein calories as fat emulsion. The utilization of fat as an energy source does not require the same degree of increased oxygen consumption and carbon dioxide production as does the use of glucose.[49]

Hepatic Dysfunction

One complication associated with parenteral nutrition is an alteration in liver function tests (LFT) and changes in hepatocyte structure. Despite our increasing knowledge of metabolic events, hepatic dysfunction during nutritional support therapy remains a concern.

Hepatic dysfunction may range from asymptomatic and transient elevations of LFT to progressive hepatic failure and coma. Physical changes within the hepatocytes may involve cholestatis, fatty metamorphosis, hepatocellular necrosis, fibrosis, and cirrhosis. These changes in the structure of the hepatocytes usually are severe only in the neonate and young child. The clinical picture in adults is benign and usually reversible.[52] Elevation of LFT occurs in the majority of adult patients who receive TPN for longer than two weeks. The rise in LFT may be self-limiting. In a study of 100 patients, serial comparisons of LFT (pre-TPN and during TPN) demonstrated that serum glutamic-pyruvic transaminase (SGPT) increased to 5.4 times the baseline, serum bilirubin increased to 2.3 times the baseline, and lactic dehydrogenase (LDH) increased to 1.5 times the baseline value. These LFT elevations lasted from 4 to 10 days.[53]

Patients with preexisting hepatic disease may show marked progression of LFT changes. Liver biopsies taken during periods of LFT elevations demonstrate fatty infiltrates of the hepatocytes and increased glycogen stores, but no inflammatory or cholestatic changes, as is often seen in neonates. Those receiving prolonged TPN may, at a later date, again exhibit LFT changes, this time accompanied by inflammation of the hepatocytes.[53]

The cause of these hepatic alterations is unclear. At one time or another all of the macronutrients have been implicated. Early elevation of LFT is thought to be caused by the initiation of refeeding during a time of hepatic enzyme and metabolic inactivity. Essential fatty acid deficiency has also been implicated. There is a consensus that provision of excessive glucose calories or an inappropriate calorie:protein ratio plays a major role.[52] In both animal and human studies, reversible fatty infiltration of the liver has been shown to be related to concentrated infusions of glucose. Burke et al. have suggested that an upper limit of glucose utilization exists, especially in the hypermetabolic patient.[54] Delivery of glucose above this level results in the conversion of glucose to intrahepatic fat. The diagnosis of TPN-related hepatic dysfunction is largely by exclusion since biliary disease, sepsis, malignancy, anesthesia, and hepatoxic drugs all cause alterations in hepatic function.

Treatment of hepatic dysfunction during TPN administration includes: (1) the provision of adequate but not excessive calories; (2) a decreased reliance on glucose alone as the nonprotein calorie source; (3) the provision of an adequate calorie:protein ratio (e.g., no higher than 200:1); and (4) the cycling of TPN during the course of a 24-hour period.

Cyclic TPN involves the provision of the patient's daily nutrient requirements over a period of less than 24 hours. Typically the patient receives TPN for 8–16 hours each day and, if needed, glucose-free fluids during the remaining hours of the day. During this rest period from glucose infusion, the liver is able to clear itself of the accumulated glucose. Cyclic TPN must be performed cautiously since hepatic dysfunction also affects glucose tolerance.

Protein-Related Complications

Azotemia

Complications related to protein intake were identified during the early use of nutritional support therapy. Gault et al. described a tube-feeding syndrome consisting of hypernatremia, azotemia, and dehydration. Blenderized tube feedings relied heavily on protein content. It was common for the daily protein intake to reach levels greater than 210 g.[3]

Although the etiology of this syndrome is a high concentration of protein instead of carbohydrate, the sequence of events and potential clinical outcome are similar to HHNC. Metabolism of exogenous protein results in the production of large amounts of urea, which is manufactured in the liver and transported to the kidneys for excretion. The increased urea production sends an increased solute load to the kidney. Increased urine production and excretion are required for urea disposal. The main contributors to renal solute load are protein (urea), sodium, potassium, and chloride. Blenderized tube feedings frequently contain large amounts of all these components. In the case of elderly or other patients with renal dysfunction, the kidney may not be able to adapt to such additional demands.

Patients receiving TPN may also be at risk for azotemia. Amino acid concentrations as high as 11 percent are used for compounding parenteral nutritional solutions. Clinicians studying the effects of nutritional support on the critically ill have emphasized the need for a lower protein:calorie ratio (80:1) as opposed to the traditional 150:1 ratio.[17] High protein intakes in this patient population must be closely monitored since acute renal failure frequently occurs as a part of the primary disease process.

Hyperammonemia

Hyperammonemia is not a common complication of TPN in adults. It was reported in infants who received TPN solutions containing protein hydrolysates. Increased blood ammonia levels in the infants were attributed to the free ammonia found in the hydrolysate solution. Crystalline amino acids contain less free ammonia than protein hydrolysate solutions.[55] Hyperammonemia in infants who received TPN solutions manufactured with crystalline amino acids, however, has also been reported. Insufficient quantities of arginine in the TPN solution also have been implicated in the development of hyperammonemia, since arginine is essential for the deamination of ammonia via the urea cycle.[55]

Acid Base Imbalance

Protein hydrolysate solutions have a high buffering capacity and may lead to metabolic acidosis, especially in patients with pulmonary and renal dysfunction. Crystalline amino acids have a weaker buffering capacity, but may also lead to a metabolic acidosis because of the presence of increased cation amino acids (arginine, histidine, and lysine) as compared with anion amino acids.[56]

A hyperchloremic metabolic acidosis has also been reported. Glomerular filtration of chloride is increased in response to increased chloride infusion. The chloride is reabsorbed by the renal tubules along with sodium ions. Less than normal amounts of hydrogen ions are secreted in exchange for the sodium ions, leading to a metabolic acidosis. Acetate, lactate, or phosphate salts may be substituted for chloride salts when TPN solutions are compounded to prevent acid-base imbalances due to chloride ion abnormalities.[34]

Amino Acid Imbalance

The quantity and quality of amino acids utilized in various disease states has received increased attention. The first disease-specific study included patients with renal failure. In question was the ability to manufacture nonessential amino acids within the body if only essential amino acids were provided. This was the basis for the "renal failure solutions" used in the past. It is now recognized that both essential and nonessential amino acids are needed exogenously during renal failure and that dialysis should be used, whenever possible, to ensure that the protein needs of the patient can be more easily met.[13]

The ratio of plasma amino acids is of concern as a potential cause of hepatic encephalopathy. Patients with hepatic dysfunction have decreased ability to metabolize the aromatic amino acids, in particular, tryptophan and phenylalanine. They continue to utilize the branched-chain amino acids, leucine, isoleucine, and valine, that are metabolized by skeletal muscle. Plasma ratios of aromatic amino acids rise, while the ratios of branched-chain amino acids fall. It is theorized that the aromatic amino acids cross the blood-brain barrier in increased numbers and enter into false neurotransmitter reactions, which are thought to be the etiology of the central nervous system symptoms of hepatic encephalopathy. Provision of solutions containing an increased percentage of branched-chain amino acids have been shown in some instances to decrease hepatic encephalopathy, resulting in less somnulence and lethargy. Controversy exists, however regarding whether eventual patient outcome is altered.

Current study of the traumatized, hypermetabolic, critically ill patient has led to further investigation of the role of the branched-chain amino acids. Cerra et al. demonstrated an improved utilization of the branched-chain amino acids, especially leucine, in this patient population. The relation of improved metabolism of amino acids to final patient outcome, however, is still a controversial issue.[17]

Fat-Related Complications

Despite the demonstrated safety of currently available fat emulsions, concern over potential complications still exists. The overloading syndrome noted to occur during the use of cottonseed oil emulsion, however, has not been observed with currently available emulsions. During clinical use, both in Europe and the United States, the use of soybean or safflower oil emulsions has not been problematic, although there have been reports of adverse effects during the use of soybean or safflower oil emulsions. Some have suggested, however, that other physiologic events related to the patient's underlying disease state may contribute to the observations.[52]

Prior to hydrolysis, intravenous fat emulsions are taken up by the liver and spleen. Final clearance is via the reticuloendothelial system in the Kupffer cells of the liver. Changes in Kupffer cell pigmentation have been observed but appear to be reversible and without pathologic effect once the fat emulsion has been discontinued.[52]

Infusion of 500 ml of 10% soybean oil emulsion produced a decrease in the pulmonary diffusion capacity of healthy young men, but these changes were no greater than those observed during postprandial lipemia.[57,58] Pulmonary congestion has been attributed specifically to the infusion of fat emulsion, but similar observations have been reproduced by infusing excessive quantities of normal saline.[57] Ventilatory and perfusion defects were observed in 8 preterm infants who died after soybean oil infusions. But these infants died from unrelated causes, and there is little evidence to indicate that the fat accumulation noted in their lungs was responsible for the deaths.[59]

Alterations in erythropoiesis have been observed, but these observations are inconsistent and at times contradictory. Hypercoagulability has been reported, but further studies have failed to confirm this observation. Soybean oil does appear to produce a reduction in platelet adhesiveness, lasting several hours after the infusion has been stopped, but prolonged infusion has demonstrated no effect on platelet count.[57]

Plasma clearance of fat emulsions has been observed, even in critically ill patients and those with liver dysfunction. This observation has been attributed to the metabolic preference for fat as an energy source during sepsis.[60] Other researchers, however, question the critically ill patient's ability to utilize exogenous fat emulsion as an energy source. Pediatric patients can clear the fat emulsion from their plasma, but the use of fat emulsions has been shown to elevate serum bilirubin levels in neonates.[61] Cholestasis during extended courses of TPN has also been reported. The etiology of this is believed to be injury to the bilirubin transfer mechanism in the liver.[62] Lipids support the growth of bacteria and fungi and potentially may enhance the risk of infections in susceptible patients.[63]

These reports of adverse reactions to the administration of fat emulsions should alert one to the need for careful monitoring whenever parenteral fat emulsions are used. Use of the recommended daily dose of 2–4 g/kg should be well-tolerated by most patients.[60] Serum triglyceride levels before and routinely during administration should be assessed. Observations of the patient's serum for lipemia should be made, as lipemic serum can alter other chemistry values (i.e., a false hyponatremia). Some argue that normal serum triglyceride values may not indicate adequate plasma clearance. The triglycerides may have been degraded to free fatty acids, high levels of which have been noted to be irritating to pulmonary alveoli (i.e., palmitic acid). Unfortunately, clinical laboratories do not have the facilities to measure free fatty acids on a routine basis. Drugs such as tetracycline have been implicated as a cause of impaired plasma clearance of triglycerides.[60]

Micronutrient-Related Complications

The fluid- and electrolyte-related complications outlined in Table 7-5 can easily be prevented with close laboratory monitoring and daily rewriting of nutritional support orders. Confusion may result in under- or overprescription when many physicians are involved in the patient's care and all order according to their perceptions of patient requirements. The nurse can be a key figure in coordinating the fluid and electrolyte orders of the patient by keeping up-to-date on the actual amount of each received by the patient when all treatments are reviewed.

The increased need for trace element replacement has been well-studied, especially in relation to those trace elements frequently lost when excessive GI losses occur or malabsorption is present (i.e., zinc, chromium, magnesium). Increased attention to trace element requirements is required during long-term nutritional support. The reader is referred to Jeejeebhoy's review of micronutrient requirements.[39]

METABOLIC MONITORING BY NUTRITIONAL SUPPORT NURSES

Laboratory Monitoring

Many laboratory parameters are monitored during nutritional support therapy. "TPN profiles" or standing laboratory orders are not uncommon during the use of TPN. The need for similar laboratory monitoring during enteral nutritional support has been emphasized. The need for such close monitoring has become more apparent as disease-specific nutritional support solutions and formulas have become available. The most frequently ordered laboratory tests are listed in Table 7-7. Concern about cost has caused nutrition support teams to reevaluate the need and frequency of these tests in order to determine whether test results would alter their use of nutritional support. Once a patient's nutritional support prescription has been stabilized, many of these tests may be obtained on an "as needed" basis. Baseline testing, however, is important to adequately observe trends during the course of therapy.

When reviewing laboratory reports the nurse might ask the following questions:

- Is the BUN rising in response to the increased protein intake?
- Has the blood glucose remained under control?

Table 7-7
Frequency of Laboratory Parameters Monitored During Nutrition Support

Test	Frequency (after baseline)
Blood glucose	Daily until stable, then M,W,F
Serum electrolytes	Daily until stable, then M,W,F
(Na+, K+, Cl−, CO$_2$)	
Creatinine, blood urea nitrogen	Daily or every other day while protein load increasing, then M,W,F
Plasma osmolality	As indicated by electrolyte results
Chemistry Profile	At least twice weekly until stable, then once/week
(Total protein, albumin, bilirubin SGOT, SGPT, LDH, alkaline phosphatase, calcium, phosphorus, magnesium)	
Complete blood count	Weekly
Trace elements	Baseline if losses or need suspected, then as indicated
Triglycerides	M,W,F if fat emulsions used
Folate, B12 levels	If supplemented
Hematology studies	Dependent on CBC and
(Fe, TIBC, ferritin)	laboratory capability
Prothrombin time	Weekly
Urine electrolytes	As indicated
Blood gases	As indicated
Plasma amino acid profile	As indicated
Prealbumin, transferrin	

- Is the fall in serum sodium a dilutional result of the delivery of large amounts of fluid, necessitated by the use of the peripheral lipid system?
- Is the rise in serum potassium due to the potassium content of the enteral formula, or is the patient also receiving medication such as penicillin that may contain a large amount of potassium?
- Should serum zinc be measured, since the patient's diarrheal losses have dramatically increased?
- Has the patient's renal or hepatic function diminished, as evidenced by changes in creatinine, BUN, and liver function tests?
- Have serum phosphorus levels fallen with the use of high concentrations of glucose?

Developing a "trend" sheet can help the nurse easily observe changes in laboratory values, especially in those situations when patient charts are forever "being thinned."

Since one of the goals of therapy is to maintain the patient in a positive nitrogen balance, 24-hour collections of urine and sometimes stool for nitrogen balance studies are commonly ordered to assess the adequacy of the nutritional support therapy. For trace element analysis, 24-hour collections of urine and stool may be important in those particular patients who have excessive GI losses. Unfortunately, the results of 24-hour collections are often dismissed due to poor collections. The nurse has a major role in ensuring that specimens are collected accurately and on time. Obtaining three consecutive 24-hour collections so that the outlier value can be discarded during test interpretation has proven beneficial.[64]

Patients At Risk

An accurate generalization is that many of the metabolic complications relate, in one way or another, to fluid and electrolyte homeostasis. The nurse must therefore be able to identify those patients who because of age, disease, or treatment are at particular risk for fluid imbalance.

Although the human body is primarily composed of water, very little margin exists against the consequences of major fluid shifts. The percentage of body water changes throughout life as a function of age and sex. Infants are composed of approximately 70% water. When infants lose fluid, as with watery diarrhea, they lose proportionally more water than electrolytes. Under such conditions physiologic states of hypertonicity develop at a rapid rate. As one ages, lean body mass, which contains water, is replaced by dense adipose tissue, which contains less water. Older women, who generally have a higher proportion of adipose tissue, are only 50% water by composition. They represent one group that poorly tolerates fluid shifts.

Renal function diminishes as a normal part of the aging process. The ability to concentrate urine, even in the presence of sufficient antidiuretic hormone, is decreased. The elderly may be prone to excretion of large amounts of dilute urine despite the need to preserve body water.

The presence or absence of thirst is an important parameter indicative of the state of one's hydration. If the hypothalmic center has been altered because of neurologic disease, or if the patient is unable to express thirst, as in the case of the unconscious or intubated patient, a crucial defense mechanism has been lost. Some patients, knowing they are NPO (receiving nothing by mouth), do not complain of thirst. These patients expect to be thirsty and do not sense thirst as an altered state. An important role for the nurse is that of patient education. The patient must be made aware that increased thirst should be reported.

Fluid balance can easily be altered. Those patients at particular risk for fluid imbalance include the very young, the elderly, and those with glucose intolerance, renal dysfunction, neurologic damage, or excessive losses such as fistula output or secretions. Patients who are intubated or receiving steroids, diuretics, or calorically dense formulas must also be carefully monitored.

Patient Assessment and Observation

Nursing actions such as documentation of intake and output, weights, vital signs, and urine testing should not be considered routine. The importance of these simple activities will be more meaningful if the nurse understands the relationship of these activities to metabolic monitoring.

Many of the nurse's bedside monitoring activities are intended to assess fluid and electrolyte balance. Accurate intake and output records must include an estimation of insensible fluid losses and calculation of daily, as well as cumulative, fluid balance. Although an accurate measurement of all outputs may not be possible in all cases, an estimation of loss should be made. Descriptions of loss as "small," "medium," or "large," however, are meaningless unless standard definitions for each term have been devised. Intake and output forms often do not contain adequate space to properly document all the different types of intake a patient may be receiving. Figure 7-4 illustrates a Daily Fluid Record that I have used effectively. Not only can fluid balance be easily determined, but essential information needed to calculate actual calorie and protein intake is available. Such an intake and output sheet also provides a quick, visual reference for the accuracy of the infusion control device being used. Comparison of the prescribed hourly rate of infusion with what actually was infused may highlight unidentified infusion control problems.

A standard routine for weighing patients is also mandatory. The weighing of patients has always been an unpopular task. It is time-consuming and the weights obtained often are questioned as inaccurate despite frequent calibration of the bed scales. Weighing schedules for patients receiving nutritional support should be standardized. Patient weights should be part of nursing standards of care and not require a physician's order. Any patient who is critically ill or has a potential for fluid and electrolyte imbalance should be weighed daily. Otherwise, those requiring bed weights can be weighed on a Monday-Wednesday-Friday schedule. Although nutritional support nurses are cognizant of the importance of weights in the management of a patient's fluid and electrolyte balance, this importance needs to be underscored to those on the nursing team who may be doing the actual weighing. It must not be viewed as only a mandatory nursing chore. Nutritional support teams can often assist the nursing department by providing written justification for the purchase of enough bedscales so their availability is not an issue in their use.

Temperature and vital signs should be obtained every 4 hours unless the patient's condition is very stable. Signs of fluid overload or dehydration may be detected by changes in pulse and blood pressure readings. Chronically starved and hypometabolic patients such as those with anorexia nervosa are often hypotensive and bradycardic on admission. Refeeding may potentiate conges-

Fluid Intake and Output
Summary Record

DATE	TIME	INTAKE									OUTPUT				
		ORAL	TUBE FDG.	HYPER AL.	LIPIDS	PAREN TERAL	BLOOD	H.L.	TOTAL	URINE	EMESIS/ SUCTION	OTHER	OTHER	TOTAL
	7-3													
	3-11													
	11-7													
	TOTAL													

Fig. 7-4. Fluid intake and output summary record.

tive heart failure if nutritional support therapy is not initiated cautiously. The critically ill patient who is being monitored hemodynamically may require the use of very concentrated nutritional support solutions if changes in pulmonary wedge pressure, cardiac output, or central venous pressure document fluid overload or cardiac insufficiency. The effects of malnutrition and refeeding on cardiac muscle and function are receiving increased clinical attention and investigation.[65]

Urine testing for the presence of glucose or ketones has been previously discussed. Patients receiving continuous infusions of nutritional support solutions should have their urine tested every 6 hours, not according to the usual "before meals and at bedtime" schedule. The accuracy of urine testing may be altered by drugs, the freshness of the testing materials and the urine, or the patient's renal function. Whenever possible, testing should be done with double-voided specimens. Initial correlation of blood glucose and urine glucose may be needed to determine the patient's renal threshold for glucose excretion. Patients with a high or very low renal threshold may require sliding-scale insulin coverage, based on frequent blood sampling. The use of chemstrips has decreased our total reliance on urine testing for monitoring glucose tolerance.

Documentation of blood sugar results, urine testing results, and the frequency of sliding-scale insulin administration on the same flowsheet is beneficial. Correlation of the clinical signs of the patient and the treatment rendered can be better assessed so errors in management are less likely to occur.

The nurse should monitor the infusion control of the nutritional support solution or formula on a half-hour to hourly basis, despite the use of infusion control devices. When multiliter containers are being used for parenteral nutritional delivery, volumetric control is mandatory. Many hospitals now control enteral formula administration via an infusion control device. If the staff nurse understands the potentially dangerous consequences of "catch up" of the TPN rate, especially in the patient who is glucose-intolerant, or "fluid bolusing" in an elderly patient, better compliance with infusion control will occur.

TPN bottles and multiliter bags should be labeled as to actual volume. The nurse should not have to guess whether the container is "overfilled." Administration containers for enteral formulas frequently contain volume calibrations that are difficult to read. Graduated containers should be available so that the nurse can accurately measure the filling and/or remaining enteral formula volume.

Clinical observations of the patient should correlate with laboratory data. For example, if the patient is in negative fluid balance, is complaining of thirst, and has a serum sodium of 150 mEq/dl, one would question the accuracy of the weighing procedure if the patient's weight has increased. In another example, a weight gain of more than 0.5 lb/day most likely represents fluid retention and may be associated with hyponatremia, pulmonary congestion, or peripheral edema.

Daily physical assessment of the patient by the primary nurse provides valuable information. During the physical assessment the nurse should focus particularly on the neurologic, cardiopulmonary, and renal systems, in addition to the GI tract. The following section provides some examples of how the patient's nutritional status can influence the nurse's clinical observation and assessment of the patient.

The nurse should assess the patient's mental status and level of consciousness. When admitted, the elderly may appear mentally confused and moribund, possibly because of a terminal illness, but more often because of fluid and electrolyte imbalance or malnutrition. Correction of these imbalances should improve the patient's mental status. If a patient is treated successfully for hepatic encephalopathy, increased mental alertness is anticipated. A patient with hypophosphatemia may appear lethargic or encephalopathic.

During the physical assessment, the nurse should listen to the patient's lungs and the quality of the breath sounds. Accumulation of fluid because of early congestive heart failure is assessed by listening for rales in the lower lobes. Decreased breath sounds may indicate fluid consolidation.

If dehydration is suspected, the nurse should examine the patient's skin and mucous membranes. Is the tongue moist, dry, or cracked? Is the skin dry, moist, resilient to touch? Does it "tent"when pinched? Is there any edema? The lower extremities are commonly the site of edema, but sacral edema is more common in the bedridden patient.

If a patient is gaining excessive weight and no edema is evident, accumulation of fluid in the cardiopulmonary system might be suspected. One might expect the urine to be concentrated and have a high specific gravity. If the patient is severely hypoalbumenic, generalized anasarca may be present. Fluid overload can occur, particularly when the peripheral lipid system is being used. Use of the peripheral lipid system usually requires a fairly large fluid load for the desired caloric intake to be administered.

The nurse should determine if there is evidence of increased fluid loss such as excessive tracheal secretions or a large draining wound. What other insensible losses may be altering fluid balance?

Telfer and Persoff studied fluid and electrolyte problems in the elderly and found that clinical determinations of the initial state of hydration often were misleading. Subsequent changes in hydration, however, could be followed by determination of the rate and degree of small vein filling. To test for small vein filling, one occludes a small hand or foot vein at a distal point using finger pressure. The small vein is emptied of its blood supply by stroking the vessel proximally with another finger. When the pressure on the vein is released, the rate and degree of blood return is observed and compared to a preestablished scale, similar to that used to estimate the presence of edema.[66]

Assessment of GI function may be difficult if the patient's primary disease involves the GI tract. Is the abdomen soft, distended, or tender? Is it tympanic or dull to percussion? Does the patient complain of nausea, fullness, or general

Table 7-8
Standard Nursing Actions for Monitoring Patients Receiving Nutrition Support

Daily physical assessment:
 • Changes in mental status,
 • State of hydration,
 • Cardiopulmonary function,
 • Renal function,
 • Gastrointestinal function.
Intake and output records with fluid balance calculated.
Patient weights daily or M,W,F.
Urine testing for sugar/acetone every 6 hours.
Temperature and vital signs every 4 hours.
Monitor infusion control every ½–1 hour.
Monitor abnormal laboratory parameters (keep "trend" Record).
Identify patients "at risk".

malaise? Is the tube-fed patient receiving medications that may cause GI distress?

If the patient has diarrhea, is it related to eating, the initiation of tube feeding, or medications? A patient receiving an elemental diet may be concerned over the lack of a daily bowel movement. The use of chronic antibiotic therapy may result in alterations in intestinal flora causing diarrhea. Above all, the nurse needs to make an independent judgment about the presence and amount of diarrhea, because self-reporting by the patient may be influenced by previous experience and expectations.

The presence or absence of bowel sounds should be determined each shift. A tendency now exists to resume tube feeding on the first postoperative night, especially in those patients who did not undergo an abdominal operative procedure. This aggressive use of nutritional support, although warranted, needs close monitoring.

The previous comments regarding physical assessment are not meant to be all-inclusive. The intent is to highlight those areas of usual concern. During the physical assessment the nurse experienced in the assessment of the malnourished patient may identify the subtle signs of micronutrient deficiencies.

Table 7-8 lists the nursing actions involved in metabolic monitoring. Most of those listed are routine nursing activities and should be initiated whenever a patient is receiving nutritional support therapies.

SUMMARY

Frequent metabolic monitoring ensures that potential metabolic complications will be prevented or documented and treated. As the most frequent person at the bedside, the nurse is in a key position to monitor for changes in metabolic and nutritional status. Minor changes in clinical status may or may not correlate with laboratory data, but their observation and treatment can prevent continuation of an eventually irreversible metabolic problem.

Nurses are often data collectors, measuring vital signs, recording intake and output, and so on. They must also be able to interpret the data collected, identify patients at risk, and correlate all this with the consequences of nutritional support therapies. An understanding of nutrient composition and expected as well as potential untoward physiologic responses will aid the nurse in the interpretation of collected data.

The nurse has an important role in the monitoring of patients receiving nutritional support therapy. Ready access to information concerning the nutritional support prescription, the availability of efficient forms for data documentation and follow-up, and modern equipment such as easy-to-use bedscales and glucometers are needed. This attention to detail will enhance the ability of the nurse at the bedside to observe and accurately report changes in the patient's condition that may potentiate or cause metabolic complications related to nutritional support therapy.

REFERENCES

1. Dudrick SHJ, MacFadyen BV, VanDuren CT, et al: Parenteral hyperalimentation: Metabolic problems and solutions. Ann Surg 176(3):259–264, 1972
2. Weinsier RL, Bacon J, Butterworth CE: Central venous alimentation: A prospective study of the frequency of metabolic abnormalities among medical and surgical patients. JPEN 6(5):421–425, 1982
3. Gault MH, Dixon ME, Cohen WM: Hypernatremia, azotemia and dehydration due to high protein tube feeding. Ann Intern Med 68(4):778–791, 1968
4. Engle FL, Jaeger C: Dehydration with hypernatremia, hyperchloremia and azotemia complicating nasogastric tube feeding. Am J Med 17:196, 1954
5. Kubo W, Grant M, Walike B, et al: Fluid and electrolyte problems in tube-fed patients. Am J Nurs 76(6):912–916, 1976
6. Vanlandingham S, Simpson S, Daniel P, et al: Metabolic abnormalities in patients supported with enteral tube feeding. JPEN 5(4):322–324, 1981
7. Pareira MD, Conrad EJ, Hicks W, et al: Therapeutic nutrition with tube feeding. JAMA 156:810–816, 1954
8. Cuthbertson D: Historical background to parenteral nutrition. Acta Chir Scand 498(suppl):1–11, 1980
9. Elman R: Urinary output of nitrogen as influenced by intravenous injection of a mixture of amino acids. Proc Soc Exp Biol Med 37:610–613, 1937
10. Krey SH, Crocker KS, Procelli KA, et al: Prolonged use of modular enteral hyperalimentation. Nutri Clin Prac 1(3):140–145, 1986
11. Rose WC: The significance of the amino acids in nutrition. Harvey Lectures 30:49–65, 1934–1935.
12. Wretlind A: History and overview of parenteral nutrition, in Human Nutrition,

Clinical and Biochemical Aspects. Proceedings of the 4th Arnold O. Bechkman Conference in Clinical Chemistry. 1980, pp 323–351

13. Valgeirsdotter K, Munro HN: Protein and amino acid metabolism, in Fischer J (ed): Surgical Nutrition. Boston, Little, Brown, 1983, pp 127–164

14. Anderson GH, Patel DG, Jeejeebhoy KN: Design and evaluation by nitrogen balance and blood annigrams of an amino acid mixture for total parenteral nutrition of adults with gastrointestinal disease. J Clin Invest 53(3):904–912, 1974

15. Bergstrom J, Bucht H, Furst P, et al: Intravenous nutrition with amino acid solutions in patients with chronic uremia. Acta Med Scand 191(4):359–367, 1972

16. Fischer JE, Bower RH: Nutrition support in liver disease. Surg Clin N Am 61(3): 653–660, 1981

17. Cerra FB, Lipson D, Angelico R, et al: Branched chains stimulate postoperative protein synthesis. Surgery 92(2):192–199, 1983

18. Matarese LE: Enteral alimentation, in Fischer J (ed): Surgical Nutrition. Boston, Little, Brown, 1983, pp 719–755

19. Asatoor AM, Cheng B, Edwards KD, et al: Intestinal absorption of two dipeptides in Hartnup Disease. Gut 11(5):380–387, 1970

20. Hellier MD, Holdsworth CD, Perrett D, et al: Intestinal dipeptide transport in normal and cystinuric subjects. Clin Sci 43(5):659–668, 1972

21. Fischer JE, Freund HR: Central hyperalimentation, in Fischer J (ed): Surgical Nutrition. Boston, Little, Brown, 1983, pp 663–702

22. Cooper DR, Iob V, Coller FA: Response to parenteral glucose of normal kidneys and of kidneys of postoperative patients. Ann Surg 129:1–13, 1949

23. Dudrick SJ, Wilmore DW, Vars HM, et al: Can intravenous feeding as the sole means of nutrition support growth in the child and restore weight loss in the adult? An affirmative answer. Ann Surg 169(6):974–984, 1969

24. Gudmand-Hoyer E, Dahlquist A, Jarnun S: The clinical significance of lactose malabsorption. Am J Gastroenterol 53(5):460–473, 1970

25. Rhoads JE, Vars HM, Dudrick SJ: The development of intravenous hyperalimentation. Surg Clin N Am 61(3):429–435, 1981

26. Third JLHC, Bremner WF: Lipid and lipoprotein metabolism, in Fischer J (ed): Surgical Nutrition. Boston, Little, Brown, 1983, pp 213–240

27. Jeejeebhoy KN, Anderson GH, Nokooda AF, et al: Metabolic studies in total parenteral nutrition with lipid in man. J Clin Invest 57(1):125–136, 1976

28. Long JM III, Wilmore DW, Mason AD Jr, et al: Effect of carbohydrate and fat intake on nitrogen excretion during total intravenous feeding. Ann Surg 185(4):417–422, 1977

29. Recommended Daily Allowances. National Research Council, Food and Nutrition Board (ed 9). Washington DC, National Academy of Sciences, 1980, pp 137–165, p 178

30. Guidelines for essential trace element preparations for parenteral use: A statement by an expert panel. AMA: Department of Foods and Nutrition. JAMA 241(19): 2051–2054, 1979

31. Wolman SL, Anderson GH, Marliso EB, et al: Zinc in total parenteral nutrition: Requirements and metabolic effect. Gastroenterol 76:458–467, 1969

32. Alpers DH, Clouse RE, Stenson WF: Manual of Nutritional Therapies. Boston, Little, Brown, 1983

33. Pestana C: Fluid and Electrolytes In The Surgical Patient. Baltimore, Williams & Wilkins, 1977

34. Grant JP: Handbook of Total Parenteral Nutrition. Philadelphia, WB Saunders, 1980

35. Coburn JW, Klein GL: Metabolic Bone Disease in Total Parenteral Nutrition. Baltimore, Urban & Schwarzenberg, 1985

36. Berlyne GM: A Course in Renal Disease (ed 5). Oxford, Blackwell Scientific Publications, 1978, p 430

37. Travis SF, Sugarman HJ, Ruberg RL, et al: Alterations in red cell glycolytic intermediates and oxygen transport as a consequence of hypophosphatemia in patients receiving intravenous hyperalimentation. N Engl J Med 285(14):763–768, 1971

38. Silvas SE, Parpgas PD: Paresthesias, weakness, seizures and hypophosphatemia in patients receiving hyperalimentation. Gastroenterol 62:513, 1972

39. Jeejeebhoy KN: Total Parenteral Nutrition in the Hospital and the Home. Boca Raton, FL, CRC Press, 1983

40. Jeejeebhoy KN, Chu RC, Marliss EB, et al: Chromium deficiency, glucose intolerance and neuropathy reversed by chromium supplementation in a patient receiving long term total parenteral nutrition. Am J Clin Nutr 30(4):531–538, 1977

41. Shike M, Roulet M, Kurian R, et al: Copper metabolism and requirements in total parenteral nutrition. Gastroenterol 81(2):290–297, 1981

42. Baker SS, Lerman RH, Krey SH, et al: Selenium deficiency with total parenteral nutrition: Reversal of biochemical and functional abnormalities by selenium supplementation: A case report. Am J Clin Nutr 38(5):769–774, 1983

43. Caldwell MD, Kennedy-Caldwell C: Normal nutritional requirements. Surg Clin N Am 61(3):489–507, 1980

44. Freed BA, Hsia B, Smith JP, et al: Enteral nutrition: Frequency of formula modification. JPEN 5(1):40–45, 1981

45. Grant MM, Kudo WM: Assessing a patient's hydration status. Am J Nurs 75(8):1306–1311, 1975

46. Witt L: HHNC. Nursing 76(2):66–70, 1976

47. Bivins BA, Hyde GL, Sachatello CR, et al: Pathophysiology and management of hyperosmolar, hyperglycemic, nonketotic dehydration. Surg Gynecol Obstet 154(4):534–540, 1980

48. Kaminski MV: A review of hyperosmolar, hyperglycemic, nonketotic dehydration (HHNC): Etiology, pathophysiology and prevention during intravenous hyperalimentation. JPEN 2(5):690–696, 1978

49. Askanazi J, Rosenbaum SH, Hyman AI, et al: Respiratory changes induced by the large glucose loads of TPN. JAMA 243(14):1444–1447, 1980

50. McCauley K, Weaver TE: Cardiac and pulmonary diseases: Nutritional implications. Nurs Clin N Am 18(1):81–96, 1983

51. Covelli HD, Black JW, Olsen MS, et al: Respiratory failure precipitated by high carbohydrate loads. Ann Intern Med 95(5):5789–5581, 1981

52. Krevsky B, Levine GM: Hepatic complications of TPN. Nutri Supp Ser 3(5):11–14, 1983

53. Grant JP, Cox CE, Kleinman LM, et al: Serum hepatic enzyme and bilirubin elevations during parenteral nutrition. Surg Gynecol Obstet 145(4):573–580, 1977

54. Burke JF, Wolfe RR, Mullany CF, et al: Glucose requirements following burn injury. Ann Surg 190(3):274–285, 1979

55. Heird WC, Nicholson JF, Driscoll JM, et al: Hyperammonemia resulting from intravenous alimentation using a mixture of synthetic L-amino acids. A preliminary report. J Pediatr 81(1):162–165, 1972

56. Heird WC, Dell CB, Driscoll JM, et al: Metabolic acidosis from intravenous administration of mixtures containing synthetic amino acids. New Engl J Med 287: 943–948, 1972

57. Tweedle DEF: Metabolic Care. London, Churchill Livingstone, 1982

58. Greene HL, Hazlett D, Demaree R: Relationship between Intralipid-induced hyperlipemia and pulmonary function. Am J Clin Nutr 29(2):127–135, 1976

59. Levene MI, Wigglesworth JS, Desai R: Pulmonary fat accumulation after intralipid infusion in a pre-term infant. Lancet 18,2(8199):815–818, 1980

60. Freeman JB, Fairfull-Smith RJ: Physiologic approach to peripheral parenteral nutrition, in Fischer J (ed): Surgical Nutrition. Boston, Little, Brown, 1983, pp 710–713

61. Shennan AT, Cherean AG, Ansel A, et al: The effect on intralipid on estimation of serum bilirubin in the newborn. J Pediatr 88(2):285–288, 1976

62. Allardyce, DB: Cholestasis caused by lipid emulsions. Surg Gynecol Obstet 154(5): 641–647, 1982

63. Crocker KS, Noga R, Filibeck DH, et al: Microbial growth comparisons of five commercial parenteral lipid emulsions. JPEN 8(3):391–395, 1984

64. Crocker KS, Krey SH, Steffee WP: Judging the accuracy of collections of single versus consecutive 24 hour urine specimens. Poster Presentation at American Nurses Association, Denver, CO, November, 1983

65. Poindexter Sm, Dear WE, Dudrick SJ: Nutrition in congestive failure. Nutr Clin Prac 1(2):83–88, 1986

66. Telfer N, Persoff M: The effect of tube feeding on the hydration of elderly patients. J Gerontol 20(14):543–566, 1965

Christine Kennedy-Caldwell

8

Pediatric Nutritional Support

T he interrelationship of nutrition with physical and psychosocial development affects normal and hospitalized children alike. As early as the first day
of life, forces come into play that will not only impact the child's biological
existence, but personality development, social skills, and general well-being.
Because of the immediate and long-range implications, this chapter seeks to
clarify the understanding of normative behavior and the skills of feeding.
Applying this information to the child requiring specialized nutrition will enable
the nursing professional to appreciate the profound role that food and feeding
has on the sick child.

Eating is one of the earliest exposures involving human interaction in the
child's world. During feeding the infant is intimately exposed to the emotions
and attitudes of the parent or feeder. It is largely through this person-to-person
interaction that the infant begins to establish basic trust or mistrust in its world.
This early social situation serves as a foundation for rich learning experiences
and the genesis of physiologic satisfaction on satiety or, conversely, the
beginning of faulty interpersonal relationships and pathology.

It is not unusual during a hospital stay for an infant or child's normal
nutrition to be compromised because of the illness, difficulty with eating, nausea,
vomiting, or dysfunction of the intestinal tract. Nutritional support is an integral
part of the child's therapy and convalescence to promote healing, optimal
growth, the child's feeling of well-being, and to potentially shorten the hospital
stay. The child's problem is reviewed by staff nurses and pediatric nutritional
clinical nurse specialists who contribute to the decision and either supplement a
regular diet or provide alternative feeding routes such as tube feedings or
intravenous nutrition.

NUTRITIONAL SUPPORT IN NURSING
ISBN 0-8089-1889-3

233

Pediatric nurses should be competent in the advanced techniques required for specialized nutritional support. They must have thorough knowledge of all aspects of asepsis as well as skill in physical assessment. In addition, concepts of fluid, electrolyte, and acid-base balance should be completely understood. The hospitalized infant or child is especially vulnerable to nutrient deficiencies and the resultant poor health. The presence of chronic underlying disease or disability seriously interferes with adequate nutrition. Nutritional assessment studies of the hospitalized pediatric population at four major teaching medical centers revealed an incidence of 20–50 percent nutritional deficit existing in pediatric patients.[1-4] The pediatric nurse is critical in promoting health and wellness based on nutritionally sound practices.

Nutritional requirements are complex and ever-changing in the growing child. Collaborative sessions with pediatric nutritionists and pharmacists aid in identifying those nutrients necessary and utilizing commercial products appropriately designed for the child. All pediatric health care providers should seek to incorporate knowledge of developmental facets into the overall care of their patients and families.

DEVELOPMENTAL CONSIDERATIONS

The First Two Years: Premature and Normal Infants

The infant's pattern of feeding behavior begins developing very early. Its foundation lies within the neuromotor architecture of the brain and the central nervous system. This complex blend of the physical and psychosocial reflects early structural and neuromuscular development. As early as 7 weeks in utero the fetus demonstrates oral reflexes. Many of the elementary neural and muscular components of sucking and swallowing are functioning in the third to fourth prenatal month.[5] Tastebuds are present well before the middle of gestation.

The premature infant of 28 weeks' or less gestation has weak or absent sucking and swallowing reflexes. In those older than 32 weeks, reflexes are present but not adequate to maintain nutrition. These infants are generally not interested in feeding, and their appetite does not serve as a guide to nutritional requirements. Incorporation of oral reflexes and physio-psychological readiness for the feeding process is generally not well-established until close to 35–36 weeks' gestation.

Normal-term infants have a rounded mouth and special fat pads in both cheeks that help the lips pucker. The sucking reflex involves protraction and retraction of the tongue in a lick-suck pattern. The ability to suck depends on the competency of the lip structure and the relationship of the mandible to the maxilla. The initial rooting reflex is complemented by the suck-swallow, which requires adequate tone of the lip structures. Also essential is the integrity of the palatal structures with the oral reflexes of rooting, suck-swallow, gag, bite, and the asymmetrical tonic neck reflex.

At birth, peristalsis and swallowing are unstable; vigorous sucking is preceded by rooting movements but the infant may stop sucking, rest, and even sleep for brief periods during a feeding. Five behavioral stages have been delineated:[6]

1. Prefeeding: the level of arousal shown before feeding, indicating hunger.
2. Approach: the predominant physical mode of reaching out to food.
3. Attachment: activities enacted during nipple engagement and nursing.
4. Consummatory: the act of sucking and swallowing
5. Satiety: acts that indicate saturation.

By 3 months sucking is stronger and is no longer preceded by rooting movements. At this point, the infant shows excitement at the sight of food and sucks or "mouths" fingers and anything held in the hands. By the time the child is 5 months of age, the lips can approximate a cup and the extension reflex (a tongue reaction were excessive foods are pushed out of the oral cavity) becomes voluntary.

Sick or premature infants should be assessed for potential feeding disorders. Preventive nursing care is usually indicated when the infant requires tube or parenteral nourishment. Simple procedures such as the use of pacifiers during gavage feeding appear to enhance growth and gastrointestinal (GI) function in these infants. In one study, investigators found nonnutritive sucking (NNS) in premature infants shortened the time for completion of initial feeding and transitions to total nipple feeding as well as GI time. Increased weight gain in the NNS group suggests that its use may influence nutrient absorption or energy expenditure.[7]

Feeding reflexes may be absent, delayed, or impaired, and deviant oral-motor patterns may develop. With prolonged tube feeding, infants can develop increased oral sensitivity and abnormal tongue movements.[8] Persistent rooting may lead to excessive head motion and interfere with feeding. The sucking reflex and infantile suck-swallow may not extinguish. Lack of coordination between jaw and tongue can result in ineffective swallowing.

These early feeding patterns are so closely linked to development of future speech patterns that any abnormality may affect the child's attempts to babble and later make articulate sounds. Nursing consults with speech therapy practioners can individualize programs for specific infants and establish protocols for the overall care of these high risk patients.

Both in the hospital and home setting, nursing plans should address the parent-child and family interaction. Food is highly symbolic, frequently equated with love and caring in our culture. A mother's image of herself as well as the image she projects to others is often strongly colored by her role in the feeding situation. Moore describes eating as human and feeding as maternal; the mother's self-esteem is deeply involved.[9] Failure to accomplish the task of feeding the child brings into question the mother's basic competency in our society.

Feeding problems can develop very early with these alternatively nourished infants—by failure to enact the feeding behaviors and, conversely or jointly, the failure of the reciprocal feeder/parent to react to the infant's behavior.

Parents and nursing staff need to be in tune with their babies to recognize components of the feeding behavior cues. Failure to recognize developing individuality or faulty interpretation of the message cues communicated by a child can lead to inappropriate action on the part of the parent or caretaker and confusion for the infant. Nurses' powers of observation and understanding of normative development should be shared with the parents so that responses to verbal or conceptual communication answer the child's actual needs.

The second stage in the feeding process begins normally between 4 to 6 months of age with demonstration of the readiness of fine and gross motor skills. The tongue, initially concave and flat, gradually forms a central depression during sucking, and food is more effectively carried back to the pharynx. The child learns to adjust the degree of mouth munching. Munching appears to evolve from a combination of the primitive phasic bite reflex and the sucking pattern. The food is mashed against the hard palate and mixed with saliva.

Infants on total parenteral feedings—if at all possible—should be allowed some type of oral sustenance, even if it is minimal. Besides the potential (as yet unsubstantiated) positive trophic effect enteric stimulation may offer, it serves also to decrease the likelihood of adverse food reactions such as rumination when food is no longer medically contraindicated. Although there are no studies in the literature to date, my clinical experience is that these total parenteral nutrition (TPN) infants later demonstrate feeding and speech difficulties if unable to experience some oral stimulation during this critical early period, as described by Illingsworth and Lister.[10]

Also important during this period is the beginning coordination between eye and body movements. Older infants explore the world with eyes, fingers, hands, and mouth; by 4 months they learn to reach their mouths with their hands; by 6 months they will be able to feed themselves biscuits. This second stage of the sensorimotor period, as described by Piaget, reflects the infant's learning through moving, touching, and feeling. Our techniques of nutrient provision thus should ideally not alter these experiences. Nevertheless, it is a common practice for infants and toddlers that are tube-fed or have central line catheters to have either their hands or movement restrained as demonstrated in Figure 8-1.

The caveat for nursing practice is clear—although nursing interventions must address the child's safety—restraints that inhibit movement and self-exploration impede the development of trust, which is vital for this age group. Techniques that "limit mobility and opportunity for discovery and social interchange will affect all other phases of the developmental process."[11] All too often nurses assume volition in these young children when they find a tube or dressing undone; actually the infant is seeking visual stimulation or tactile

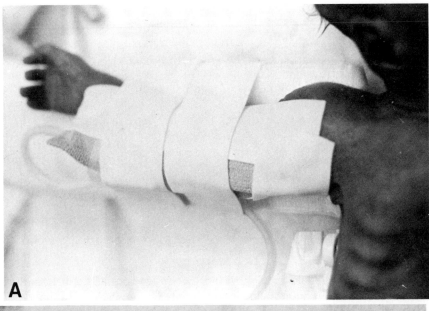

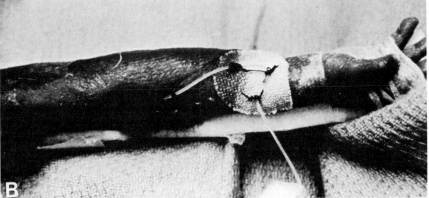

Fig. 8-1. (A) Peripheral bulky intravenous line dressing with restraint of elbow. (B) Central intravenous line inserted peripherally with taping restraint of fingers.

experiences. It is normal for infants to chew on fingers and toes. If you immobilize part of their body, it should be no surprise that they will seek other objects to manipulate and chew. An alternative is demonstrated in Figure 8-2.

Early Childhood

Progression to self-feeding is a hallmark development in the yearling stage. Children at this time begin to demonstrate their awareness of self as distinct from others. They learn by exploring and testing limits with their new-found mobility

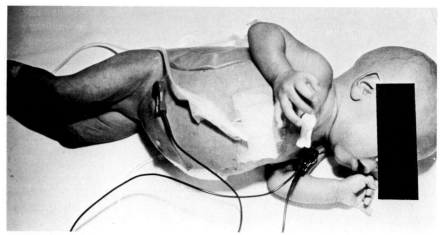

Fig. 8-2. Subclavian central venous line which allows mobility of upper torso.

and its attendant "independence." Achieving self-feeding skills enhances early self-image. This requires good finger and thumb flexor muscles, arm-hand and eye-hand coordination, palmar grasp, and intact oral-motor skills.

During this period, provision of specialized nutrition must be incorporated into the child's struggle for autonomy. An issue often at stake among hospitalized children is the loss of their new-found control. If not addressed, frustration and anger at painful procedures and confinement will erode or block confidence derived from the achievement of a sense of autonomy. If independence and autonomy are fostered, the child can proceed to develop initiative.

One 6-year old girl illustrates this point. After being home on TPN for a month, she was referred to our follow-up clinic. She was unusually withdrawn and quiet. The physical examination and family history revealed no problems, but in exploring the family's management of their TPN regimen, it was revealed that during her nightly 12-hour cycling, she was needing to void frequently. Since she had been instructed by her parents not to touch any of her heavy intravenous (IV) equipment and so was unable to get out of bed to go to the bathroom, she was having "accidents" in bed. The parents, frustrated by this development, took to diapering her. Diapers, when they must be worn beyond the age of 2-1/2 or 3 years old, become an embarassment to children, especially when they have previously achieved continence. This loss of control upset the 6-year-old girl and resulted in her depression and loss of self-esteem. A more concentrated solution to decrease total TPN volume, a change to a portable IV unit, and establishing a routine whereby her parents helped her to the bathroom before they retired for the night, resulted in the termination of any incontinence.

Lack of interest in food and erratic food jags are common in this age group. Patterns of food intake, food preferences, and management of mealtime behavior are all significant issues at this time. Superimpose chronic illness, hospitalization, or unusual routes of feeding and problems are bound to arise. Jeter explains that, "Young children are likely to perceive that the parts of their body that receive the most attention must be the most important. If these 'most important' organs are damaged, they may feel wholly inferior."[12] With their transductive thinking—whereby cause and effect are directly related—and fertile imaginative processes, young children frequently assume they are to blame when something goes wrong. Illness or therapeutic intervention can then be perceived as punishment for being "bad" or for harboring some unknown secret thought.

Children who require prolonged tube feedings, gastrostomy, or parenteral feedings frequently have numerous hospitalizations and may have endured several operative procedures. The effects of the chronicity of their conditions on overall development have generally gone unrecognized. Chronic illness, interspersed with frequent periods of crisis, keeps the family in a prolonged period of disorganization and uncertainty. This is aggravated by the extreme separation and despair characteristic of long-term hospitalization. Parents can become overwhelmed by the complexity of the child's physical problems and dependence on technology for survival: "They often cope with their feelings by avoiding the child and/or adopting a parenting technology associated with the child's disease. The result of both coping strategies is the failure to relate to the 'real' child. . . ."[13]

In an effort to achieve normalcy, increasing numbers of children are being sent home with specialized nutritional procedures and requirements. Teaching skills to parents thus assumes increasing significance. An organized and methodical program of home care will need to address both technique and psychodynamic issues to ensure the child's optimal growth and development.

Late Childhood

Late childhood and puberty are periods when the child increases dealings with people outside the immediate family. Food is frequently associated with a social setting and companionship, especially with peers. School and its related activities normally take up a significant amount of the child's day, providng not only academic training but also important social interactions. Conformity in appearance and bodily privacy are sensitive issues at this stage. For some chronically ill children, developmental delay has been traced to insufficient social stimulation during multiple hospitalizations.[14]

School-age children requiring specialized nutrition respond well to nursing interactions that facilitate the child's adaptation to intrusive procedures.

Oncology nurse specialist E. T. Wear and colleagues state, maintenance of autonomy includes providing the child with opportunities to control as many of the conditions before, during, and after the procedure as is realistically possible. Having these opportunities affords the child a safe, positive way to adapt to the stress of the procedure and reduces the threat of doubt and shame inherent in losing all control.*

At this age children are active learners whose understanding is facilitated by manipulation of objects. Opportunities to handle and experiment with procedure equipment thus benefit their development. They are often interested in the purpose of a procedure and demonstrate great curiosity about the world around them and their bodies.

In both hospital practice and parent home-management, we have found it useful to incorporate children's desires to exert control and do things for themselves. By establishing a set routine, encouraging them to prepare any equipment possible (cut tape, open alcohol pads, etc.), one minimizes postponing request and problems (i.e., laying still during dressing changes, etc.).

Wear et al. state that "Because meeting expectations of themselves and adults can be so important . . . they also benefit from a description of the behaviors required during the procedure. Relating these behaviors to situations they have experienced can help them understand and comply."[15]

Limitations such as restrictions on participation in sports, parties, and other group activities decrease the child's opportunity for group recognition—an important determinant in self-esteem. Plans should be made with staff and family to incorporate activities that allow the child to experience successful group interactions and feedback.

SPECIALIZED NUTRITION

Approaches to Nourishing

Scientific developments in specialized nutrition via enteral and parenteral routes have expanded our ability to deal with starvation and illness in both the hospital and home environment. Concomitantly, technological advances in pediatric care and neonatal intensive care have reduced morbidity and mortality for infants and children, enhancing the survival capabilities of the pediatric population.

Pediatric conditions involving specialized nutrition present an extraordinary challenge to the nurse. This section will review approaches to nourishing children, nutrient requirements, and requisite nursing care. Below are listed those conditions that are common indicators for enteral nutrition intervention:

1. Prematurity of generally less than 34-weeks' gestation.
2. Inability to suck or swallow (e.g., developmentally delayed children).

---

* From Wear ET, Covey J, Brush M: Facilitating children's adaptation to intrusive procedures, in Fochtman D, Foley GV (eds): Nursing Care of the Child with Cancer. Boston, Little, Brown, 1982, p 69. With permission.

Table 8-1
Pediatric Feeding Tubes*

Name	Material	Sizes tube caliber/size infant 3.5 Fr <1.5 kg 5.0 Fr 1.5–12 kg 6-8 Fr >12 kg	Length
Argyle PVC (Sherwood Medical, St. Louis, MO)	Polyvinylchloride	3.5 Fr 5 Fr 6 Fr	12" 16"
Argyle Indwell	Polyurethane	5 Fr	20" and 36"
Argyle Quest Duo-tube		5 Fr 6 Fr	40" 40"
Accumark (Concord Labs, Keene, NH)		5 Fr	15", 20", 40"
Biosearch Pediatric, Dobbhoff & Entinflex (Biosearch Medical Products, Somerville, NJ)		6 Fr	20"
Corpak Nutrition (Corpak Co., Wheeling, IL)	Polyurethane	6 Fr 8 Fr	22", 36" 22", 36"
Ethox (Buffalo, NY)	Polyurethane	5 Fr	42"
Keofeed-Ivac Corp. (San Diego, CA)	Polyurethane	6 Fr	variety

3. Congenital anomalies (e.g., esophageal atresia, tracheo-esophageal fistula, and some types of cleft palate).
4. Hypermetabolic states (e.g., cardiac disease, severe respiratory distress, thermal burns, severe trauma, cancer).
5. Need for continuous infusion of partially digested nutrients (e.g., recovery from severe diarrhea or in short bowel syndrome).
6. Inability to absorb adequate nutrients (e.g., cancer and cystic fibrosis).
7. Refusal to eat (e.g., anorexia nervosa).
8. After intestinal resection.

Enteral feeding routes include: the mouth for simple supplementation; nasogastric, naso-duodenal, and jejunal (transpyloric); gastrostomy and jejunostomy. Indications, contraindications, insertion, and nursing care techniques are similar in principle to procedures for adults (see Chapter 5). Table 8-1 lists available tubes and pediatric sizes.

For pediatric nasogastric insertion, the nurse should gently but steadily

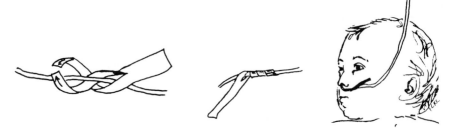

Fig. 8-3.   Preferred taping of nasogastric tube.

thread the tube through the nostril to the predetermined point. There should be no resistance; however, the child will experience gagging. Periodically, swallowing sips of water or sucking on a pacifier may help the child pass the tube more easily. Infants must breathe through their mouths. Don't constantly block this airway with a pacifier. Difficult passage, resistance, choking, coughing, or color change are indications for withdrawing the tube for reinsertion.

Secure the tube in place with clear nonallergic tape or paper tape only. The tube should be taped flat as it leaves the nares. Under no circumstances should the tube be pulled up and against the tip of the nares or against nasal mucosa where it will cause irritation and tissue breakdown. Narrow adhesive tape fits around the tube and across the cheek in one strip, thereby preventing the tube's slipping out of place. Use of tincture of benzoin is not recommended in infants and children to help secure the tape and tube but may be applied before taping if tape alone has proven unsuccessful (Fig. 8-3).

In children with difficulty passing transpyloric tubes, 0.1 mg/kg (< 6 years old) or 2.5–5 mg (6–14 years old) metoclopramide (Reglan; A. H. Robins, Richmond, VA) IV should be administered every 6 hours for 3 doses to increase gastric motility. It has been shown to facilitate passage into the small bowel.

For children receiving gastrostomy feedings, elevate the head of the bed 50 degrees or hold the child in an upright position. Allow an infant to suck on a pacifier during feeding. If infant cannot be held, position him or her on the right side with the head elevated 30 degrees. Aspirate gently to check for stomach contents. If aspiration is not accomplished easily or resistance is met, reposition the child and try again. General guidelines for greater than normal residual are as follows:

- Premature infants up to 3 months: > than 30 cc
- Infants 3–12 months: > than 45 cc
- Children over 1 year or on a bolus schedule greater: > than 60 cc

Follow irrigant with feeding. Feeding should run in slowly by gravity over 20–25 minutes. The nurse administering any enteral feedings should be familiar with the complications listed in Table 8-2.

Table 8-2
Potential Problems Associated With Pediatric Enteral Tube Feedings

Mechanical
1. Respiratory compromise
   · Indwelling nasogastric—partial upper airway obstruction
   · Intermittent nasogastric—severity and frequency of apnea induced by vagal stimulation
   · Oralgastric—apnea induced mucous production necessitating frequent suctioning and retaping
   · Oralgastric—displacement of tube by tongue movements
2. Material related
   · Gastrointestinal perforation with stiffening after 3-day usage
   · Nasal trauma with improper insertion and taping technique

Metabolic
1. Dumping syndrome—usage of hyperosmolar solutions (>300 mOsm)
2. High intestinal losses of potassium and fats—transpyloric route

Psychosocial
1. Absence of or loss of normal feeding behaviors

Enteral Feedings

The formulas appropriate for the full-term infant under one year of age are listed below.[15] The products listed are suitable for the full-term infant when a cow's milk formula of normal dilution or a calorically concentrated formula is desired. Nutrient distribution is essentially the same as human milk, and there is no significant difference in composition among these products.

Normal Dilution (20 kcal/oz)

- Enfamil (Mead Johnson & Co., Evansville, IN), with and without iron
- Similac, (Ross Laboratories, Columbus, OH), with and without iron

Concentrated Caloric Density

- Enfamil® 24 kcal/oz, with iron only
- Similac® 24 kcal/oz, with and without iron
- Similac® 27 kcal/oz, without iron only

Formulas designed for the premature infant with an immature GI tract necessitate manipulation of all three major nutrients. Lactose is found in human milk and may therefore have special significance; however, the low birth weight (LBW) infant's lactase activity does not reach that of the full-term infant until the ninth month of gestation. Therefore, in these formulas only 40–50 percent of the carbohydrate is available as lactose. This mixture of carbohydrates facilitates utilization because multiple digestive and absorptive pathways are involved. The whey:casein ratio (60:40) of human milk is incorporated in these formulas because (1) whey forms smaller, more digestible curds, avoiding lactobezoar formation, and (2) it offers a more appropriate amino acid composition that is higher in cystine, which may be essential to the LBW infant, and lower in tyrosine, an amino acid that a LBW infant may not have the metabolic pathways to handle. LBW infants frequently are unable to digest long-chain saturated fats that form insoluble calcium: fatty-acid complexes resulting in impaired absorption of fats, calcium, and other minerals. This poor digestion is thought to be related to low bile acid pools and poor reabsorption of the bile acids, thus medium-chain tryglycerides (MCT) oil has been utilized. None of these formulas are fortified with iron, nor are they available outside the hospital without prescription. The LBW infant still requires supplementation with a multivitamin preparation with the following products.

Similac Special Care® (20 kcal/oz and 24 kcal/oz)

- Requires approximately 8–10 oz/day to meet calcium needs

Premature Enfamil® (20 kcal/oz and 24 kcal/oz)

- Requires approximately 12–14 oz/day to meet calcium needs

"Preemie" SMA (Wyeth Laboratories, Philadelphia, PA) (24 kcal/oz)

- Requires approximately 16–18 oz/day to meet calcium needs

Formulations with low renal solute load are often used when the infant's status requires a low sodium intake (containing approximately half the sodium of other infant formulas). Both formulas have often been used with the premature infant secondary to their whey:casein ratio (60:40) and have been well-tolerated. They have less than optimal features for the premature infant, however, because the carbohydrate content is 100% lactose and the levels of folic acid, calcium, and vitamin E are inadequate. These Formulas are listed below:

- SMA® 20 kcal/oz, 24 kcal/oz, and 27 kcal/oz; all with iron
- PM 60/40 (Ross Laboratories, Columbus, OH) 20 kcal/oz without iron

Formulas with manipulations of carbohydrate source secondary to allergy or disaccharidase deficiency are designed for the full-term infant and are iron-fortified. Most come as concentrate liquid and powder form that can be easily mixed to increase kcal concentration. These Formulas are described below:

- Isomil (Ross Laboratories, Columbus, OH) (20 kcal/oz) has a soy protein base and is lactose-free. Hypoallergenic soy protein isolate is used when cow's milk allergy is diagnosed. It is lactose-free for the management of lactose intolerance due to diarrhea, primary lactose intolerance, and galactosemia. Use in the premature infant can induce phosphous deficiency rickets.

- Prosobee (Mead Johnson, Evansville, IN) (20 kcal/oz) is a lactose- and sucrose-free soy protein base. The indications listed for Isomil are also applicable. In addition, it is appropriate when chronic or transient diarrhea also causes a sucrose deficiency and can be used in gluten sensitivity.
- Nursoy (Wyeth Laboratories, Philadelphia, PA) (20 kcal/oz) is a lactose- and corn-free soy protein base for use when corn allergy is diagnosed.

Nutramigen (Mead Johnson, Evansville, IN) and Pregestimil (Mead Johnson, Evansville, IN) are hypoallergenic protein hydrolysates for easy protein digestion. Further details are as follows:

- Nutramigen® (20 kcal/oz) is indicated primarily in cow's milk allergy or other protein-allergic sensitivity, severe or multiple food allergies, severe or persistent diarrhea, or other GI disturbances. It is also used as a maintenance diet during elimination-diet testing and in galactosemia.
- Pregestimil® (20 kcal/oz) is appropriate for idiopathic defects in digestion or absorption, intestinal resection, intractable diarrhea, cystic fibrosis, steatorrhea, and food allergies. It contains 40 percent of fat kilocalories as MCT oil. It is iron-fortified and an ideal elemental formula for infants.
- Portagen (Mead Johnson, Evansville, IN) (20 kcal/oz) is a modified fat source and should be used when significant steatorrhea occurs in the following conditions: cystic fibrosis, intestinal resections, pancreatic insufficiency, lymphatic anomalies (intestinal lymphangiectasia, etc.), celiac disease, and biliary atresia. Available only in powder form, it is iron-fortified and contains 86 percent of fat kilocalories as MCT oil.

Oral electrolyte solutions for maintenance of fluid and elecrolyte balance during mild to moderate diarrhea and in recovery from diarrhea contain a balanced formulation including electrolytes, calories, and water in proportions needed to prevent metabolic deficits. These solutions are listed below:

- Pedialyte (Ross Laboratories, Columbus, OH) (6 kcal/oz) is glucose with 3 mEq Na: 2 mEq K: 3 mEq Cl, mOsm = 368.
- Lytren (Mead Johnson, Evansville, IN) (9 kcal/oz) is glucose and sucrose with 3 mEq Na: 2.5 mEq K: 2.5 mEq Cl, mOsm = 267.

RCF (Ross Laboratories, Columbus, OH) (24 kcal/oz) is for infants with metabolic disorders. It is used for dietary management of infants or children unable to tolerate disaccharides or other carbohydrates. Specific indications include intractable diarrhea and glycogen storage disease. The concentrate does not provide a completely balanced formula unless diluted with table sugar, dextrose, polycose (glucose polymers) or corn syrup. It allows flexibility in the type and amount of carbohydrate that can be tolerated. It also contains soy protein to avoid symptoms of cow's milk allergy or sensitivity and is iron-fortified.

MSUD (Mead Johnson, Evansville, IN) (20 kcal/oz) is for the management of branched-chain ketoacidemia. It is an amino acid mixture free of the branched-chain amino acids that also contain the fat, carbohydrate, vitamins, and minerals essential for the infant. It can be used as the sole diet until plasma levels of leucine, isoleucine, and valine return to normal range. Supplementation with an infant formula or milk to provide sufficient branched-chain amino acids to meet minimal requirements is necessary as soon as plasma levels return to normal.

Lofenalac (Mead Johnson, Evansville, IN) (20 kcal/oz) is for the management of infants with phenylketonuria. It contains 11 mg phenylalanine per 100 ml, which is not adequate to meet the total daily requirement of the growing infant. Sufficient phenylalanine from other sources such as infant formula, breast milk, or cow's milk may be added to Lofenalac® to meet the patient's minimum requirements for growth and development.

Some formulas provide a complete diet without lactose (for children over 1-year old. (Table 8-3). These diets are appropriate for patients with normal gut function or slight dysfunction of the GI tract. They contain normal nutrient distribution with an optimal nonprotein kcal:N ratio of 150–200:1 and are available in a ready-to-use form. Used in hypermetabolic states, head and neck injuries (i.e., radiation to these areas or wired jaws), coma, burns, protein-calorie malnutrition, inflammatory bowel disease, celiac disease, and mild pancreatic insufficiency, these formulas contain intact nutrients that require normal digestion and are not suitable in the presence of severe pancreatic insufficiency, a short or damaged intestine, or when the patient needs bowel rest (i.e., during treatment of intestinal fistulas). All require additional free water secondary to solute load. Unless otherwise indicated, all products are unpalatable when taken orally, contain no lactose, gluten, or oxalate, and are very low in purine, cholesterol, and residue content. Most provide 1 kcal/cc. Certain formulas indicate nasojejunal (NJ) or jejunal (J) as an acceptable, well-tolerated route of administration and as such should usually be given as continuous infusions.

Parenteral Feeding

Conditions that may require TPN are listed in Table 8-4. The preferred route of parenteral nutrition in those children who are going to be alimented for greater than 7-days' duration and in whom growth and development is a desired goal is by central access. Placement of long-term parenteral nutritional catheters is indicated in those children who require home parenteral nutrition, those who have short-bowel syndrome, or require TPN for greater than one month.

The other route for intravenous nutrition is by peripheral infusions. Most newborn infants with respiratory problems are begun on peripheral parenteral alimentation until feedings are tolerated. An occasional postoperative infant that is expected to recover in a rapid fashion can also be supported with peripheral TPN. The major complication with prolonged therapy is the development of soft-tissue skin sloughs. This is likely to occur in a small premature baby who is receiving a prolonged course of peripheral venous nutrition via a pump driving at a high pressure with glucose concentrations exceeding 10 percent. To prevent

Table 8-3
Tube Feedings, Without Lactose

Formula	Route*	Indications
Complete B Modified	NG, G, bolus	To be used when a home-blenderized diet is anticipated. Contains moderate amounts of fruit and plant fiber. Lactose-containing version is still available (with dry skim milk) and may be beneficial when a higher residue diet is needed. Contains purines.
Isocal (Mead Johnson, Evansville, IN)	NG, G, NJ, or J, bolus	Contains intact sources of nutrients (protein isolates)—with exception of fat—of 37%, 30% is soy oil, 7% MCT oil. Can be used as a home blenderized diet and is isotonic.
Osmolite (Ross Labs, Columbus, OH)	NG, G, NJ, or J, bolus	Is very similar in composition to Isocal except a greater % kcals come from MCT oil (16%) and therefore may be helpful in the management of patients with fat malabsorption. Also isotonic.
Portagen (Mead Johnson, Evansville, IN)	NG, G, NJ, or J	Unique in that 34% of total come from MCT oil. Product should be used when fat absorption is impaired as may occur in the following clinical conditions: pancreatic insufficiency, bile acid deficiency, some intestinal resections, and lymphatic anomalies. It needs to be ordered as 1 kcal/ml because it is also available as an infant formula. Requires mixing.

this complication, peripheral catheters should be rotated every 72 hours and secured with clear tape so that the infusion site can be examined frequently. Should any signs of an early slough develop, the catheters should be promptly removed.[16] Contrary to recommendations for immediate excision and grafting, it has been found in the pediatric population that local care to these particular sloughs with saline wet-to-dry dressing or Silvadine rarely produces a long-term problem.[17,18]

A higher complication rate exists in patients having central catheters in place, but when one takes into account the length of therapy that such patients receive, the per diem risk rate for peripheral and central routes are largely the

Table 8-3
Continued

Formula	Route*	Indications
Tube Feedings/Oral Supplements Without Lactose		
Precision (Doyle Pharmaceutical, Minneapolis, MN)	P.O., NG, G, bolus	Slightly lower fat content at This p.o. supplement has been well-tolerated particularly with inflammatory bowel diseases. Orange and vanilla flavors available. Isotonic. Requires mixing.
Ensure (Ross Labs, Columbus, OH)	P.O., NG, G, bolus	Because it is slightly hypertonic it should be sipped slowly to avoid diarrhea and is not suggested as a transpyloric feeding. Multi-flavored: vanilla, chocolate, and strawberry. All but chocolate are purine free.
Ensure Plus (Ross Labs, Columbus, OH)	P.O., continuous G or NG	Contains less than optimal nonprotein kcal:nitrogen ratio, but is actually more palatable than Ensure 1 kcal/cc. It is particularly important to sip slowly (600 mOsm H_2O) and is not recommended as a transpyloric feeding. Flavors as above.
Magnacal (Organon, West Orange, NJ) 2 kcal/cc	P.O., continuous NG or G	Particularly useful in fluid restrictions or when patient is unable to ingest adequate volumes of food (i.e., oncology patients). Transpyloric feedings are not recommended. Available in bland vanilla so a variety of flavors can be added. As product is a concentrated source of nutrients, fluid balance must be closely monitored.

same (Table 8-5). In a large series assessing the relative risk of each mode, little difference was noted.[19] This study emphasized the fact that a higher glucose and fat solution can be administered centrally, and that this higher caloric intake is associated with a concomitant higher weight gain. On the basis of these studies, it can be seen that the caloric requirements and estimated caloric needs of the patient are the only real criteria to decide whether the patient should be alimented peripherally or centrally when parenteral alimentation is necessary.

The subclavian venous route is beneficial because of the ease of performing the catheterization, comfort and ease of activity for the patient, and the fact that

Table 8-3
Continued

Formula	Route*	Indications
Elemental Diet Without Lactose		
Vital (Ross Labs, Columbus, OH)	Continuous NG, G, P.O. when flavored	Indicated when significant GI dysfunction is present, such as that found in steatorrhea secondary to severe pancreatic insufficiency, radiation therapy to the bowel, and short gut syndrome. Also indicated for treatment of intractable diarrhea, exudative enteropath, bowel rest, and lower intestinal fistulas. Because it is absorbed proximally and has a low residue content, it is appropriate as bowel prep. Note that it contains an adequate % of linoleic kcal to prevent fatty acid deficiency. Not suggested as a transpyloric feeding secondary to its high osmolality (460 mOsm).

From Zitarelli MB, Healy M, Lechner D, et al: Indications for Commercial Tube Formulas and Indications For Commercial Tube Feedings and Supplements (in part). Philadelphia, Children's Hospital of Philadelphia, 1982. With permission.
*NG = nasogastric, G = gastric, NJ = nasojejunal, J = jejunal, P.O. = by mouth

repeated catheterizations from the right to the left side can be performed without causing the loss of any major vessels. Individual cases may require utilization of other, less accessible veins such as the internal jugular. Use of this vein, however, severely limits head movement by the child, and it is difficult to maintain dressings in this area. The preferred route for insertion of a Broviac catheter is to use either the external jugular technique or the facial vein by cutdown, passing the catheter through the internal jugular vein and down into the superior vena cava.[20,21] This catheter is likewise tunneled out onto the chest. For children over age five, percutaneous insertion of the catheter can be accomplished using strict aseptic technique in a treatment room. Younger children, especially premature infants, should have placement done in the operating room or intensive care unit because of the small size of the vein. Alternatively, a percutaneous Broviac (Evermead, Kirkland, WA) catheter can be inserted using a modified Seldinger technique with a 5- or 8-Fr peel-away sheath.[22] See Table 8-6 for a list of lines commercially available.

Table 8-4
Common Indications for TPN in Pediatric Patients

Surgical
  Omphaloceles
  Intestinal atresia
  Tracheoesophageal fistula
  Diaphragmatic hernia
  Volvulus and malrotation
  Short bowel syndrome
  Gastroschisis
  Meconium ileus and peritonitis
  Hirschsprung's disease
Medical
  Chylothorax
  Low birth weight ($<$ 1500 g)
  Necrotizing enterocolitis
  Failure-to-thrive 2°:
    Anorexia nervosa
    Cardiac cachexia
    Cystic fibrosis
    Intractable diarrhea
    Tumor burden and/or chemotherapy
  Inflammatory bowel disease
  Pancreatitis
  Chronic idiopathic intestinal pseudo-obstruction syndrome
  Chronic malabsorption 2° congenital deficiencies (metabolic)
  Hypercatabolic states 2°:
      Trauma
      Burns
      Severe infection–sepsis
  Renal failure
  Hepatic failure
  Secretory diarrhea

Catheter Care

The basic principles of catheter care for adults discussed elsewhere in this book (see Chapter 6) also apply to pediatric patients. Aseptic technique is even more critical in the neonatal population, however, because of the patients' relatively immature immunologic status. LBW infants in particular are most susceptible to bacterial infections. Boettcher and Pereira[23] cite 4 faulty mechanisms: (1) deficient supply of neutrophils,[24] (2) decreased bacteriocidal activity of leukocytes,[25,26] (3) impaired chemotaxis of neutrophils and monocytes,[27,28] and (4) deficient supply of complement.[29] Additionally, malnutrition compromises these infants' immunologic defense systems.

The second pediatric subgroup also at higher risk is the child with oncologic

Table 8-5
Potential Problems Associated With Pediatric TPN

Mechanical
  1. Placement of catheter or needle
  2. Duration of invasive device
Infection
  1. Local topical injection
  2. Early or late systemic primary sepsis
Metabolic
  1. Carbohydrate Disorders
      Hyperglycemia
      Glycosuria
      Osmotic diuresis
      Hyperosmolar coma
      Hypercarbia
      Rebound hypoglycemia
  2. Amino Acid Disorders
      Hyperammonemia
      Amino acid imbalance
      Prerenal azotemia
      Hyperchloremic metabolic acidosis
  3. Lipid Disorders
      Hypertriglyceridemia
      Enhanced indirect bilirubin deviation
      Impaired white cell function
      Impaired lung function for oxygen transport
      Thrombocytopenia
  4. Fluids
      Overload
      Refeeding edema
Psychosocial
  1. Separation from family
  2. Food aversions—rumination
  3. Developmental delay

problems. Infections are a significant cause of morbidity and mortality.[30] Chemotherapy, radiotherapy, and antineoplastic therapy compromise the child's already inadequate white cell response. Infection risk varies with the type of neoplasm—lymphoproliferative malignancies being greater than solid tumors. The reader is referred to an extensive review of this subject by the Association of Pediatric Oncology Nurses.[31]

Many useful techniques have been designed by nurses to circumvent the technical problems encountered in adapting equipment for pediatric use. Fortunately, the commercial market is beginning to address some of these problems with the manufacturing of pediatric products (Figs. 8-4 and 8-5).

Table 8-6
Pediatric Central Line Catheters

Name	Material	Sizes	Insertion	Removal
Broviac	silastic	4 Fr/infant	percutaneous	cutdown
(Evermed, Kirkland, WA)		8 Fr/ped	or cutdown	
Centrasil	silastic	16 g	percutaneous	straight
(Travenol, Deerfield, IL)			or cutdown	
Hemed	silicone	4 Fr	cutdown	cutdown
(GISH Biomed Inc.,		6.6 Fr		
Santa Ana, CA)		7.0 Fr	double lumen	
Intramedicut	polyvinyl	14 g	percutaneous	straight
(Sherwood Medical,		16 g		
St. Louis, MO)		18 g		
		20 g		
Pediatric Racif				
(Quinton Instrument Co.,				
Seattle, WA)				

Because of their limited ability to self-report difficulties, children and especially infants require careful nursing observation and assessment. Monitoring parameters to include in a nursing care plan should include at least the following:

1. Vital signs: every four hours. If the vital signs are unstable, TPR and BP should be taken every hour.
2. Strict intake and output. Skin turgor and mucous membranes should be assessed for hydration.
3. Growth Parameters: (a) Daily weight should be taken at the same time each day, with the same scale, amount of clothing, and/or equipment. Infants who gain more than 30 g/day indicate retention of water. (b) Length should be measured recumbent weekly for infants. (c) Height should be measured monthly for children. (d) Head circumference should be measured weekly for infants and monthly for children less than 2 years of age.
4. Urine: glucose, protein, ketones, specific gravity, and pH. Urine determinations are necessary to be sure the child is able to tolerate the solutions and also to assess nutritional status. They should be done: (a) every four hours for the first 24 hours after the initiation of therapy and for the 24-hour period after an increase in glucose concentration or substantial increase in the volume of the solution feeding, (b) every 8 hours after this initial phase of therapy when all urine studies are within normal limits, (c) every 24 hours once at home on feeding.
5. Hematologic values: (a) Daily when stable: glucose, Na, K, Chl, CO_2. (b)

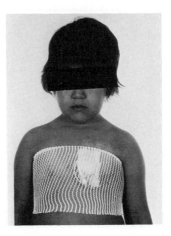

Fig. 8-4. Tubular style alternative to chest wall taping of central venous line.

Weekly: BUN, creatinine, calcium, phosphorus, magnesium, total and direct bilirubin, alkaline phosphatase, serum glutamic oxaloacetic transaminase (SGOT), serum glutamic pyruvic transaminase (SGPT), total protein and albumin, free fatty acid. (c) Monthly: zinc,* copper,* selenium.* (d) When imbalance is chemically suspected: biotin, chromium,* managanese,* iodide,* folate, B_{12}, NH_3, Fe.

Nutrients

Although the dietary requirements for most nutrients taken by mouth are fairly well established, empirical information pertaining to parenteral requirements is less available. Nowhere is this lack more apparent than in the case of premature infants. In the absence of exact knowledge of parenteral requirements, extrapolations have been made from enteral data.

The following sections briefly review guidelines of daily nutrient requirements. A number of excellent review articles have been written describing nutritional requirements of preterm infants, older infants, and children.[8,23,32–35]

---

* Requires metal-free syringe and storage tubes.

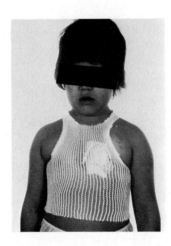

Fig. 8-5.   T-shirt style alternative to chest wall taping of central venous line.

Fluid

Fluid requirements are based on replacement of ongoing normal losses and can be altered by numerous situations:[36] (1) environmental temperature, including incubators, phototherapy warmers, ambient temperature, drafts, heat shields, and humidity level, and (2) medical status, including respiratory distress syndrome, hypermetabolic state, fever, diarrhea, renal olguria, glycosuria, and medications.

Daily maintenance in neonates range as listed below:

- First week of life: 40–60 ml/kg/day
- 1–2 weeks: 100–200 ml/kg/day
- 3–12 weeks: 130–140 ml/kg/day

Maintenance for term infants and children is delineated below:

- 1–10 kg: 100 ml/kg/day
- 11–20 kg: 1000 ml + 50 ml/kg for each kg >10
- >20 kg: 1500 ml + 20 ml/kg for each kg >20

Tables 8-7, 8-8, 8-9 list enteral requirements for this population.

Table 8-7
Recommended Dietary Allowances

| Age | Weight | | Height | | Protein | Energy Needs | |
years	kg	lbs	cm	in	g	kcal	(w/range)
0.0–0.5	6	13	60	24	kg × 2.2	kg × 115	(95–145)
0.5–1.0	9	20	71	28	kg × 2.0	kg × 105	(80–135)
1–3	13	29	90	35	23	1300	(900–1800)
4–6	20	44	112	44	30	1700	(1300–2300)
7–10	28	62	132	52	34	2400	(1650–3300)

Adapted from Recommended Dietary Allowances, ed 9. Washington DC, National Academy of Sciences, revised 1980.

Table 8-8
Recommended Vitamin and Mineral Dietary Allowances

VITAMINS

| Age | Weight | | A | D | E | C | Folacin | B_3 | B_2 | B_1 | B_6 | B_{12} |
years	kg	lbs	IU	IU	IU	mg	mcg	mg	mg	mg	mg	mg
0.0–0.5	6	13	2100	400	4	35	30	6	0.4	0.3	0.3	0.5
0.5–1.0	9	20	2000	400	6	35	45	8	0.6	0.5	0.6	1.5
1–3	13	29	2000	400	7	45	100	9	0.8	0.7	0.9	2.0
4–6	20	44	2500	400	9	45	200	11	1.0	0.9	1.3	2.5
7–10	28	62	3500	400	10	45	300	16	1.4	1.2	1.6	3.0

MINERALS

| Age | Weight | | Calcium | Phosphorus | Iodine | Iron | Magnesium | Zinc |
years	kg	lbs	mg	mg	mg	mg	mg	mg
0.0–0.5	6	13	360	240	40	10	50	3
0.5–1.0	9	20	540	360	50	15	70	5
1–3	13	29	800	800	70	15	150	10
4–6	20	44	800	800	90	10	200	10
7–10	28	62	800	800	120	10	250	10

Adapted from Recommended Dietary Allowances, ed 9. Washington DC, National Academy of Sciences, revised 1980.

Table 8-9
Estimated Safe and Adequate Daily Dietary Intakes of Additional Selected
Vitamins and Minerals*

	VITAMINS			ELECTROLYTES		
Age	K	Biotin	Pantoth. Acid	Sodium	Potassium	Chloride
years	µg	µg	mg	mg	mg	mg
0.0–0.5	12	35	2	115–350	350–925	275–700
0.5–1.0	10–20	50	3	250–750	425–1275	400–1200
1–3	15–30	65	3	325–975	550–1650	500–1500
4–6	20–40	85	3–4	450–1350	775–2325	700–2100
7–10	30–60	120	4–5	600–1800	1000–3000	925–2775

TRACE ELEMENTS†

Age	Copper	Manganese	Fluoride	Chromium	Selenium	Molybdenum
years	mg	mg	mg	mg	mg	mg
0.0–0.5	0.5–0.7	0.5–0.7	0.1–0.5	0.01–0.04	0.01–0.04	0.03–0.06
0.5–1.0	0.7–1.0	0.7–1.0	0.2–1.0	0.02–0.06	0.02–0.06	0.04–0.08
1–3	1.0–1.5	1.0–1.5	0.5–1.5	0.02–0.08	0.02–0.08	0.05–0.1
4–6	1.5–2.0	1.5–2.0	1.0–2.5	0.03–0.12	0.03–0.12	0.06–0.15
7–10	2.0–2.5	2.0–3.0	1.5–2.5	0.05–0.2	0.05–0.2	0.1–0.3

Adapted from Recommended Dietary Allowance, ed 9. Washington DC, National Academy of Sciences, 1980.
*Because there is less information on which to base allowances, these figures are not given in the main table of the RDA and are provided here in the form of ranges of recommended intakes.
†Since the toxic levels for many trace elements may be only several times usual intakes, the upper levels for the trace elements given in this table should not be habitually exceeded.

Calories

A balanced parenteral solution includes both carbohydrate and fat. Metabolism of each potential energy substrate has a respiratory quotient (RQ) defined as the ratio of carbon dioxide produced to oxygen consumed. RQs near 1.0 tend to reduce respiratory reserve capacity and may be detrimental in the acutely ill child with pulmonary insufficiency. Fat emulsions can serve as a source of nonprotein calories and are associated with less CO_2 production than isocaloric amounts of glucose. Children who weigh 50 pounds or more can have their actual RQ and resting energy expenditure measured by indirect calorimetry to ascertain their exact caloric requirements.

Neonatal caloric expenditure can be computed as follows:

Minimal (non-growing) Expenditure:

Resting	50
Intermittent activity	0–15
Occasional cold stress	0–10
	50–75 total cal/kg/24-hr

Additional Expenditure with Growth:

Specific dynamic action	10
Fecal losses	10
Growth	25
	45 total cal/kg/24-hr

Total Caloric Expenditure: 90–120 cal/kg/24-hr

Term infants should be provided with calories estimated by the Harris Benedict equation:

Basal energy expenditure (BEE) (term infants) $= 22.10 + 31.05W + 1.16H$

where W = weight in kg, H = height/length in cm. Calories can also be estimated by the following chart:

Age (yrs)	cal/kg/24-hr
0–1	90–120
1–7	75–90
7–12	60–75
12–18	45–60

Caloric requirements are increased in the following situations:

- Fever: 12% for each degree >37°C
- Cardiac failure: 15–25%
- Major surgery: 20–30%
- Burns: up to 10%
- Severe sepsis: 40–50%
- Long-term growth failure: 50–100%
- Protein-calorie malnutrition: 125–140% infants (twice basal requirements for children)

Intravenous protein requirements in children are estimated to vary from 1.5 to 3 g/kg/day. The catabolism of each gram of protein administered results in approximately four calories. Infused proteins should not be counted as a source of utilizable energy, however, but as a source of nitrogen for protein synthesis and formation of new tissue necessary for growth.

Protein Requirements

Protein requirements for pediatric patients are listed below:

- Premature and term infants: 2.0–2.5 g/kg/day
- Older infants: 2.5–3.0 g/kg/day
- Older children: 1.5–2.5 g/kg/day

When providing protein intravenously, it is necessary to maintain a ratio of 1 g nitrogen (which is contained in 6.25 g protein) to a minimum of 150–250 nonprotein calories in order to prevent protein catabolism.

In addition, premature infants may require cysteine. Recommended supplementation is 75 mg/kg/day. Currently, not all of the commercial solutions contain this amino acid, so it may need to be ordered as a supplement to the parenteral nutrition. Tables 8-10 and 8-11 provide information about intravenous vitamin, mineral, and electrolyte requirements.

Infants weighing less than 1500 g may require the following adjustments in their TPN: one half of the total sodium as the acetate salt, the other half as the chloride salt to reduce chloride load; calcium gluconate at 2 g/500 ml TPN to provide 40 mg elemental calcium/kg/day. The maximum amounts of calcium and phosphorus that can be given in the same solution are limited by their

Table 8-10
IV Vitamin Requirements*

Vitamins	Multivitamin† for IV use for under 11 yrs	Multivitamin for IV use for over 11 yrs
A (retinol), IU	2300.0‡	3300
D, IU	400.0§	200
E (α tocopherol), IU	7.0	10.0
K₁ (phylloquinone), mg	0.2	
C (ascorbic acid), mg	80.0	100.0
Folacin, μg	140.0	400.0
Niacin, mg	17.0	40.0
Riboflavin, mg	1.4	3.6
Thiamin, mg	1.2	3.0
B₆ (pyridoxine), mg	1.0	4.0
B₁₂ (cyanocobalamin), μg	1.0	5.0
Pantothentic acid, mg	5.0‖	15.0
Biotin, μg	20.0‖	60.0

Adapted from Nutrition Advisory Group of Department of Food Nutrition, AMA: Multivitamin preparations for parenteral use statement by the Nutrition Advisory Group. JPEN 3:260, 1979.
*Adapted from Tables 1, 2, 4, Guidelines for multivitamin preparations for parenteral use, AMA, 1095.
†May be provided in appropriate salt or ester form in equivalent potency.
‡700 μg of retinol.
§As ergocalciferol or cholecalciferol.
‖RDA not established; amount = 20 × 100 kcal human mil.

Table 8-11
Mineral and Electrolyte Requirements

Mineral	Amount/kg/24-hours
Sodium	3–5 mEq
Chloride	3–5 mEq
Potassium	2–3 mEq
Magnesium	0.25–0.5 mEq
Calcium	0.5 mEq (10 mg)
Phosphorus	1 mM (1.47 mEq)

solubilities. Six factors enter the equation: (1) pH, (2) temperature, (3) amino acid concentration, (4) calcium salt used, (5) dextrose concentration, and (6) order of calcium and phosphorus addition.

Trace Elements

The trace elements recognized for parenteral use are zinc, copper, chromium, manganese, selenium, molybdenum, and iron. Pediatric requirements set by the AMA for zinc, copper, chromium, and manganese are listed below:

Zinc:
300 mcg/kg/day (prematures < 1500 g–3 kg)
100 mcg/kg/day (full term infants–5 years)
2.5–4.0 mg/day (children > 5 years)
Copper: 20 mcg/kg/day
Chromium: 0.14–0.2 mcg/kg/day
Manganese: 2–10 mcg/kg/day

Suggested dosages of selenium and iron for children who are on long-term TPN with little p.o. intake or low serum levels are listed below:
Selenium:
25–30 mcg/day
Iron (for initial restoration dose):

$$0.3 \times \text{body wt. in lbs.} \times \left(\frac{\text{Hgb observed} \times 100}{\text{Hgb desired}} \right) = \text{mg iron}$$

For children less than 13.6 kg consult titrating schedule in Physicians' Desk Reference.

As with vitamins, trace elements should be provided daily. Patients with large volumes of intestinal fluid loss are at increased risk for zinc deficiency, since a large proportion of zinc excretion from the body is normally through the GI tract. Postgastrointestinal surgical infants have been found to require doses of zinc two to four times the recommended normal dose.

SUMMARY

Nutritional and technological advances in the past 20 years have changed the practice of pediatric nursing irreversibly. Hand-in-hand with these advances are new profound ethical issues that the nurse must face. Never has this been more in the public domain than with the recent Baby Doe controversies.[37–41] Possibly more difficult are the issues brought into play with the increasing number of high-risk premature and LBW infants surviving today.[42,43]

Ethical dimensions of nursing are reflected in day-to-day clinical practice, and the nursing literature has begun to address issues such as human rights, nursings' contract with society, confidentiality, consent, codes, and so on. In our society, however, nourishment is regarded as a basic human right. At what, if any, point in the progressions from oral sustenance to invasive parenteral provision does feeding become a medical intervention? Curtin questions,

> This point is important or it becomes important when physicians order the discontinuance of artificial means of feeding. Is providing food by whatever means legitimately within the medical prerogative? Do the rights of persons to adequate nutrition depend on their degree of debility or dependancy? Do physicians have the moral and legal authority to withhold nutrients?[44]

These questions have far-reaching implications for the nurse involved in specialized pediatric nutrition. We must prepare ourselves to examine our values and positions and to articulate and act on them.

References

1. Merrit RJ, Suskind RM: Nutritional survey of hospitalized pediatric patients. Am J Clin Nutr 32:1320, 1971
2. Parson HG, Francoer TE, et al: The nutritional status of hospitalized children. Am J Clin Nutr 33:1140, 1980
3. Cooper A, Jacobowski D, et al: Nutritional assessment—An integral part of the preoperative pediatric surgical evaluation. J Pediatr Surg 16:554, 1981
4. Mize C, Cunningham C, Teitell B, et al: Undernutrition of pediatric inpatients: Repeated nutrition status evaluation. Nutr Supp Serv 4(4):27–39, 1984
5. Gesell A, Ilg FL: Feeding Behaviors of Infants. Philadelphia, JB Lippincott, 1937
6. O'Grady R: Feeding behavior in infants. Am J Nurs 71(4):736, 1967
7. Bernbaum J, Pereira G, Watkins J, et al: Enhanced growth and gastrointestinal function in premature infants given nonnutritive sucking. Abstract. Society Pediatric Research, April 1981
8. Pipes PL: Nutrition in Infancy and Childhood. St. Louis: CV Mosby, 1981, p 282
9. Moore HB: The meaning of food. Am J Clin Nutr 5(1):79, 1957

10. Illingworth RS, Lister J: The critical or sensitive period, with special reference to certain feeding problems in infants and children. Pediatrics 65(6):839–848, 1964

11. Jeter KF: The pediatric patient: Ostomy surgery in growing children, in Broadwell DC, Jackson BS (eds): Principles of Ostomy Care. St. Louis: CV Mosby, 1982, p 497

12. Jeter KF: The pediatric patient: Ostomy surgery in growing children, in Broadwell DC, Jackson BS (eds): Principles of Ostomy Care. St. Louis: CV Mosby, 1982, p 506

13. Schraeder BD, Donar ME: The child with chronic respiratory failure: A special challenge, in Miller K (ed.): Neonatal and Pediatric Critical Care Nursing. New York, Churchill Livingstone, 1983 p 139

14. Wear ET, Covey J, Brush M: Facilitating children's adaptation to intrusive procedures, in Fochtman D, Foley GV (eds) Nursing Care of the Child with Cancer. Boston, Little, Brown, 1982, p 61

15. Zitarelli MB, Healy M, Lechner D, et al: Indications for Commercial Infant Formulas and Indications for Commercial Tube Feedings and Supplements (in part). Philadelphia, Childrens Hospital of Philadelphia, 1982

16. Howell CG: Parenteral feeding: Route, risks, and complications. Lecture at Nutritional Support of the Child, Children's Hospital of Philadelphia, April 1982

17. Yosowitz P, Ekland DA, Shaw RC, et al: Peripheral intravenous infiltration necrosis. Am Surg 182:553, 1975

18. Brown AS, Hoelzer D, Piercy S: Skin necrosis from extravasating intravenous fluids in children. Plast Reconstr Surg 64:145, 1979

19. Zeigler M, Jacobowski O, Hoelzer D, et al: Route of pediatric parenteral nutrition: Proposed criteria revision. J Pediatr Surg 15:472, 1980

20. Dudrick SJ, Groff DB, Wilmore DW: Longterm venous catheterization in infants. Surg Gynecol Obstet 129:805, 1969

21. Zumbro GL, Mullin MJ, Nelson TG: Central venous catheter placement utilizing common facial vein. Am J Surg 125:654, 1973

22. Gauderer MW, Stellato TA, Izant RJ Jr, et al: Broviac silastic catheter insertion in children: A simplified direct subclavian approach. J Pediatr Surg 17(5):580–584, 1982

23. Boettcher MD, Pereira GR: Nutritional management of the critically ill neonate, in Miller KS (ed) Neonatal and Pediatric Critical Care Nursing. New York. Churchill Livingstone, 1983

24. Christensen RD, Rothstein G: Exhaustion of mature marrow neutrophils in neonates with sepsis. J Pediatr 96:316, 1980

25. Wright WC Jr, Ank BJ, Herbst J, et al: Decreased bacteriocidal activity of leukocytes of stressed newborn infants. Pediatrics 56:579, 1975

26. Stoerner JW, Pickering LK, Adcock EW III, et al: Polymorphonuclear leukocyte function in the newborn infants. J Pediatr 93:862, 1978

27. Weston WL, Carson BS, Barkin RM, et al: Monocyte-macrophage function in the newborn. Am J Dis Child 131:1241, 1977

28. Schuit KE, DeBiasio R: Kinetics of phagocyte response to group B streptococcal infections in newborn rats. Infect Immun 28:310, 1980

29. McCracken GH Jr, Eichenwald HF: Leukocyte function and the development of opsonic and complement activity in the neonate. Am J Dis Child 121:120, 1971

30. Saver S, Atwood P, Sohner D: The challenge of physical care, in Fochtman D, Foley G (eds) Nursing Care of the Child with Cancer. Boston, Little, Brown, 1982
31. Fochtman D, Foley G (eds): Nursing Care of the Child with Cancer. Association of Pediatric Oncology Nurses. Boston, Little, Brown, 1982
32. Kennedy-Caldwell C, Caldwell M: Pediatric enteral nutrition, in Rombeau J, Caldwell M (eds): Enteral and Tube Feeding. Philadelphia, WB Saunders, 1984
33. Forlaw L: Parenteral nutrition in the critically ill child. Crit Care Quart 3:7, 1981
34. Avery GB, Fletcher AB: Nutrition in Avery GB (ed): Neonatalogy. Philadelphia, JB Lippincott, 1981
35. Pereia GR, Glassman M: Parenteral nutrition in the neonate, in Caldwell M, Rombeau J (eds) Clinical Nutrition Vol 2: Parenteral Nutrition. Philadelphia, WB Saunders, 1984
36. Kerner JA: Fluid requirements. Manual of Pediatric Parenteral Nutrition. New York. John Wiley and Sons, 1983
37. Jonsen AR: Critical issues in newborn intensive care: A conference report had a policy proposal. Pediatrics 55(6):756, 1975
38. Frost N: Ethical issues in the treatment of critically ill newborns. Pediatr Ann 10(10): 16, 1981
39. Robertson JA, Frost N: Passive euthanasia of defective newborn infants: Legal considerations. J Pediatr 88:883, 1976
40. Nondiscrimination on the basis of handicap relating to health care for handicapped infants. 45CFR Part 84 Federal Register Part III, 48(129), 1983
41. President's commission for the study of Ethical Problems in Medicine and Biomedical and Behavioral Research: Seriously ill newborns. Deciding to forego life-sustaining treatment: Ethical, medical and legal issues in treatment decisions. Washington DC: US Government Printing Office, March 1983, Chapter 6
42. Wegman ME: Annual summary of vital statistics—1980. Pediatrics 68:755, 1981
43. Lee KS: Neonatal mortality: An analysis of the recent improvement in the United States. Am J Pub Health 20:15, 1980
44. Curtin L: Case studies XI and XII: Hyperalimentation—The distribution of a scarce resource, in Curtin L, Flaherty MJ (eds): Nursing Ethics—Theories and Pragmatics. Bowie, MD: Robert J Brady, 1982

Mary C. Hoppe
Carla S. Bour

— 9 —————————————————

Psychological and Social Responses to Nutritional Support

Advances in alternative methods of nutritional support have been heralded as significant contributors to the treatment of many patients who otherwise would die of malnutrition. The use of parenteral and enteral nutrition has concurrently generated new psychosocial stresses for patients and their families. Just as we need to recognize the need to use nutritional support to prevent or repair nutrient deficits in our patients, so do we need to recognize their psychosocial responses to these therapies to assist their adaptation.

The purpose of this chapter is to explore the psychological and social responses seen in patients receiving nutritional support therapies. This first section includes a brief review of psychological reactions to stress and illness in order to obtain a better understanding of the variety of usual responses. This will be followed by a discussion of the psychosocial effects of enteral and parenteral nutrition and special considerations for the home patient.

Although many specific psychosocial responses are peculiar to nutritional support therapies, an individual's reaction generally is based on previous state of health, past experience with illness, and usual coping mechanisms. A patient's understanding of illness is based on various cultural, ethnic, and social beliefs. We must remember, however, that each response is unique in that it relates to our patients' particular self-concepts, priorities, and plans in life.

Stress occurs when the patient is unable to cope effectively with a given situation. The inability to adapt may be due to the situation's extreme circumstances or the individual's limited resources. To restore balance, the person will attempt to utilize *defense mechanisms* (ego adaptive mechanisms) that have been successful in the past. Defense mechanisms are used to provide a respite

NUTRITIONAL SUPPORT IN NURSING
ISBN 0-8089-1889-3

263

while the individual attempts to reorganize and integrate changes, to keep emotions within certain boundaries during periods of sudden change, or to deal with an "unresolvable conflict".[1] Various mechanisms utilized may include denial, regression, repression, displacement, and sublimation. Specific defense mechanisms are by themselves not considered maladaptive (although some are believed healthier than others). Maladaptive defense mechanisms are inflexible and lead to avoidance of the conflict rather than to its resolution. Such maladaptive coping can be accompanied by considerable regression.[1] Effective coping permits the individual to emerge from the conflict with self-concept intact.[2] Assistance by the health care professional may be required to support the patient's ability to cope.

Eating has a significant role in our lives. Loss of the ability to eat can be a key factor in a patient's adjustment to nutritional support. The psychology of eating involves a study of the complicated relationship between our social and cultural selves. Each individual has particular eating patterns and food preferences that are based on lifelong habits and experiences. When we eliminate or restrict an individual's ability to eat, we can therefore anticipate a complex set of responses based on the disruption of an activity that has profound social, psychological, and cultural meaning.

From birth, eating occurs within a social framework, for unlike sleeping, it involves two persons.[3] Mealtimes continue as a social activity as the child grows. Meals can be a pleasurable experience, a time for the family to discuss daily activities and make plans for tomorrow. Children become socialized into their families. Within it, one can feel supported and loved. But meals can be a negative experience as well, a time for discipline and discord, with little socializing among family members. Additionally, foods can be used to reward or soothe and pacify the child.[4] These experiences become ingrained and can continue into adulthood as we eat both to celebrate and to ease feelings of depression.

The cultural aspects of eating also come into focus during childhood. Cultural and ethnic heritage determines what foods are appropriate to eat, how we should prepare them, and when we should eat them. For example, in some cultures animal blood is ingested to increase strength and promote aggression, while in others blood must be removed from meats prior to eating. Milk, believed essential in our culture for proper growth and development, is viewed with distaste in others.[5] Cultural food preferences can have far-reaching political and environmental repercussions as well. Consider the ongoing conflicts between environmental groups and Japanese and Soviet whaling rights advocates, for example.

Food symbolizes friendship and peer acceptance. It plays an integral part in our national and religious celebrations, as well as in our daily social obligations. It has also been shown that we accept foods more readily from persons we know and with whom we feel comfortable. We are also more willing to try new foods or accept suggestions on food preparation from those for whom we feel an affinity.[5]

Age is also an important consideration in any discussion of the psychology of eating. Adolescence is a stressful period of enormous change. Adolescents are experiencing rapid physical growth, sexual maturation, and the development of value systems, role differentiation, and pressure to plan for the future. They often are unprepared for this onslaught of developmental tasks. Reflecting these inner conflicts, moods vary dramatically, self-consciousness is heightened, and body image is altered. As a result, food is often used in an attempt to regain control. Boys may become overly concerned with muscle development and weight gain. Girls may become obsessed with thinness. An extreme desire for control can lead to two psychiatric disorders, *anorexia nervosa* and *bulimia*. These disorders primarily affect adolescent females, and their incidence is on the rise.[6]

The elderly patient experiences a change in eating behavior as metabolic activity declines. The demand for food decreases as changes in levels of activity along with alterations in taste and smell occur. Chronic illness with prescribed dietary restrictions can lead to decreased interest in food. In addition, social factors of isolation and limited income restrict the elderly's opportunity for the enjoyment of food. It may become increasingly difficult to ensure adequate nutrient intake in this age group.

Although brief, the previous discussion describes the highlights of the psychosocial considerations of eating. This background should provide a basis for understanding the additional psychosocial issues associated with parenteral and enteral nutritional support therapy.

ADAPTATION TO NUTRITIONAL SUPPORT

Enteral Nutritional Support in Hospitalized Patient

Enteral feedings, as previously described, are delivered to the patients via either a temporary or "permanent" tube. This method of feeding can result in significant psychosocial reactions. These are discussed in the following sections.

Factors That Influence Acceptance of Feeding Tubes

Enteral feedings now are as common in the hospital setting as chest X-rays. They are considered routine, safe therapy for those patients with a functioning gastrointestinal (GI) tract who, for a myriad of reasons, are unable to take and assimilate food orally.

Mention tube feedings to any nurse and the picture that frequently comes to mind is that of the elderly medical patient with organic brain syndrome. This patient refuses every meal and therefore requires a feeding tube, which is inserted amid much protesting. We need to remove this stereotyped view of the tube-fed patient and remember the developmentally disabled infant, the adolescent with Crohn's disease, and the middle-aged man with head and neck cancer, all of whom cannot voluntarily ingest food orally. As a result, the psychological and emotional responses to enteral nutrition support are as varied and complex as the individuals receiving this therapy.

The success of any therapy hinges on the patient's acceptance and cooperation. Psychological responses, as mentioned earlier, are an inevitable consequence of the stress of the illness, hospitalization, and its concomitant therapies. The nurse must recognize each response and then help the patient to cope effectively to regain equilibrium. Adequate coping can facilitate ready acceptance of the enteral nutritional regimen.

Factors that influence the patient's acceptance of the feeding tube include the type of tube, its location, the physical discomfort caused by the tube, ability to eat, educational preparation, and the nursing staff's attitude toward the therapy itself.

The type of tube used for feeding has implications for patient acceptance in regards to both comfort and aesthetics. Although a number of small-bore polyurethane transnasal feeding tubes are available, many institutions continue to inappropriately use the larger polyvinyl chloride (PVC) "salem" tubes. The rationale given is that PVC tubes are safer (no guidewires), easier to insert, and less traumatic for the patient, especially if one is already in place for gastric suctioning. The smaller-bore tubes, on the other hand, are softer and more flexible so they cause less mucosal irritation and necrosis. They also are weighted, permitting transference into the small intestine. Being smaller, they are more aesthetically appealing. The disadvantage is that they may not permit administration of viscous formulas or crushed medications.

The *location of the tube* is significant in that it can affect the appearance of the patient, therefore causing alterations in body image and self esteem. The transnasal tube is visually obvious on initial contact with the patient and can be particularly unsightly if good personal hygiene has not been practiced. The enterostomal tube is easier to conceal from others as it can be rolled up, taped to the skin, and hidden under clothing. The patient, however, can be concerned about the effect of the appearance of stoma and tube on the spouse or significant other.

Enterostomal tubes generally are preferred for long-term therapy because of their relative permanence, improved safety factors (decreased risk of dislodgment or aspiration), and ease of concealment.

Padilla, et al.[7] discussed the subject of physical discomforts caused by nasogastric feedings in their study of 28 hospital patients. The most frequent complaints included thirst, sore nose and mouth, dry mouth, and runny nose. Other complaints mentioned that carry implications for patient care were GI-related such as nausea, vomiting, abdominal cramping, and diarrhea. They found that physical discomforts may be better tolerated if the patient knows they are temporary. Therefore, these complaints may have even greater implications in the patient on long-term therapy. As minor as these complaints may seem on initial examination, they can be compounded by adjunctive therapies, as well as the length of the therapy itself.

Enteral feedings will also be better accepted by patients if they retain the ability to take some foods or liquids orally or have some hope for doing so again in the future. The earlier discussion on the psychology of eating explains the importance of this factor. The patient who is deprived of any oral intake merits special attention by the nurse to develop a means of adjusting to this change in lifestyle.

The patient's first glimpse of the feeding tube may occur when the nurse walks into the room to insert it. If the tube is to be inserted during an operative procedure, the patient may not see it until after it is in place. The insertion period is an anxious time for the patient. Anxiety can be reduced by adequate and properly timed educational preparation of the patient. Acceptance of the tube can be maximized by providing the patient with an understanding of the reason for tube feeding and all events associated with it.

Nurses can unknowingly influence acceptance of the feeding tube through their attitudes and their preparation of the patient for the therapy. Rains[8] noted in her interviews with 10 home patients that while hospitalized, they viewed feeding more as a procedure than as a meal. Technically, enteral nutritional support is a procedure, but the nurse's delivery of the formula can impact the patient's view. For instance, a nurse can run in and out of the patient's room to empty a can of formula into a feeding bag without any interaction with the patient. This behavior is not only insensitive, but also increases the patient's sense of isolation. Frequently, feeding schedules are for the convenience of the staff and may not correlate to "normal" mealtimes or to the desires of the patient. Alternatively, the nurse can attempt to schedule enteral feedings at mealtimes and take the opportunity to talk with the patient during the administration. This can emphasize that the patient is "eating."

Causes of Nonacceptance of Enteral Nutritional Support

A patient's nonacceptance of feeding tubes and enteral therapy may be due to a variety of causes, including oral deprivation, negative body image, dependency, and negative family and peer reaction. These all contribute to a patient's view of the quality of life.

Oral deprivation in the tube-fed patient has been discussed in studies by Padilla et al.[7] and Rains.[8] The patient receiving enteral feedings exclusively lacks the opportunity to taste, chew, and swallow foods. In the Padilla et al. study, patients ranked "having an unsatisfied appetite for certain foods" as significant as being away from home and family. Rains' subjects identified the loss of favorite foods as one of their most frequent problems. Padilla et al. suggest allowing the patient to ingest favorite foods unless medically contraindicated or permit them to satisfy their oral needs by tasting and chewing foods, but not swallowing. Mouth rinses, ice chips, chewing gum, or hard candy are other alternatives to ease the cravings.

Some patients may be so disturbed by the sight and smell of food that they pull the curtains around their bed or, in the case of home patients, retreat into another room during meals. While this may be necessary in some cases to ease stress, it serves to lessen social and family relationships and advances the feelings of isolation.

Body image can be defined as patients' perceptions of themselves, which in turn leads them to perceive how others view them. Negative body image can result from the appearance and presence of the feeding tube. Some individuals may perceive the surgical procedure of implanting the enterostomal feeding tube as very threatening to their self concept. They opt to replace a transnasal tube daily for nocturnal feedings. The tube then can be removed the next morning on completion of the feeding. They thus retain control over the feeding and the tube, which is temporarily placed, and leave their body image unaltered. Others may choose a surgically placed tube in place of a tube visible on the face.

A negative body image threatens an individual's self-concept, producing further psychological stress. Unless the patient can adapt and resolve this conflict, enteral feedings will be unacceptable. Patients can also reject the tube because they believe enteral feeding places them in an excessively dependent relationship to family or medical personnel.

The length of therapy is another important factor in acceptance of tube feedings. Patients may be more accepting of a therapy if they know it is only temporary, particularly when it occurs within the confines of a hospital room. Acceptance of home enteral therapy requires acceptance that one is chronically ill, which means reorganizing one's self-concept.

Feelings of hope, family and community support, purposefulness, and worth all contribute to the quality of life. Hospitalized or chronically ill patients analyze these aspects of their lives and compare them to the negative aspects of their illness: despair, loss of control, and dependency on others. When the level of the quality of life no longer is acceptable, compliance with treatments or willingness to begin new ones will end. These feelings need to be identified and explored with the patient and family.

Common Psychological Reactions to Enteral Nutritional Support

Psychological responses to tube feeding are similar to those seen in illness and are dependent on the patient's usual responses to stressful situations. The patient's goal is to regain the equilibrium (by altering or reforming self-concept) lost with the introduction of an alternate method of eating. It should be remembered that these are normal, even expected, responses but can cause maladaption if unsolved.

Anxiety and fear are immediate reactions to situations perceived as dangerous, whether they be physical or psychological threats. Both may be related to possible complications of the feeding, to reactions of family and friends, to the prognosis of the illness, and, in the case of the home patient, the fear that the procedures are too difficult to learn and cope with daily.

Patients often are angry. The anger is usually in response to attempts to answer the question, "Why me?" Patients may become angry for being dependent on others, for being unable to cope as they would like, or for no known specific reason. Anger can be displaced onto others, namely, staff and the family. We must not personalize such anger but rather attempt to understand it and assist the patient and distraught and confused family members with coping with the behavior. Often the energies generated by the anger and hostility can be used in a positive way to motivate self-helping activity.

Depression is the most common response and can be the most difficult one with which to cope. It can cause the individual to withdraw and give up.

Feelings of ambivalence may occur early in the therapy. The patient may recognize the benefits of enteral nutrition but be angered by the impact on lifestyle. Patients may not have had time to comprehend the full implications of the loss of food yet feel they must comply with the medical regimen. Ambivalence may lead to further confusion and a vague sense of loss of control along with some feelings of guilt.

Nursing Interventions in Care of the Enteral Nutritional Support Patient

To assist the patient in accepting tube feeding, the nurse first must identify those factors that will influence the response. This process being during the initial assessment of the patient's usual coping styles. How have they dealt with other life stresses? Is there a history of psychiatric disorders? How are they coping with the present illness? Is the illness chronic or acute? What family supports are available? To what extent has the illness altered family roles?

This information is then integrated into the general plan of care as well as into the educational plan. By presenting tube samples, pictures of individuals with feeding tubes who are receiving feedings, and allowing the patient and family to talk with other people receiving enteral nutrition, the nurse can help to decrease anxiety by reducing fear of the unknown. By remembering that excessive anxiety interferes with the learning process, the thorough evaluation of learning then becomes very significant. During the teaching sessions, the nurse can explore the fears and concerns of the patient and family. The nurse can also assist them in identifying their own coping strengths and family support systems, as well as strategies for problem solving.

Psychological responses should be discussed with the patient and family to reassure them that certain behaviors, while possibly disturbing, are normal reactions to stress. At the same time, however, the nurse should be able to recognize maladaptive behaviors and seek the advice and assistance of more specially-trained personnel if necessary. The assessment of psychosocial responses and evaluation of nursing interventions is an ongoing process. Based on knowledge of the patient's coping patterns, the nurse can provide psychological support during various feeding procedures.

The nurse can also assist patients in regaining a sense of control by permitting them to make decisions regarding delivery of the feeding. In the case of intermittent feedings, allow the patient to choose administration times. Although this policy of self-care may seem alien to many nurses, it often is necessary in the case of the hospitalized "home" patient. While some patients will gladly relinquish their tube feeding responsibilities for the duration of hospitalization, others will resent the nurse for removing one of their normal functions. Conflicts may arise between the staff and some patients with regard to proper procedures. Such patients have integrated the tube feeding into their pattern of daily life and might feel threatened by a possible alteration of their accustomed role, much the same as they did when the tube feeding was initiated.

The nurse should be aware of the discomforts that can be caused by the tube itself, the feeding, and the resulting oral deprivation. The nurse also should be sensitive to the patient's needs for privacy if desired during administration, yet mindful that it may lead to increased social isolation.

Parenteral Nutrition Support in the Hospitalized Patient

Parenteral nutritional (PN) support is the delivery of essential nutrients via the intravenous route. Patients receiving this support therapy may exhibit significant psychosocial responses because it deviates greatly from normal feeding.

Factors Contributing to Acceptance of PN Support

Factors that contribute to the acceptance of PN in the hospitalized patient include the patient's perception of intravenous therapy, the acuteness of the illness, the level of physical discomfort experienced, and whether the patient retains the ability to eat.

The public today, through the media and personal experience, is fairly sophisticated in its knowledge of common medical terminologies and therapies. Most people are familiar with the term IV (intravenous) and have seen mock IV setups in either television or films. Many have received intravenous therapy or know others who have had this experience. IV feeding is considered a common therapy in hospitalized patients and not viewed as an extremely threatening component of the hospital experience. Others may have personal or anecdotal knowledge of painful arm swellings or intravenous needles that were difficult to insert. Those with previous negative experiences may have more difficulty initially accepting intravenous nutrition.

In the case of the acutely ill hospitalized patient, the patient and family's immediate focus is on the patient and the condition: "How are they?"; "Are they going to be all right?" The focus then shifts to the seriousness of the illness and the level of physical discomfort it causes. Major treatment modalities such as surgery also may become a concern at this state. The patient and family require time and support from staff to adjust to the illness, its nature, and impact on the future. Anxiety, fear, and confusion are common psychological reactions at this time.

The ability to eat may become an issue as the recovery progresses. If the patient retains a functioning gut or hopes to regain function, PN is regarded as a temporary treatment, therefore more easily acceptable. If loss of gut function is permanent, however, acceptance may be more difficult as the patient attempts to reconcile the loss. Denial and anger are common reactions. For example, a patient may reveal denial and display anger in making statements such as "I could eat if I weren't getting so much of that stuff."

Causes of Nonacceptance of PN

The intravenous catheter (and additional apparatus) may be the cause of negative body image in much the same way as the feeding tube in enteral nutrition. In addition to the catheter, the loss of bowel function may also cause nonacceptance of the therapy, particularly if the individual is unable to resolve the loss and to overcome the alteration of body image.

Fear of dependency on machines also may cause nonacceptance for several reasons. First, the pump may be perceived as an extension of the individual during infusion, altering body image. The pump also symbolizes further loss of control of daily activities. The patient may fear a malfunction of the pump, which would cause physical complications and a setback in recovery.

Hospitalized patients are very vulnerable. They are existing in an unfamiliar environment with no voice in its rules. Often they are not even aware of all the rules; even the language is foreign. To become healthy again, the patient is forced into a dependent role. Throughout the experience, the family and friends remain an important link with the familiar. Their support and understanding of therapies are crucial. Nonacceptance on their part places a severe strain on the patient and could be responsible for the patient's own nonacceptance.

In the hospitalized, terminally ill patient, quality of life issues raise many ethical concerns and can cause great conflict and stress within the patient and family. Some view PN in these patients as "merely feeding" them and consider it a component of routine care and comfort measures. Others see it as a "heroic" therapy that prolongs life unnecessarily and postpones the inevitable death. Each patient, family, and situation is different. Each family operates from its own belief system. The nurse can assist the patient and family to explore their feelings, so when the decision is made to terminate therapy, it can be done with a minimum of conflict and guilt.

Common Psychological Reactions to PN

Psychological phenomena related to PN can be grouped into those that represent disturbance in brain function (organic brain syndromes) and those that are efforts to cope with disease and its treatment.

Malcolm et al.[9] delineated several syndromes that appeared to have an organic basis. Delirium was the most common, appearing generally in elderly patients and associated with previous drug use, low hemoglobin, fever, and electrolyte imbalances. Delirium is characterized by clouding of consciousness and confusion, in which may be added agitation, bizzare behavior, and visual hallucinations. Another group of patients presented with ". . . apathy, slowed mentation, irritability with handling, saddened mood and insomnia." Age did not seem relevant, but all were found to be protein-depleted on nutritional assessment. They noted these symptoms cleared within 48 hours to 1 week after initiation of PN. Lastly, impotence, primarily considered psychological in origin, may be due to zinc deficiency.[10]

Gulledge et al.[11] also found acute organic brain syndromes to be common. (The term *acute brain syndrome* is equivalent to delirium). Symptoms included decreased ability to acquire and comprehend new information and decreased attention span that produced further anxiety. Causes for the syndrome included sepsis, electrolyte imbalance, hyper-anal hypovolemia, and a variety of medication. The staff, not recognizing the organic cause of such cognitive and behavioral symptoms, had labeled these symptoms as anxiety problems, inadvertently placing too many demands on the patients. This increased both the frustration of the staff and of the patients.

Psychological coping responses to PN are complex and are dependent on the specific illness, the circumstances surrounding the need for PN, and/or the prognosis for recovery. Once again, the most common reactions are depression, fear, anxiety, anger, and ambivalence.

Many of the disease states treated with PN are chronic such as inflammatory bowel disease, cancer, and anorexia nervosa. Each has its own implications for care. Other diseases are sudden and unanticipated such as major trauma or burns, short bowel syndrome secondary to mesenteric infarct, or congenital or premature neonatal conditions.

Frequently, those with chronic illness respond positively to PN and the feeling of well-being it offers. Conversely, patients suffering from an acute incident respond less positively as they must adapt to a sudden change in lifestyle along with the PN.

Depression is a frequent response. The patient has to face the temporary or permanent loss of bowel function and of normal eating patterns. These losses are further affected by the loss of control to make decisions about one's life, on being dependent on others, as well as being tied to machinery. As stated previously, metabolic imbalances and the effects of malnutrition complicate and can intensify depression. Severe chronic pain and multiple hospitalizations and surgeries also are a source for depression. The intensity and duration of the depression may become quite severe, requiring psychotherapy and medication.

Fear of the future and of the unknown can produce high states of anxiety. Patients may be fearful of reoccurrence of the illness and death. They may fear having to rely on others, while at the same time worry about losing the support of the hospital staff. They may fear being faced with a serious complication and not responding correctly. Lastly, there can be significant concern over the financial ramifications of PN therapy.

Although we may view PN support as a "life saving" procedure, often patients may be unable to separate the procedure from the disease state as the cause of their hospitalization. The PN is a constant reminder of the disease and the limitations it imposes. These feelings can produce much anger until the person resolves the conflict and regains some measure of autonomy.[12] Thus, we should not be surprised that many patients may resent the very procedures that are keeping them alive.

Circumstances that engender anger in one patient can cause ambivalence in another. For example, strivings for autonomy can be counterbalanced by needs to remain dependent out of fear of losing staff guidance. A wish to take control of one's treatment may be in conflict with a desire to be looked after.

Parents of infants on PN can also experience anxiety, anger, depression, and ambivalence. We must remember that parents will often feel responsible for the illnesses of their children. These feelings should be explored with the family, along with methods of coping and adapting to potential changes in lifestyle.

When assessing the patient for negative responses and identifying coping strengths, the nurse may wish to consider the following issues.

General Psychological Factors

- usual response to stressful events and coping style
- past experience with hospitalizations/illness and reactions
- level of growth and development
- individual's definition of sick role
- other stressful life situations that are also occurring
- social support, i.e., family and friends

Illness Specific Factors

- usual coping style associated with illness
- past psychiatric history
- level, duration, and frequency of depressive episodes
- past experience with disease
- professional treatment for reactions
- psychotherapy or medications included in treatment
- family members included in treatment

The nurse then uses the information obtained in the assessment to assist the patient and family in identifying coping strengths. The nurse also may use the information when planning other aspects of care. For example, if body image has been identified as a major concern, the nurse may want to include the patient in the decision as to where the catheter should be placed. This action also returns some sense of control back to the patient, thus increasing independence.

The nurse can help to decrease the patient's anxiety and fears through anticipating which situations provoke anxiety and providing educational learning experiences beforehand. It should be remembered, however, that anxiety can decrease the ability to absorb new information. Explanations may have to be repeated many times. If the patient continues having difficulty in learning, the nurse should reassess the ability to learn, teaching methods, or causes of anxiety. If the patient is unable to concentrate because of other fears, these will have to be addressed first before learning can take place. The possibility of a disturbance in brain function will also need to be considered.

The third step in the process involves evaluating the patient and family's response to your interventions. The nurse should assess whether anxiety was alleviated through teaching or if needs were not properly identified.

HOME NUTRITIONAL SUPPORT: SPECIAL CONSIDERATION

Home nutritional support (HNS) has been proven a safe and cost-effective means of providing alternate methods of nutrition at home to a select group of individuals. This success has been achieved through advanced technology and improved pharmaceutical and medical equipment. It has permitted persons to carry on normal, productive lives that otherwise may have been characterized by numerous hospitalizations, pain, and malnutrition.

Factors Influencing Acceptance of Home Nutritional Support

Price et al.[13] noted in their study of 19 permanent HNS patients a distinct difference in the coping patterns between those who had chronic bowel disease and those who suffered a sudden, unanticipated bowel trauma. Those patients with chronic problems adjusted more easily to home therapy than did those with the acute problem. Price et al. theorized that the chronic patients already had resolved the loss of bowel function and were willing to exchange their present lifestyle, characterized by much pain and discomfort, with one that included machine-controlled infusions.

The acutely ill patient, on the other hand, had to cope with unexpected illness, hospitalization, loss of bowel function, and resolution of the conflicts involved with long-term therapy and changes in lifestyle. The chronically ill individual could perceive some of the benefits, while the acutely ill person could only see loss.[13] Hall et al.[14] found in their study of long-term PN patients that those who suffered an "acute loss of bowel function" (gunshot wounds, stabbings, or infarction) were more likely to have psychiatric disturbances than those individuals with previous histories of mental disorders prior to initiation of PN.

The importance of family and peer support in the hospitalized patient has already been noted. In HNS, family involvement is even more critical to the success of the therapy. The earliest reactions to HNS are anxiety and fear, discussed in a previous section. The patient will require much support from family and friends. To reduce many of these fears and to reduce the patient's sense of isolation, at least one family member should be designated "secondary caregiver" and receive training along with the patient.[14] The two can support each other during the training period. Once home, the patient can feel secure that another trained person is available to assist if necessary. This is not only helpful from a psychological view, but also from a safety one. In the event of an emergency and the patient is unable to respond, the family member is competent to respond appropriately.

In the hospitalized individual, body image usually is not a major concern unless the possibility of long-term therapy exists. In the home patient, negative body image can have a significant impact on sexual functioning. The person may feel unattractive and highly anxious about a catheter protruding from the chest. Other factors such as old incisions or ostomy stomas may reinforce the negative image.[15] The patient becomes very concerned about the reaction from the spouse or significant other. The uninvolved person can be concerned about the impact on future relationships.

The ability of the individual to learn complex procedures in order to safely and competently administer HNS is also a consideration. While intellectual ability is important to assess, even patients with low to normal intelligence have been taught the necessary procedures utilizing behavioral analysis and behavioral modification techniques. For example, Lansky et al.[16] reported on two individuals who frequently failed at tasks during the learning process because of an inability to memorize complex steps. Their failures contributed to increased anxiety and lowered self esteem, which in turn contributed to further failure. These women eventually succeeded by using individual index cards with one specific instruction on each instead of the more complex training manual. These techniques certainly have implications for use with other patients, particularly the elderly who may have short-term memory loss.

Prior to discharge, the HNS patient will begin to focus, with good reason, on the economics of the situation. The financial burdens of HPN can be enormous. In some areas, home parenteral nutrition has been estimated to cost $70,000 or more per year. Private insurance carriers may cover the majority of the costs, provided the patient's policy offers such coverage. Medicare will pay for 80 percent of the costs for those who are over 65 or those who qualify as "disabled" if the diagnosis is appropriate. Many persons do not have supplemental insurance to cover the remaining 20 percent, and in the case of the disabled person, coverage begins after two years of disability. Large debts may be incurred as a result. The most frustrating problem may occur in younger Medicare patients who become well enough to begin working yet risk losing their benefits if they do so. Furthermore, these individuals generally are considered poor risks by third-party insurance payers.

The psychological ramifications for patients and their families may be severe. Young patients may feel they face a future devoid of employment and financial security. The head of a household may worry about the future of spouse and children. The added stress results in depression, anxiety, and lowered self esteem and may cause interpersonal conflicts.

Patients' usual coping styles also play a role in acceptance of HNS. Unlike hospital therapy, home patients assume a tremendous responsibility. Although medical professionals will provide continued support and the patient will be monitored through frequent check-ups, they still assume many new roles at home. They must be competent at fairly complex procedures and be able to respond correctly to various metabolic and mechanical complications. This can be tremendously overwhelming to the patient and family.

Individuals whose usual style is to respond with overdependence or depression, face a tremendous hurdle in HNS. Dependent individuals may have difficulty accepting all the responsibility that HNS entails. This places added pressure on family members who must assist or take over as the primary caregiver. Depressed patients often have compliance problems. They may become lax and careless with aseptic technique, increasing the risk for infection or other complications.

Psychological Adaptation to Home Nutritional Support

The ability to eat impacts adaptation to long-term HNS. Many patients in the initial stages of adaptation report missing the pleasures of meals and social events where food plays an important role.[17] They may exhibit an usually increased awareness of foods in magazine or television advertisements.[18] By disrupting their own routine meals, families suffer if they attempt to compensate for the other member's inability to eat. This can lead to feelings of guilt and resentment. In a study of nine HNS patients by MacRitchie,[18] three individuals stated they never felt hunger, and the remaining six were able to relieve hunger pains with sips of water. The majority were able to sit down with the family during mealtimes and take small quantities of food and sips of fluid.

The family should be encouraged to maintain their usual meal routines as much as possible. HNS patients, if able, should join the family and take orally what they can. The benefits to patient and family include relief of oral deprivation and prevention of social isolation.

Achievement of a "near-normal" lifestyle is the goal of HNS. As strength and feelings of well-being return, the greater likelihood of adaptation to HNS. Those patients who had lengthy recovery periods (because of severe metabolic imbalances or other surgeries) have been found to take longer to adapt to HNS.[18] This can be attributed to the time required for physical strength to return, as well as to adjustments in family dynamics and the sick role.

Many home patients suffer from sleep disturbances, particularly if they infuse fluids during the night. They are anxious and fearful of mechanical/pump failures, kinking or disconnecting of the tubing, or dislodgement of the catheter. Also, as they may be receiving large quantities of fluid over a 10–12-hour period, they may need to void as often as every two hours. Lack of sleep can cause irritability, fatigue, and contribute to depression and anxiety. This may contribute to prolonging the "sick role."

As we have seen, when a family member becomes ill or is hospitalized, the family dynamics are disrupted. Roles must be altered to adjust for the loss of the member. When the member returns, the family may encounter hesitancy or resistance to returning to old roles if they believe they will have to revise their problems again. Most healthy families are able to manage these role revisions.

Sexual dysfunction is a problem for many patients adapting to HNS. As stated earlier, negative body image has an impact. The person's previous sex life also impacts adaptation. For those with a history of chronic illness and diminished sexual drives, some will feel threatened and pressured by spouses who assume a normal relationship will resume when health returns. Patients to whom HNS offers a life free from pain often enjoy improved sexual relationships. Unattached persons may have fears of never establishing a normal relationship. Others may feel inhibited by the presence of cumbersome equipment and may fear dislodging the cathether or kinking the tubing. Others may complain of the lack of spontaneity as they attempt to plan sexual activities around the time of infusion. Although it may take months, most people who had satisfying sexual relationships prior to HNS are able to make reasonable adaptations.

Nursing Assessment

The selection of patients and families appropriate for HNS is possibly the most important and difficult task in the process. As has been shown, the stress of HNS can intensify every dysfunction in the person's life. The nurse plays a crucial role in this assessment process.

Nurses generally spend the greatest amount of time with patients and their families. The nurse can observe their daily interactions and note their usual coping styles and manner of relating to each other. As nurses develop a trusting relationship with the family, the family often will "open up" regarding their home situations and family problems. The nurse then is able to offer real insight into their home environment.

Psychological assessment of patients and their families should be routine for those considering HNS. Obviously not all problems can be anticipated. But if psychologically-related problems are revealed during the assessment and if the patient is selected for HNS, these areas can be monitored closely during future assessments.

'Areas that should be considered in assessment are listed below:

Factors influencing learning:

- High anxiety states or depression
- Advanced age
- Poor physical condition (from effects of malnutrition, multiple surgeries, prolonged illness)
- Organic brain syndrome

Family support system:

- Availability of secondary caregiver
- Psychological status of this individual

Usual coping styles that might interfere with adaptation:

- Severe depression
- Overdependence
- Denial

History of substance abuse:

- Chemical
- Alcohol

History of psychiatric illness

Careful assessment and planning contributes to the success of the HNS program. It is also a dynamic process, one that must be transferred to the nurse caring for the patient in the home.

The results of these assessments must be evaluated and implemented in the plan of care. Close communication must be established between the patient's physician and the nurse monitoring the patient in the home. Should the nurse find that the patient fails to adapt, evidenced by continuing manifestations of anxiety, fear, or depression and by noncompliance, a referral to a psychiatric social worker may be needed.

It is important to note in conclusion that the long-term patient can potentially experience psychological relapses caused by both physical or mental stresses. This indicates that continuing nursing support of this patient is mandated for the duration of HNS therapy.

SUMMARY

The patient who benefits physically from nutritional support therapies can demonstrate a need for psychosocial support to prevent potential psychological problems. Nursing, both within the hospital and in the home, can be key to the overall success of this mode of therapy if potential problems are anticipated, identified, and treated.

References

1. Bowden CL, Anxiety, defenses, and adaptation, *in* Bowden C, Borstein A (eds): *Psychosocial Basis of Health Care.* Baltimore, Williams and Wilkins, 1983
2. Nahigan EG: Effects of illness on the schoolage child, *in* Scipien GM, Barnard MV, Chard MV, et al (eds): *Comprehensive Pediatric Nursing* (ed 3). New York, McGraw-Hill, 1986
3. Gretchell EL, Howard RB: Nutrition in development, *in* Scipien GM, Barnard MV, Chard MV, et al (eds): *Comprehensive Pediatric Nursing* (ed 3). New York, McGraw-Hill, 1986
4. Werner-Beland JA: The Psychosocial aspects of illness, *in* Beland IL, Passos JY (eds): *Clinical Nursing.* New York, MacMillan, 1975
5. Williams SR: Cultural, social, and psychological influences on food habits, *in* Williams SR (ed): *Nutrition and Diet Therapy (ed 5).* St. Louis, CV Mosby, 1973
6. Bayer LM, Bauers CM, Kapp, SR: Psychosocial aspects of nutritional support, *Nursing Clin North Am, March, 1983*
7. Padilla GV, et al: Subjective distresses of nasogastric tubefeeding. JPEN 3(2):53–7, 1979
8. Rains BL: The non-hospitalized tube fed patient. Oncol Nurse Forum 8(2):8–13, 1981
9. Malcolm R, et al: Psychosocial aspects of total parenteral nutrition. Psychosomatics 21(2):115–25, 1980
10. Dudrick SJ, Englert DM: Total care of the patient receiving total parenteral nutrition. Psychosomatics 21(2):109–10, 1980
11. Gulledge AD, et al: Home parenteral nutrition for the short bowel syndrome. Gen Hosp Psychiatry 2(4):271–81, 1980
12. Robinovitch AE: Home total parenteral nutrition: A psychosocial viewpoint. JPEN 5(6):522–5, 1981
13. Price BS, Levine EL: Permanent total parenteral nutrition: Psychological and social responses of the early stages. JPEN 3(2):48–52, 1979
14. Hall RC, et al: Psychiatric reactions to long-term intravenous hyperalimentation. Psychosomatics 22(5):428–433, 1981
15. MacRitchie KJ: Parenteral nutrition outside hospital: Psychosocial styles of adaptation. Can J Psychiatry 25(4):308–13, 1980
16. Lansky D, Doerr H, Ivey, M: Teaching home parenteral nutrition to patients with limited compliance skills. JPEN 6(2):160–2, 1982
17. Perl M, et al: Psychiatric effects of longterm home hyperalimentation. Psychosomatics 22(12):1047–1463, 1981
18. MacRitchie KJ: Life without eating or drinking. Can P Assoc J 23, 1978

Deann M. Englert
Millie Lawson

10

Ambulatory Home Nutritional Support

The science and technology for providing safe and effective long-term nutritional support have been modified and improved steadily during the past several decades.[1] Patients previously faced with a poor or even fatal prognosis secondary to inadequate or compromised gastrointestinal (GI) function can now be maintained for prolonged or indefinite periods of time by using a variety of feeding techniques. Of the unfortunate patients whose nutrient requirements cannot be obtained via the gut, most can be nourished optimally by ambulatory continuous or intermittent (cyclic) infusion schedules. Less dramatic, but equally important, is the genesis and development of a number of portable enteral feeding systems simplistically designed for use in the home.

These exciting and innovative forms of lifesaving nutritional and metabolic support have signficantly impacted clinical judgments made in the management of seriously or chronically ill patients. Not only have the vast majority of these afflicted individuals recovered dramatically from their primary disease process, but they have been discharged from the hospital to return to normal or near-normal lifestyles and productive roles in society. A 1986 national survey has shown that as many as 45,000 patients are currently receiving some form of home nutritional support.*As the number and complexity of patients continue to escalate each year, these new modalities of therapy have revolutionized the concepts and methods of delivering outpatient services in the community.

Much of the success of a home nutritional support program is attributed to persistent cooperation and interaction of highly skilled professional nurses. Expertise in this clinical specialty of nursing combines knowledge, patience,

---

* From Susanne Loarie, Travenol Laboratories, Inc., September 1, 1986. Personal Communication.

NUTRITIONAL SUPPORT IN NURSING
ISBN 0-8089-1889-3

persistence, and, above all, a close collaborative working relationship with other members of the multidisciplinary health care team.

The purposes of this chapter are to (1) review the historical development of ambulatory infusion systems, (2) consider the indications for ambulatory home nutritional support, (3) describe the process of a successful training program for the patients and their families, (4) discuss follow-up care after discharge and maintenance of quality assurance program in the home setting, and (5) explain the typical patterns of psychosocial adjustment to home nutritional support.

HISTORICAL MILESTONES IN AMBULATORY INFUSION SYSTEMS

The first patient fed entirely by vein at home was a 56-year-old woman with widespread metastatic carcinoma of the ovaries who was discharged from the Hospital of the University of Pennsylvania in 1968.[2] Although her case is a notable milestone, this homebound patient merely traded her hospital bed for the one at home, where she was able to be with her husband and four young children for six months prior to her demise.

Scribner and his colleagues initiated the first formal program to feed patients intravenously outside the hospital.[3] Using the established technology of their sophisticated home renal dialysis unit at the University of Washington, they designed a Dacron-cuffed silicone rubber central venous catheter (CVC) and an ingenious infusion system.[4] The delivery apparatus consisted of a 2-liter bottle of nutrients suspended from a counterbalanced beam scale with a built-in alarm to warn the patient when the infusion was near completion (Fig. 10-1A). A lightweight, peristaltic volumetric pump (Holter®, Extracorporeal, Inc., King of Prussia, PA) was used to propel the fluid at the prescribed rate using either alternating current from an electrical outlet or direct current from self-contained rechargeable batteries for as long as 6 hours. The daily nutrient ratio was usually infused over a 10- to 18-hour period at night while the patient was sleeping, and the feeding catheter with its distal Luer-lock connection was heparinized to free the patient from the infusion equipment for the remainder of the day. As technological advancements have been made, these premier pioneers in the field have subsequently modified and improved their mechanical system, but have retained their basic principles and techniques with outstanding clinical success.

Jeejeebhoy and coworkers in Montreal, Canada, devised a somewhat different administration system for intermittent infusions at home.[5] A series of three 1-liter plastic bags filled with nutrient solution were delivered to the patient by attaching a carbon dioxide cylinder to three fabric sleeves containing rubber bladders into which the bags were placed (Fig. 10-1B). As the carbon dioxide slowly filled the inflatable rubber bladders, the plastic bags containing the nutrient infusate were compressed, forcing the fluid into the patient's central vein

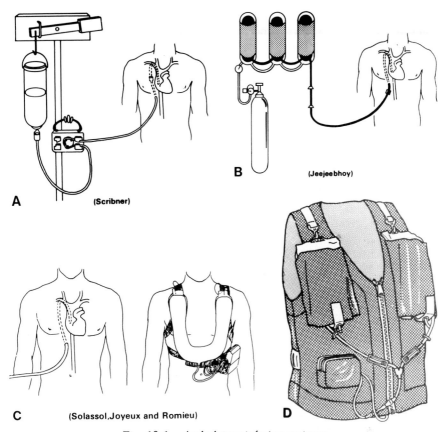

A (Scribner)

B (Jeejeebhoy)

C (Solassol,Joyeux and Romieu)

D

Fig. 10-1. Ambulatory infusion systems.

at an infusion rate related to the release of carbon dioxide from the cylinder. This method of delivery is analogous to the mechanism used to pump blood rapidly into the patient with hypovolemic shock and severe hypotension. The major advantage of the pneumatic cuff system was that it did not require a pump or source of electrical power and was therefore rather portable.

In Montpellier, France, Solassol and Joyeux developed the first technique and apparatus for truly ambulatory home nutritional support in 1967.[6] A U-shaped, 3-liter silicone rubber fluid reservoir, suspended from the patient's neck like a halter, was connected by intravenous tubing at its most dependent point to a compact battery-operated roller pump attached to a belt worn around the waist (Fig. 10-1C). The nutrient container was not only heavy and bulky, but it had to be cleaned and resterilized before each infusion cycle. When the patient was confined to bed, the infusion bag was hung at the bedside and the infusion regulated by a rheostatic pump plugged into a wall electrical outlet. Using this innovative feeding technique, many cancer patients in France received chemotherapy and/or a combination of treatment modalities while still being nourished optimally with minimal confinement in the hospital.

Maenab was the first in 1976 to use an ambulatory infusion system to feed children in England through a nasogastric tube.[7] A waistcoat was fabricated containing a plastic bag filled with enteral formula and a miniature peristaltic roller pump in pockets positioned on the back of the waistcoat similar to a camping backpack.

A prototype of an ambulatory hyperalimentation vest was designed in 1976 at the University of Texas Medical School at Houston and Hermann Hospital (Fig. 10-1D).[2] The vest was tailored to each patient using lightweight, polyester mesh fabric. A pocket over each breast, adjusted using hook-and-loop velcro fasteners, varied with the size of the patient. In infants, 100-ml bags were used; in children, 250-ml bags were used; in women and small men, 500-ml bags were used; and in larger adults, 1000-ml bags were used. The Viaflex® (Travenol Laboratories, Deerfield, IL) plastic bags were connected by specially constructed Y-tubing to a miniature volumetric pump carried in a zippered pocket in one of the lower quadrants of the vest. The 6-foot length of administration tubing was coiled and placed into one of the pockets while the vest was worn. While the patient was sleeping or not wearing the vest, it could be conveniently placed on a clothes hanger and suspended nearby to allow the patient a range of motion up to 6 feet with the tubing uncoiled. The ambulatory test was comfortable, practical, and could be concealed if desired under loose-fitting clothing.

In 1978, a 31-year-old woman who was receiving total parenteral nutrition (TPN) to heal a colocutaneous fistula following a small bowel resection was initially pleased and relieved with the pospect of continuing her TPN therapy at home rather than in the hospital.[8] The patient, however, had ambivalent feelings about wearing the rather conspicuous vest in public and felt that the infusion apparatus called attention to her health problem, thus comprising her effectiveness as an administrator in the county welfare department. With her strong desire to carry out professional responsibilities and personal commitments as unobtrusively as possible, she and her mother conceived the idea of carrying the infusion bag, tubing, and pump in a fashionable purse or tote bag, which was less cumbersome and more consistent with normal appearance. They designed an attractive drawstring purse of durable lined corduroy that allowed each component of the infusion system to be positioned and secured without compromising safety or effectiveness. The morale and spirit of the patient dramatically improved during the remainder of the outpatient treatment as a result of this personalized approach to her problem.

Although there were minimal patient complications, none of the ambulatory infusion pumps to date had safety features incorporated into their design characteristics. In late 1986, a new ambulatory peristaltic rotary volumetric pump (Pancretec® Provider 4000+ Pancretec, Inc., San Diego, CA) utilizing microprocessor control with audible feedback was introduced into the marketplace to deliver continuous or intermittent (cyclic) TPN. The pump weighs only

660 g and has the desired safety systems including air-inline detection, occlusion detection, low battery alarm, Keep Vein Open capability, and Patient Lock-Out to allow the option of a tamperproof device for those patients who would benefit at home.

The pump is worn in a variety of ways according to specific requirements and individual preferences of the patient. Various belts, slings, shoulder straps, and harnesses have been invented, modified, and/or adapted for use with the pump to meet the personal needs of each patient. These and other similar developments have allowed the vast majority of home nutrition support patients to resume normal activities of daily living with minimal compromise and embarrassment and maximal effectiveness.

For home patients receiving intermittent (cyclic) TPN, the newly created pumps have taper procedures incorporated into their operational performance. Numerous studies have demonstrated that TPN solutions can be delivered safely and effectually over a 10- to 18-hour period in selected patients with normal renal and hepatic function.[9] Reactive hypoglycemia with occasional hyperkalemia and rebound hypoglycemia occur in the stressed, hospitalized patient and rarely pose a problem in the stable, nonhypermetabolic individual.[9]

Patients are generally placed on intermittent (cyclic) infusion regimens over a 2- or 3-day period while they are hospitalized. Each day, the hypertonic dextrose infusion is discontinued in 4-hour increments until the patient is tolerating the desired schedule with no untoward effects as evidenced by serum glucose levels. Although some procedural differences exist among nutrition support teams, taper-on and taper-off practices are recommended for all patients receiving intermittent (cyclic) TPN to allow sufficient time for adaption to the high glucose load of the TPN infusate. One such device, the HomePro® pump (Travenol Laboratories, Inc., Deerfield; IL), has a TPN infusion profile which includes the following:

- A taper-on infusion time of 8 percent of the time of infusion;
- A taper-on infusion volume of approximately 5 percent of the total volume of infusion;
- An initial taper-on infusion rate beginning at 60 ml/hour and increasing to the desired maintenance infusion rate over 8 percent of the total infusion time;
- A maintenance infusion time comprising 84 percent of the total time in infusion;
- Maintenance infusion rate calculated by the pump if volume and time of total infusion is selected;
- A taper-off infusion time of 8 percent of the total time of infusion;
- A taper-off volume of approximately 5 percent of the total volume of infusion; and
- A taper-off infusion rate gradually decreasing to 40 ml/hour over 8 percent of the total infusion time.[10]

These and other comparable advancements promise to continue to revolutionize the technology in this exciting field of endeavor.

CANDIDATES FOR HOME NUTRITIONAL SUPPORT

The technique of ambulatory home nutritional support has become a common adjunctive treatment for many patients who require extended or lifelong nutritional and metabolic supplementation (Table 10-1). More recently

Table 10-1
Indications for Home Nutritional Support

Enteral	Parenteral	
Head and neck cancer	*Chronic*	*Acute*

Chemotherapy, radiation therapy	Short bowel syndrome
	  Mesenteric vascular
	    catastrophe
	  Venous thrombosis
		Active inflammatory
		  bowel disease
		  Crohn's disease
		  Ulcerative colitis
		  Infectious enterocolitis

Central nervous system disorders	Arterial occlusion	

Dysphagia	Congenital atresia	Antineoplastic therapy
		  Chemotherapy
		  Radiation

Anorexia nervosa	Crohn's disease	Immunotherapy Operation
Depression	Retroperitoneal neoplasia	Combination therapy
Coma	Major abdominal trauma	Incomplete bowel obstruction

Organic brain disease	Postoperative or
	  postirradiation complications
		Miscellaneous disorders
		  Chronic dialysis

Cervical fracture	Gangrenous volvulus
	  Radiation enteritis
		Hepatic insufficiency
		  Relapsing pancreatitis

Severe arthralgias	Fistulas	

Some types of
  inflammatory bowel
  disease, short gut
  syndrome, malabsorption,
  high intestinal fistulas,
  pancreatitis
	Malnutrition and
	  malabsorption syndromes	

All "wasting diseases" in
  patients who have a
  functioning GI tract below
  the ligament of Treitz		

during the diagnosis related grouping (DRG) era of the 1980s, patients are being treated for even shorter periods of time in the home. Outpatient enteral nutrition is indicated for any condition in which adequate oral intake is not possible, but the GI tract is functioning and can be used safely. On the other hand, there are many poorly understood chronic malnutrition and malabsorption conditions in which the use of the alimentary tract for optimal nourishment of a patient can be supplemented or fed entirely by vein to maintain adequate nutritional status until their primary disorder can be relieved or corrected.

It has been recently estimated that there are approximately 9000 chronic home TPN patients with some degree of GI dysfunction.* In addition, at least 10,000 cancer patients are now receiving intravenous nutrition at home for treatment periods ranging from three to six months between or during courses of antineoplastic therapy.* Projections indicate that the home enteral market is expected to grow at an annual rate of 20 percent, while the home TPN patient population is likely to increase 5 percent each year.* As increasing knowledge and experience are gained in the techniques of home nutritional support, applications will inevitably be expanded and extended to virtually every medical discipline within the next several years.

PATIENT AND FAMILY TEACHING

The single most critical factor that determines the success of home nutritional support may be the training program for the patient and family members. Educational preparation for outpatient TPN has traditionally required 2–3 weeks, depending on the logistics of the treatment regimen and the patient's physical, intellectual, and emotional capabilities.[11] With the major trend toward home health care today, some patients can now learn the theory and practice of home TPN or tube feeding as outpatients without being admitted to the hospital. Other patients who are hospitalized for reasons related to their primary disease process are being discharged earlier, often before completion of the teaching/learning program. In this chaning milieu, the nutrition support nurse in the hospital must collaborate closely with the home care nurse to coordinate the continuation of the educational process and facilitate a smooth and uneventful transition into the home setting.

Assessment

Prior to catheter insertion and after informed consent has been granted, the nurse assesses the patient and close family members to determine their learning needs. Variables that are considered include motivation, manual dexterity, fine

---

* From Susanne Loarie, Travenol Laboratories, Inc., September 1, 1986. Personal communication.

motor coordination, mental aptitude, home environmental considerations, psychological and social support systems, and any other factors that might affect the feasibility, safety, and efficacy of the treatment.

The patient is primarily responsible for the technical care of the CVC apparatus whenever possible. When a patient lacks the necessary cognitive and motor abilities needed for these functions, however, a family member or close friend must be designated as the primary caregiver. Ideally, at least one additional family member should become adept in the skills and procedures to provide back-up support in case the patient becomes ill and unable to continue self care.

Indeed, the education and support of family members and friends is undoubtedly important for positive patient outcome. When relatives are informed of the patient's basic pathophysiology, medical management, and progress, they tend to be more helpful, less anxious, and more satisfied with the quality of health services provided. The patient's loved ones should certainly be familiar with, but acknowledge the limitations and constraints imposed by the nutrient therapy.

Several learning barriers common among nutritional support patients deserve special mention. First, the learning ability of an emaciated patient is inherently compromised by the pathophysiology of malnutrition. According to the degree and severity of nutritional and metabolic derangements, the patient may be afflicted with chronic fatigue, inability to concentrate for long periods of time, and slow mentality. Although most cachetic patients become stronger after the first few days of nutritional replenishment, others with more severe deficiencies can require weeks or longer before there are noticeable improvements in energy level and ability to learn. In addition to the patient's physical illness and degree of malnutrition, energy level can be further compromised by psychological and social responses, the number and intensity of other stressors in one's life, and current situational and maturational crises.

Patients who are weak and unsteady in their movements may benefit from daily physical therapy until their condition improves. In other instances, the nurse may suggest squeezing a rubber ball or starting a knitting or needlepoint project for those who need to improve their fine motor coordination.

The complexity of the infusion system is often overwhelming to the patients when they are first introduced to its operation and maintenance. Mild anxiety actually strengthens learning ability, while intense anxiety, fear, and pain have the opposite effect, resulting in serious impairments in listening ability and long-term retention of cognitive information. Therefore, it is usually quite beneficial for patients to hold their feeding catheters or tubes and other infusion equipment before they begin to learn the related psychomotor skills. During this tactile experience, patients are encouraged to ask question and discuss their feelings freely and openly with the nurse in order to establish mutual rapport and a strong relationship based on trust.

Nighttime hospital routines and poor sleeping habits can deprive patients of the sleep required to learn the knowledge and procedures for home nutritional support. Patients with sleep disturbances have symptoms of irritability, apathy, lack of alterness, fatigue, anxiety, poor judgment, and increased sensitivity to pain and discomfort.[12]

The average adult has approximately 4–6 sleep cycles per night, each composed of 2 distinct phases. The second phase of the cycle, known as rapid-eye-movement (REM) sleep, is vital for learning, memory, and psychological adaptation. Not only are the day's events reviewed and categorized into the brain's storage system, but problems are solved, and the individual gains perspective and insight into troublesome or difficult matters. Excessive fear and anxiety will cause the patient to waken often during the night, thereby decreasing REM sleep and hindering learning potential.

Acute pain can also have a negative effect on learning ability. Some discomfort is relatively minor and annoying to patients, while more serious pain may preoccupy them to the exclusion of all else, including curiosity and the will to learn. Pain, whether visceral and deep or stabbing and intermittent, will always cause some degree of learning incapacitation. Narcotics sometimes relieve the pain, but of course there are side effects that have negative impacts such as drowsiness, central nervous system depression, and decreased coordination. Drug dependency in the patient who is preparing for home feeding is a serious challenge for the nurse, and often the teaching effort must be directed toward the patient's designated caregiver.

Planning

Following completion of the initial assessment, an individualized teaching plan that is well organized and sequenced is formulated to meet the learning needs of the patients and maximize their involvement in the program. On the basis of the teaching plan, a verbal or written contract is tentatively negotiated between the patient and involved members of the health care team.[8] The original contract, which specifies the estimated period of instruction, must be revised when patient objectives are either not met or only partially accomplished by tentative dates. Essentially, the contract implies that the team members, the patient, and family or involved friends identify their respective general and specific expectations, privileges, and obligations and agree mutually to adhere to these conditions during their interactions. Utilization of the contractual relationship enhances patient independence and satisfaction as the terms of the agreement are fulfilled. It minimizes patient and staff conflict and frustration, encourages open communication, and promotes a collaborative union between patient and staff with joint accountability and responsibility.

Patients learn in a variety of ways according to their level of growth and development, individual lifestyle, personality, and past experiences. Children typically learn faster than adults and are more flexible in their attitudes toward the feeding treatment. Some of the well-known characteristics of the adult learner that the nurse considers in planning the instructional program include the following:

- Self-concept changes from dependence to independence, which means that adult learners are capable of self-direction;

- The adult's life experiences are more diverse than those of a child and will impact the learning process;

- The adult's motivation is usually to solve life problems and immediately apply what has been learned;

- More time may be required for learning because adults are less confident and more uncertain of their abilities than are children.[13]

A comprehensive curriculum for patient education is developed that allows each individual the opportunity to advance at an independent rate of learning, at least to a predetermined level of acceptable competence (Fig. 10-2). Learning should be a positive, supportive experience in which the patient gains confidence and self-esteem as goals are accomplished. Instruction begins with planned activities in which the student will be able to accomplish the tasks and feel a sense of success. This is very important because adults are often self-conscious about performing a new skill, worrying that they may look "foolish" or will cause irreparable harm to the patient.

According to the patient's state of health and ability to concentrate, teaching sessions are ideally scheduled at a convenient time for no longer than one hour each day. Biorhythms explain why some people are better learners in the early morning, while others prefer the later afternoon to schedule their classes. Instructional activities are most effective in an environment that is not too complex—preferably a well lighted, comfortable classroom removed from the patient's hospital room with minimal distractions and equipped with an adequate work surface to perform the procedures.

Methodology

A variety of teaching and learning materials should be used to accommodate differences in the abilities of the individuals being taught. For pediatric patients, play therapy using descriptive animated cartoons, coloring books, dolls,

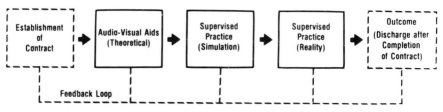

Fig. 10-2. A teaching/learning model for home nutritional support.

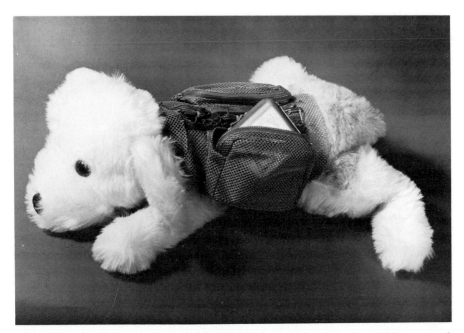

Fig. 10-3. Stuffed animals are invaluable teaching tools when the child's age and developmental status are considered.

models, and stuffed animals are invaluable teaching tools when adapted to the child's age and developmental status (Fig. 10-3). Furthermore, the teaching program may have a normalization component that enables the children to function in their usual school, play, and home environment while concurrently receiving home nutritional support. For the more mature learners who assume some accountability in the care of their lifelines, a combination of instructional strategies may be employed. These include media, printed materials, classroom learning activities, return demonstrations, and informal discussion.

Studies have demonstrated that a number of well designed audiovisual (AV) aids are equally effective in facilitating the patient's learning.[14] Dwyer proposes that 11 percent of a person's total learning experiences occur through hearing and 18 percent through sight.[14] He finds people usually remember 10 percent of what they read, 20 percent of what they hear, 30 percent of what they see, 50 percent of what they see and hear, 70 percent of what they say, and 90 percent of what they say while performing a task.

Videocassettes are popular in many home nutritional support teaching programs, especially with a cable distribution system that allows broadcast on a hospital-wide basis. With such AV equipment, the patient can view the appropriate programs at a prearranged time each day or whenever it is convenient in the hospital room. To enhance cognitive learning, the instructional aids should offer a combination of color, pictures, motion, and sound and be entertaining as well as informative to the patient and family members. Presentations are best divided into clearly defined sections, each of which informs the viewers what they are expected to know after completing the module. Titles and commentary are helpful in organizing information that they may seem somewhat confusing to the learner at first, with key points and sequences reiterated throughout the presentation of material.

Following the initial exposure to the cognitive ideas that must be learned using AV aids, patients and their alternate caregivers are encouraged to attend 1-hour group classes to learn the care of the central venous catheter. During the classroom demonstration, the instructor demonstrates how to: (1) heparinize the feeding catheter, (2) replace the heparin injection cap, (3) change the sterile protective dressing over the CVC exit site, and (4) monitor the infusion system for problems.

Learning research has shown that at least two or three exposures to new ideas and complex procedures are necessary before the content can be retained.[14] Therefore, the teacher performs the procedure in logical sequence and explains each step with its appropriate rationale. Since the learners will always attempt to mimic every detail of the teacher's actions, accuracy in technique during the demonstration is of obvious importance.

The first time patients and their caregivers practice the feeding procedures, they are usually frightened and nervous that some harm to the patient will result. Empirical evidence has shown unequivocally that the learner's anxiety level is reduced significantly when the first return demonstration is simulated in a classroom setting using a mannequin or Cath-Train® (Caremark, Inc., Newport Beach, CA). This teaching aid, a type of chest shield with an implanted catheter affixed to the anterior side, is worn like a shirt, allowing the patients to perform the TPN tasks with the catheter positioned close to their own CVC device (Fig. 10-4).

The patients and their classmates usually want to review any written materials that have been provided during the TPN teaching/learning program and to mentally rehearse the steps of the procedures before beginning a return demonstration. The nurse should encourage to continue mannequin practice until they feel comfortable and adequately prepared to care for the patient's central venous catheter. When the learners are encouraged to pace themselves, they are more likely to feel a sense of accomplishment, pride, and control over their environment as they progress from the simpler procedures to the more complex TPN skills such as operating the infusion pump and adding medications to the TPN container. Unless there is a financial motive, most patients do not become involved in the daily admixture of the TPN solutions.

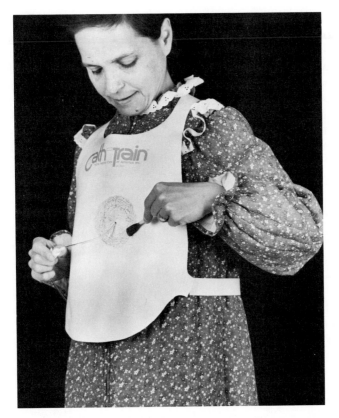

Fig. 10-4. The Cath-Train® is a teaching tool that enables simulated practice during the teaching/learning program.

Evaluation

The nurse closely supervises the patients during these practice sessions, reassuring them often that assistance will be provided if there are problems or errors in technique or judgment. Patients progress at their own pace and are encouraged to repeat each task until it has been mastered in all respects.

Feedback is provided to acknowledge the desired changes in behavior and the patient's progress toward independence and self-care. This feedback is (1) descriptive rather than evaluative, (2) specific rather than general, (3) directed toward behavior the patient can change rather than the patient as a person, and (4) provided on a timely basis after each step of the procedure.[15]

Since reinforcement is a major condition for learning, the nurse instructor explores reinforcers that are closely linked to the patient's value system. Praise, recognition, and encouragement are universally valued by all, while verbal reinforcers including recognition phrases and nonverbal reinforcers such as nodding, smiling, and moving toward the student can be equally effective for others. Incentive feedback to help the patient obtain a more tangible reward such as a daytime pass or a certificate of accomplishment signed by all involved parties at the time of discharge are also desirable rewards for most people.

The nutrition support nurse can use rating scales, checklists, or anecdotal notes to collect the appropriate descriptive evaluation data. All aspects of the contract must be completed prior to discharge, after which the patient must be followed conscientiously on an outpatient basis to document the competency, accuracy, and consistency of the nutritional support regimen.

FOLLOW-UP CARE IN THE HOME SETTING

On the same day the patient is discharged from the hospital, the assigned home care nurse receives the final verbal report from the inpatient nurse who coordinated the training program before making the first outpatient visit that same day. It is customary for patients to feel inundated when they first return home and need a great deal of support in setting up the work area and beginning the routine daily TPN procedures.

During the inpatient teaching program, the patients were expected to select the most appropriate storage and work area in their respective homes. The bedroom is likely to be the optimal storage area for supplies if it is cleaner than the bathroom and kitchen. When the rooms appear crowded and space is a problem, general department stores carry plastic shelving and drawer units that are relatively inexpensive and ideal for patients to stock the TPN supplies away from their children and pets. Sometime during the visit, the nurse reiterates the importance of keeping ceiling fans, oscillating fans, and air conditioning window units removed from the work space, and that no vacuum cleaners or brooms are to be used during the procedures. Another responsibility of the nurse is to confirm that there is sufficient space in the refrigerator for storage of the premixed TPN bags and that power sources and wall outlets in the house are adequate for the infusion equipment. If cleanliness poses a particular challenge, the nurse works closely with patients and their families to provide an improved and suitable environment for administration of home nutritional support.

Shortly after returning home, many patients seem to forget what they learned while in the hospital and exhibit signs of learning overload such as fatigue, remissness, and/or regression in previously acquired abilities. It is precisely for this reason that the instructional program must be continued in the home until the caregiver is able to demonstrate capability and voice confidence in the care of the feeding catheter. When left alone, the patients and their families must be able to perform the TPN procedures accurately and be prepared to solve any problems that might arise during the night.

Home care nurses make visits as often as necessary, usually more frequently during the early days of home therapy, until the patients become more independent. Reimbursement of nursing services is outlined and defined by the respective insurance carriers. For indigent patients, the Visiting Nurses' Association in some areas of the country has on occasion consented to make routine visits as often as needed to the patient's residence for follow-up care, teaching, and documentation of patient progress.

At least one member of the nursing team must be available to the patient 24 hours a day via a radiophone beeper system in the event of an emergency situation, and the facilities of a specially-equipped clinic or hospital must be also identified within reasonable proximity to the patient's dwelling in case more complex or potentially lethal problems present. In addition, each patient wears a Medic-Alert bracelet or necklace to provide emergency medical identification whenever necessary. This unique system of communication, which is recognized on an international basis and is well-known to Emergency Medical Technicians, consists of (1) an individually engraved emblem designed to attract attention, (2) an annual wallet card that contains personal medical information, and (3) the number of the emergency answering service for retrieval of the subscriber's medical information from a current computerized data base.

The nurse telephones the patients regularly to assess current needs and validate their physical condition and response to therapy. The patients are scheduled for return visits to the outpatient clinic for a follow-up physical examination to detect any fluid, electrolyte, and/or nutrient disorder; laboratory monitoring determinations; and a physician's evaluation prior to making changes in the feeding regimen. At the same time, the results of daily weights, temperature, and urine testing that are recorded by the patient at home on the appropriate flowsheets are reviewed. The constituents of a typical intravenous feeding unit are shown in Table 10-2. Many lifelong or long-term TPN patients have been stabilized from a metabolic and nutritional perspective without any changes in their nutrient formulation for months or even years.

The home care agency should have quality assurance programs in place for the purposes of defining and updating standards of home care and evaluating program effectiveness. Health care professionals share an important responsibility in assuring the safety, quality, and cost-effectiveness of home care. With this in mind, some of the key areas that need to be addressed are:

- the selection of appropriate patients for home care;
- the training of patients to safely self-administer nutrient formulations at home;
- the prescription or recommendation for proper nutritional formulations;
- the routine monitoring of patients to assess nutritional status and complications;
- the provision of supplies and delivery on an efficient and timely schedule;
- the coordination of transitional care from hospital to home and back to the hospital when indicated; and
- the assurance of proper reimbursement for care rendered at home.

Table 10-2
Typical Intravenous Feeding Units for Home TPN

Adult	Pediatric
Base	Base
500 ml 40–50% dextrose in water	500 ml 40% dextrose in water
500 ml 8.5–10% crystalline amino acids	300 ml 8.5% crystalline amino acids
Additives to all units	Additives
40–50 mEq sodium chloride	25–30 mEq sodium chloride
20–30 mEq potassium chloride	30–40 mEq potassium acid phosphate
15–30 mEq potassium acid phosphate	12–15 mEq magnesium sulfate
(10–20 mcg phosphorous)	25–35 mEq calcium gluconate
15–18 mEq magnesium sulfate	2 mg zinc sulfate
	0.5 mg copper sulfate
	0.05 ml Imferon
Additives to any one unit daily	2 ml MVI concentrate
10 ml MVI-12	0.5 ml folic acid
4.5 mEq calcium gluconate 10%	1.0 mg vitamin K
5–10 mg zinc sulfate	1 μg vitamin B_{12}
1–2 mg copper sulfate	1 ml Berocca-C (100 μg biotin)
0.1 ml Imferon	10 μg chromium chloride
10–20 μg chromium chloride	30 μg selenium (sodium selenate)
0.5 mg manganese chloride	
60 μg selenium (sodium selenate)	
3 mg vitamin K	Intravenous fat emulsion (10%)
	50–75 ml/kg 2–7 times weekly
Intravenous fat emulsion 10% or 20%	Infusion rate = 115 ml/kg per day
500 ml 2–7 times weekly	115 kcal/kg/day
	3 g protein/kg/day

PSYCHOSOCIAL ADAPTATION

As the methodology and equipment for prolonged home nutritional support have been improved, a new spectrum of psychological and social challenges in the last several decades have emerged. The patient's adaptation depends on the intensity and duration of their primary disease processes and their prospects for recovery from the illness and the return of adequate GI function.[16] Despite the limitations imposed by the nutrient system, it is at times somewhat miraculous to observe how well patients and their families withstand the plight of their sickness, while simultaneously maintaining a hopeful spirit and strong will to enjoy their usual lifestyles during home feeding.

Perhaps it is the persistent cooperation and interaction of a highly specialized team of professional nurses that has a profound impact on the success of long-term patient management. Through the establishment of close interpersonal relations based on mutual trust and respect, the nurse identifies environmental variables and behavioral patterns that influence the patients' adaptation to their altered health status. The provision of empathy, counseling, and psychological support are based on assessment of such factors as developmental tasks, family relationships and roles, communication skills, coping mechanisms, daily habits, and life events. Effective problem solving and objective reasoning abilities are prerequisites for each nurse on the team in order to enhance the patient's attainment of psychological equilibrium in coping with individual and other situational crises. To prevent, recognize, and treat these many-faceted psychosocial problems, the nurse has to work closely with the psychologist or psychiatrist on the nutrition support service.

Oral Deprivation

Whether the loss of the ability to eat is total or partial, the adjustment period for the patient is always difficult, perhaps because of the numerous and varied social meanings of food.[17] During the first 3–5 months of home therapy, almost all patients become painfully aware of the barrage of television and magazine advertisements inducing the consumer to eat or drink. They may even feel excluded from the daily food-related rituals and the many social and festive occasions in which food plays a major role.

When the sight and odor of food is unpleasant to the patients, they will take painstaking and sometimes drastic measures to avoid it and any activities that remind them of eating. In Rains' experience, almost 90 percent of the patients preferred to be alone during tube feeding.[18] Half of them retreated to the kitchen, when formerly they had eaten in the dining or living room. One elderly man joined in holiday greetings with his daughter and son-in-law until time to partake, when he promptly went to his bedroom.[18] The daughter explained that she and her husband ate out much of the time because the odor and sight of food bothered the patient. Price and Levine found that three-fourths of their patients chose to sit with others during mealtime.[19] Some smoked, and others chewed their food without swallowing it.

Patient coping mechanisms vary from overt defiance of medical advice with surreptitious intake of prohibited spicy and irritating foods to becoming a gourmet cook for the family. In one instance, an irresistible desire for food and obsession for water resulted in nutritional "promiscuity" for one man receiving TPN who cruised around the city visiting restaurants and fast food outlets, despite the severe diarrhea and dehydration that always followed these binges.[20] Female patients seem to satisfy their appetite vicariously by an exaggerated interest in collecting recipes or preparing meals, while men often attempt cooking responsibilities to relieve their spouse of the traditional task. The wife of one patient surrendered her domain in the kitchen angrily and regretfully after 35 years of marriage, feeling robbed on her *raison d'etre* because there was no one to cook for but herself.[19]

Patients find ingenious ways to make their feeding treatment more of a meal than a prodedure. One 22-year-old woman with Crohn's disease attached a picture of a turkey and dressing dinner to the TPN bag on Thanksgiving day. Another man, while blenderizing the food that was prepared for others in his family, talked incessantly about how much he enjoyed the taste of stew, corn bread, and buttermilk.[18] When asked why he habitually seasoned his nutrient bag with salt and pepper, he responded that his stomach was "used to it that way." Another patient and his wife felt that the tube feedings should be given in courses rather than all mixed together.[18] The meat and starch were combined, while juices, fruits, puddings, and desserts were administered separately by tube.

Home nutrition support patients need constant reassurance that they are receiving adequate nutrition, especially if they are experiencing hunger pangs. The nurse should point out the return of the well-nourished state by making the patient and his family aware of positive signs such as weight gain. A major nursing goal in the home setting is to assist the family in reestablishing the most normal food-related habits within the limitations of the patient's condition. Nursing staff encourage the patient to spend mealtimes in the usual manner in order to minimize patient isolation and derive social and family satisfaction from the associated interactions. Most patients do not have a reduced sensitivity to the aroma or taste of food and eventually regain some eating ability, though their dietary intake may be limited or of minimal nutritive value.

Fear

A universal patient response during the first few months of home nutritional support is fear of the potentially fatal complications associated with this form of invasive therapy such as air embolism, catheter infection, and pump malfunction. At times, anxiety related to the infusion apparatus and its function assumes delusional proportions. Almost all patients can relate some incident as a "horror story" or "close call" that occurred outside the hospital. One man remembers the time he was traveling in his automobile when the infusion pump inadvertently failed. Although he feels he suffered a great deal of mental anguish during the mishap, he promptly devised an ingenious way to "borrow" power from the cigarette lighter in the car. At times, patients believe the life-sustaining system is destined to fail, making death seem imminent. For instance, one patient explained, "You play with your life day-by-day. You go to bed not knowing if you'll wake up in the morning or not."[21]

If the patient is obsessed with fear of a life-threatening complication, this can interfere with usual sleep patterns or other daily routines. The caregiver often deems it necessary to sleep in the same room as the patient in order to reduce the possibility of infusion problems. The child figuratively regains the umbilical cord in the form of the somewhat restrictive feeding apparatus. Furthermore, sleep deprivation can be even more aggravated if the patient is fed 3–4 liters nocturnally. Complaining of chronic fatigue and polyuria, one woman described home TPN like ". . . bringing home a new baby . . . like getting up to feed a new baby."[19]

Even though the patient's fears can assume delusional proportions, they can usually be alleviated by the ready availability and accessibility of at least one nurse at all times and the willingness of the staff to evaluate and help solve problems during an emergency return visit to the clinic or hospital, as well as consistent emotional support and constant reassurance. In general, patients become less fearful of a catastrophic situation and more confident that they can act competently during a crisis as the duration of home nutritional support increases. When the degree of the patient's fears become manageable, overall functioning and routine daily activities can be expected to improve dramatically.

Family Relationships

Anxiety reactions vary among the patient's spouse, parents, and family members, and the quality and dependability of their support significantly affect the patient's physical, psychological, and social well-being. During the initial rehabilitation period at home, reports of marital and family difficulties are more common.[22] If there is a previously stable marital relationship, however, couples will likely continue to exhibit sharing and empathy when one partner begins home nutritional support. On the other hand, the nutrient therapy will usually add significantly to the problems of a discordant marriage.

Especially during the early months following discharge from the hospital, patients often report diminished frequence and enjoyment of sexual relations because of depression, altered body image, feelings of embarrassment, and the inconvenience, discomfort, and fear of the infusion system.[23] One documented problem, male impotence, may be of psychological origin, but it can also be a symptom of zinc deficiency or other biochemical abnormality. Inhibited sexual activity tends to be alleviated after both partners become adjusted to the new mode of feeding.

Parent/child relationships should be expected to change following the initiation of home therapy.[24] In parents of pediatric patients, intense conflict toward the child and the intravenous apparatus has been documented. Moreover, parents sometimes feel quilty about the attention they must give their afflicted child at the expense of their healthy children. They might even fear the possibility of the birth of another child, which could further compromise their ability to cope with the intravenously- or enterally-fed child. Instances have occurred in which relatives and friends have become so anxious in the presence of the delivery system that they subsequently avoid the patient. In this situation, the nurse has a responsibility to explain the treatment and its inconveniences, risks, and restraints to those involved using an approach that ameliorates rather than aggravates their fears and to support them therapeutically until normal family dynamics have been reestablished.

Leisure and social activities are an important aspect of the patient's daily activities of living. Unless the patient has an implanted venous access device, some activities such as swimming or showering could contaminate the CVC line.

Naturally, body contact sports that could interfere with catheter placement and pump function must also be restricted. Patients are encouraged to resume full-time employment unless there is a conflict with insurance coverage. The patient is encouraged to rest at regular intervals if there is a problem with fatigue and weakness.

Body Image

Distortions in body image and impairments in self-esteem are common in cachectic patients with partial or complete oral deprivation. Many nutritionally depleted persons are repulsed by their own bodies, feeling mutilated because of the external catheter, emaciation, multiple scars, ileostomy, and/or cushingoid features secondary to maintenance steroid therapy. The patients consider themselves to be very different from others, describing their body schema as "freaky," "crippled," "unattractive," "distorted," and "without sex appeal."[25]

Although true delusional thinking and loss of reality testing do not seem to occur, some patients express distorted ideas that the catheter will become dislodged, piercing the heart or eroding the body surface.[22] Female patients who have gained more weight than they desire may not comply with the feeding schedule. In a desperate attempt to assert their autonomy, they have defy the judgment and authority of the nutrition support team by decreasing the infusion rate to promote weight loss.

Before home patients can be expected to integrate their illnesses with the resulting body alterations, they must be allowed sufficient opportunity to ventilate their feelings. During the grieving period of denial, acceptance, and finally adjustment, it is crucial for the nurse to be sensitive and understanding of the patient's needs. Patients have to accept their feeding catheter just as they do a temporary or permanent ileostomy or colostomy. Since patients may not have changed their self-concepts prior to discharge from the hospital, it is often the home care nurse who facilitates this process. Appropriate interventions, which are based on the patient's adaptation to the loss, include diversional activities, group process, and the use of mirrors to increase perceptual feedback.

Depression

During the first 3–6 months of home nutritional support, about 80 percent of the patients experience a reactive-type depression with episodic sadness, dysphoria, crying spells, insomnia, loss of sexual interest, social withdrawal, and feelings of hopelessness.[21] The condition waxes and wanes and is exacerbated by increased stress, often attributed to the patient's physical condition. Mood downswings are usually brief, lasting days or weeks rather than months.

Depression at times has presented as partial denial of illness and poor compliance with the instructions of the nursing staff. Some patients have gone swimming without permission, while others have induced metabolic abnormalities and dehydration because they refused to infuse their nutrient solutions according to the prescribed schedule. Many case histories of catheter-related sepsis have been preceded by depression. The total number of patients who act indifferently or even irresponsibly toward care of their intravenous lifeline has been extremely low.

The patient who requires nutritional treatment for longer than 8 weeks is more likely to feel depressed than another whose therapy is more short term.[26] Although it seems the most serious depression occurs in patients with acute loss of bowel function, those with a previous history of depression are at an increased risk for reoccurrence. Overall, after an initial settling-in period, the majority of patients are extremely gratified with the new lease on life afforded by home TPN, and most tolerate the attendant inconveniences with a good sense of humor.

Because of this complex and many-faceted situation, each member of the nursing team must be skilled in recognizing the patient's ambivalent feelings and providing the opportunity for verbal expression and decompression. The patients' interactions are most often those of admiration, respect, and gratitude for the therapy and professional team who has kept them alive. On the other hand, patients at times may feel helpless, powerless, and at the mercy of the staff.

During the process of patient education and treatment at home, it is possible that conflicts can arise between a patient and the team members unless clear lines of authority and expectations are clearly delineated. Frequent team conferences and discussions have been beneficial to evaluate the patient's adaptation, especially during periods of maladaptation or crisis, and ongoing management of intrinsic stresses.

FINANCIAL CONSIDERATIONS

The financial burden of long-term or permanent home parenteral feeding not only induces but aggravates any preexisting depression or other psychological dilemmas. Those unfortunate patients without sufficient medical insurance must rely on hospitals, grants from pharmaceutical manufacturers, and even charitable funds established by their churches and communities. Attempts have been made at the national legislative level to obtain Medicare or other similar benefits for all home TPN patients, but these efforts to date have been futile.

Helen Meyner first introduced the House of Representatives Bill #7889 on June 20, 1977, to provide Medicare benefits to all home TPN patients, regardless of age. Although this bill was referred to the House Ways and Means Subcommittee, Medicare agreed in 1977 to assume the cost of supplies and pharmaceuticals for home TPN patients older than 65 years of age or who were otherwise eligible for Medicare after two years of total disability. Unfortunately, it has been very difficult to bear the exorbitant treatment costs for the two years prior to eligibility for Medicare disability. Moreover, a number of patients who are physically able to work forfeit eligibility for Medicare reimbursement if they procure a salary under Medicare provisions. More desirable legislation is needed to cover catastrophic illness, pay for the extraordinary medical and other costs associated with home parenteral nutrition, and allow the patient to engage in gainful employment without losing medical coverage.

Concern has been expressed that third-party support of home TPN patients would result in runaway costs similar to those incurred by the end-stage reneal disease program. Indeed, Schribner calculated in 1977 that the monthly costs of the home TPN program for a patient was $600–$1000 per month, depending on the type of amino acid solution utilized.[27] Early entry into the home TPN market has been characterized by cases of excessive profiteering by many ambitious businesses. The sale of small providers to more established national companies during a period of consolidation in the early decade resulted in numerous "get rich fast" stories. Today, it is estimated that the cost of home TPN ranges from $6000–$8000 per month.*

Whereas this consumer price increase is typical of any new industry, such a phenomenon has created grave caution regarding what is considered proper compensation for home care services. In an effort to reduce federal expenses and respond to these excessive profit margins in the home care industry, reimbursement levels are now being carefully scrutinized. Some insurance companies have even become more receptive to the provision of coverage from the time of discharge with these careful ongoing audits. These positive changes have been accelerated by major national efforts, many of which have been coordinated by the Americn Society of Parenteral and Enteral Nutrition, to accumulate the appropriate data demonstrating the cost effectiveness of this relatively new therapy.

CONCLUSION

Since 1967, outpatient ambulatory nutritional support has been shown to be a safe and effective therapeutic means of providing adequate nourishment to appropriate patients in the home and work environment. As new advances continue to be made in the technology, manufacture, and availability of miniature pumps, microprocessors, nutrient containers, administration tubings, and inline filters, it is anticipated that existing delivery systems will undergo many positive changes and modifications. No longer is it necessary or justifiable that patients with insufficient or inadequate GI function be confined to the hospital or die. Life itself can be prolonged, and the quality of living can be maintained or improved in selected individuals. Continued research in this vital area promises to yield a wealth of knowledge in the biochemical, compositional, and functional aspects of long-term or lifelong intravenously- or enterally-supported human

---

*From Susanne Loarie, Travenol Laboratories, Inc., September 1, 1986. Personal communication.

metabolism and health. Finally, the health care economic revolution of the decade with a plethora of legislation, regulation, and private initiatives will further impact this proliferating nutrition support industry.

REFERENCES

1. Schneider PJ: The home health care revolution. Nutr Clin Prac 1(4):177, 1986
2. Dudrick SJ, Englert DM, MacFadyen BV, et al: A vest for ambulatory patients receiving hyperalimentation. Surg Gynecol Obstet 148:587–590, 1979
3. Broviac JW, Scribner BH: Prolonged parenteral nutrition in the home. Surg Gynecol Obstet 139:24–28, 1974
4. Broviac JW, Cole JJ, Scribner BH: A silicone rubber catheter for prolonged parenteral alimentation. Surg Gynecol Obstet 136:602–606, 1973
5. Jeejeebhoy KN, Langer B, Tsallas G, et al: Total parenteral nutrition at home: studies in patients surviving four months to five years. Gastroenterology 71:943–953, 1976
6. Solassol C, Joyeux H: Ambulatory parenteral nutrition, in Manni C, Magalini SI, Scrascia E (eds): Parenteral Alimentation. The International Symposium on Intensive Therapy. New York, American Elsevier, 1976, pp 138–152
7. Maenab AJ: A portable infusion system for the ambulant child. J Pediatr 88:654–658, 1976
8. Dudrick SJ, Englert DM, Clague MB: Ambulatory home hyperalimentation. Kaminski MV Jr (ed) in Hyperalimentation A Guide for Clinicians New York, Marcel Dekker, 1985, pp 607–638
9. McCormick DC, Perren JB, Andrassy RJ: Benefits of cyclic parenteral nutrition. Contemporary Surgery 27:27–32, 1985
10. HomePro®: A new era in nutritional support. Travacare Home Therapy Clinical Information Bulletin 5:1–2, 1986
11. Marcin C, Misny P, Paysinger J, et al: Home parenteral nutrition. Nutr Clin Prac 1(4):179–192, 1986
12. Cunningham SG, Mitchell PH: Comfort and sleep status, in Mitchell PH (ed): Concepts Basic to Nursing, 2 ed. New York, McGraw-Hill Company 1977, pp 522–552
13. Smith CE: Patient Education: Nurses in Partnership With Other Health Professionals. Orlando, FL, Grune & Stratton, 1987, p 175
14. Dwyer FM: Strategies for Improving Visual Learning. State College, PA, Learning Services, 1978, pp. 1–20
15. Redman BK: The Process of Patient Teaching in Nursing (ed 3). St. Louis, CV Mosby, 1976, pp 88–113, 183–200
16. Dudrick SJ, Englert DM: Total care of the patient receiving total parenteral nutrition. Psychosomatics 21:109–110, 1980
17. Ladefoged K: Quality of life in patients on permanent home parenteral nutrition. JPEN 5:132–137, 1981
18. Rains RB: The non-hospitalized tube-fed patient. Oncol Nurs Forum 8:8–13, 1981
19. Price BS, Levine EL: Permanent total parenteral nutrition: Psychological and social responses of the early stages. JPEN 3:48–52, 1979
20. MacRitchie JK: Parenteral nutrition outside hospital psychosocial styles of adaptation. Can J Psychiatry 25:308–313, 1980

21. Perl M, Hall RC, Dudrick SJ, et al: Psychological aspects of long-term home hyper alimentation. JPEN 4:554–560, 1980
22. Perl M, Peterson LG, Dudrick SJ, et al: Psychiatric effects of long-term home hyperalimentation. Psychosomatics 22:1047–1048, 1050–1051, 1053–1055, 1058, 1063, 1981
23. MacRitchie KJ: Life without eating or drinking total parenteral nutrition outside the hospital. Can Psychiatr Assoc J 23:373–378, 1978
24. Perl M, Peterson LG, Dudrick SJ: Psychiatric problems encountered during intravenous nutrition, in Nutrition and the Surgical Patient, ed. 2. New York, Churchhill Livingston, 1981, pp 309–318
25. Gulledge AD, Gibson WT, Steiger E, et al: Home parenteral nutrition for the short bowel syndrome psychological tissues. Gen Hosp Psychia 2:271–280, 1980
26. Hall RC, Stickney SK, Gardner ER, et al: Psychiatric reactions to long-term intravenous hyperalimentation. Psychosomatics 22:428–429, 433–434, 437, 441, 442–443, 1981
27. Ivey M, et al: Long-term parenteral nutrition in the home. Am J Hosp Pharm 32:1032–1036, 1975

PART 11

Issues in Nutritional Support Nursing

Leah Curtin

— 11 —

Ethical Issues in Nutritional Support: Should We Feed Baby Doe?

In Phoenix, Arizona, Baby "Doe," an infant born with a severe meningomyelocele, was deprived of food and water—at her parent's request and at the order of the physician—even though she could take food by mouth.[1]

In Bloomington, Indiana, Baby "Doe," an infant born with Down's syndrome and a correctable esophageal fistula, was refused the opportunity for a corrective operation and deprived of lifesaving nutritional support by court order.[2]

In Houston, Texas, Baby "Doe," an infant with severe short bowel syndrome secondary to congenital atresia was started on intravenous hyperalimentation three days after his birth. Eleven months later, Baby "Doe," deserted by his parents but thriving on artificial life support feedings, was deprived of further nutrient therapy.

S ituations such as these poignantly illustrate contemporary ethical and legal issues in nutritional support. Although each involves both an infant and a specific feeding modality, there are significant differences among these cases. In the first instance, normal feeding was withheld because surgical correction of the infant's meningomyelocele offered no reasonable hope of survival. In the second situation, surgical intervention to correct a defect that prevented normal nutrition was denied by court order because the infant had Down's syndrome. In the third instance, intravenous nutrition was withdrawn when it became apparent to the health care team and his family that the infant's inability to absorb and assimilate food was irreversible.

Novelist Pearl Buck once commented, "I fear the power of choice over life and death at human hands. I see no human being whom I could ever trust with such power—not myself nor any other. Human wisdom, human integrity are not great enough . . ."[3] Nonetheless, nature's errors combined with biomedical advancements place such choices in human hands. Whether such choices are fearful or not for the decision-makers, "Baby Doe" situations demand decision and action. Capable or not, human beings make these decisions and enforce them on a daily basis. Each person and institution stands accountable morally and legally for his, her, or its participation in such decisions and actions.

The questions raised by nutritional life support of Baby Doe extend beyond the nursery into oncology wards, nursing homes, and inevitably to the federal government. Among the important questions raised by these three "Baby Doe" cases are the following:

1. Does withdrawal of necessary nutritional support constitute killing if this action results in the patient's demise?
2. Does imminence of death justify deliberate starvation of a person who could eat normally?
3. Does normal feeding constitute an inhumane prolongation of inevitable death?
4. Does the presence of an uncorrectable deficiency or defect (e.g., Down's syndrome) justify refusal to correct life-threatening physical defects?
5. When lifesaving surgery is not possible or has been denied for whatever reasons, should artificial life-sustaining measures be instituted or, if already instituted, should they be discontinued?
6. Does offering the patient with a hopeless prognosis for recovery a nutritional life support system constitute an inhumane prolongation of inevitable death?
7. After its initiation, can nutrient therapy legitimately be withdrawn when its removal causes death?
8. Does parental permission for a minor constitute a *sufficient* as well as a *necessary* rationale for withholding or withdrawing parenteral and enteral feeding?

The ethical, moral, and legal issues raised by these questions deserve particular emphasis and consideration.

DOES WITHDRAWAL OF NECESSARY NUTRITIONAL SUPPORT CONSTITUTE KILLING IF THIS ACTION RESULTS IN THE PATIENT'S DEMISE?

This question is far more complex than it appears at an initial glance and cannot be answered simplisticly. Unfortunately, the withdrawal of artificial nutrient life support systems often tends to be considered under the general rubric of withdrawal of medical life support measures. This tendency adds to the confusion surrounding the issue because it fails to take into account the aspects that are unique to decisions involving termination of parenteral and enteral nutrition.

It is one thing to decide not to resuscitate a terminally ill patient; it is, on the other hand, quite another to starve a person to death regardless of whether the afflicted has any hope or chance of survival. Among those aspects unique to or exacerbated by questions of continuing nutritional and metabolic life support are:

1. Possible violations of basic sustenance rights are protected by both moral and legal sanctions. Sustenance rights are founded in fundamental and universal human needs.[3] Among such needs is the need for adequate nourishment. In short, while every patient does not require cardiopulmonary resuscitation, a ventilator, or an artificial heart, liver, or kidney to exist, every human being has to have adequate nourishment. The very universality of the need therefore forms a just claim (a right) to have the need fulfilled.
2. While maintaining adequate nutrition is an appropriate part of any medical regimen, adequate nourishment itself is not solely within the medical prerogative. That is, it is not a medical option in the ordinary sense. Although the use of artificial ventilation, medications to sustain normal body functions, cardiac defibrillation, and the like is initiated and discontinued by medical prescription, nourishment is not.
3. Withholding or withdrawing medical life support measures usually is justified on the basis of futility or humanitarian concern. It is extremely difficult, perhaps even impossible, to argue that feeding is futile or that starvation is a humanitarian undertaking.

Surely, to deprive a person of ordinary sustenance is to kill. The members of the health care team thus have a duty to feed. As the means to providing sustenance have become more sophisticated during the past several decades, however, what is included in this duty has become less clear. While few persons would consider bottle feeding an infant or spoon feeding a debilitated or geriatric adult to be moral options, each is an artificial means of feeding and should be acknowledged as such. A premature neonate may have insufficient strength to suck and thus need a special nipple for bottle feeding. A weak patient who is unable to masticate or ingest normally may need a pureed diet. Are such minor adjustments in the feeding process really optional? From these examples, it is not difficult to compare the use of enteral tube feedings for premature infants who lack the suck reflex or for patients too sick to swallow. Is tube feeding a medical option or a moral imperative? Intravenous nourishment is undoubtedly the most effective means of feeding when the patient has permanent or temporary gastrointestinal dysfunction. Is total parenteral nutrition morally and legally required?

At least in this type of situation, some broad although clear distinctions are certainly possible. When adequate nutrition can be accomplished by mouth (e.g., bottle feedings with or without a special nipple, spoon feeding whether or not the food is mashed), to deliberately withhold or withdraw nutritional support constitutes killing. Neither the technology nor the financial and human cost is excessive for these patients.

In another sense, however, the use of enteral tube feedings and parenteral nutrient supplementation provides limited options. What constitutes these limits—the scope of morally and legally acceptable decisions, the distinction between killing and allowing to die—is not always clear. Indeed, some argue for the elimination of all distinctions between killing and allowing to die. While a strong case can be made for voluntary mercy killing, this case justification is not valid when the patients are incompetent or unable to make decisions pertaining to their health care (e.g., a newborn, severely retarded, or comatose patient).[4]

DOES IMMINENCE OF DEATH JUSTIFY DELIBERATE STARVATION OF A PERSON WHO COULD EAT NORMALLY?

If a person has any rights at all, he or she has a right to life, even in the face of imminent death. If the right to life means anything at all, then it means one has the right not to be killed. According to Rawls, a right not to be killed entails a right to aid "when one is in serious need or jeopardy when such aid can be rendered without excessive risk or loss to another."[5] Providing normal sustenance to a dying patient imposes no excessive risk or loss to anyone. Whether the care giver is a professional nurse or family member, whether the patient is hospitalized or at home, bottle feeding an infant or spoon feeding a malnourished adult is not an excessive burden. However, the adequacy of the nutrition and the route of feeding may vary depending on the patient's condition, prognosis, and volition.[6] A terminal patient may be fed on demand, and then only those foods he/she particularly desires,[7] and a dying infant may be fed on demand only enough to keep him or her comfortable. In the face of inevitable death secondary to another cause such as a birth defect or cancer, nourishment is used to provide comfort—and any means of feeding that produces more discomfort than comfort can be eliminated. In these instances, patients can clearly inform the caretakers what they want, while in other cases, the health team must rely on their own judgments. In all cases, however, the goal is optimal comfort for the patient.

DOES NORMAL FEEDING CONSTITUTE AN INHUMANE PROLONGATION OF INEVITABLE DEATH?

Every person must die; some individuals sooner than others, some with more pain than others, and some more "naturally" than others. But how a person dies is not without moral significance. Surely, if a living being can feel anything at all, suffering from dehydration and starvation must be among the most agonizing ways to die. To attempt to end suffering by inducing death through a painful means (e.g., malnutrition) is morally repugnant. Although a philosophical case could be made for mercy killing through rapid and painless means (a quick overdose), such a case disintegrates totally when the means are both slow and painful. Moreover, lest there be any misunderstanding, it must be stressed that direct mercy killing by deliberate starvation of a person who could eat normally or by deliberate overdosage is illegal.

DOES THE PRESENCE OF AN UNCORRECTABLE DEFICIENCY OR DEFECT (E.G., DOWN'S SYNDROME) JUSTIFY REFUSAL TO CORRECT LIFE-THREATENING PHYSICAL DEFECTS?

Federal law prohibits discrimination against any person solely by reason of handicap. Consequently, the Department of Health and Human Services (HHS) promulgated the "Baby Doe Regulation" that required the posting of a notice and established a Handicapped Infant Hotline (Fig. 11-1). Judge Gerhard Gesell ruled the Baby Doe regulation invalid because HHS had not followed proper procedures in promulgating it.[8] (See Appendix, Editor's Note #1, following Chapter 15.) George Annas, in commenting on Judge Gesell's ruled, asserted that:

> Treatment should be denied to a handicapped infant for only one reason: that the treatment is not in the infant's best interests. Withholding treatment in the interests of others (e.g., parents or society) would be monumental and unjustified change in the law, and runs contrary to child abuse and neglect statutes.[9]

The President's Commission for the Study of Problems in Medicine and Biomedical and Behavioral Research in its report, *Deciding to Forego Life-Sustaining Treatment*, offers some guidelines for determining an infant's best interests and handling conflict situations (Table 11-1). By no means are an infant's best interests always served by an operation. When surgical repair is possible for something as basic as normal feeding, however, the courts (and, for once, most ethicists agree) generally have mandated surgery. If treatment decisions must be taken to court or are the occasion of disagreement, effective artificial means of providing nutritional life support should be maintained at least until the issue is resolved.

WHEN LIFESAVING SURGERY IS NOT POSSIBLE OR HAS BEEN DENIED FOR WHATEVER REASONS, SHOULD ARTIFICIAL LIFE-SUSTAINING MEASURES BE INSTITUTED OR, IF ALREADY INSTITUTED, SHOULD THEY BE DISCONTINUED?

All common measures should be undertaken to ensure comfort and solace for the patient and the family. Certainly, any infant who could be fed by mouth should be fed on demand. When patients cannot be fed by mouth, it seems

NOTICE

DEPARTMENT OF HEALTH AND HUMAN SERVICE
Office for Civil Rights

DISCRIMINATORY FAILURE TO FEED AND CARE FOR HANDICAPPED INFANTS IN THIS FACILITY IS PROHIBITED BY FEDERAL LAW, SECTION 504 OF THE REHABILITATION ACT OF 1973 STATES THAT

"NO OTHERWISE QUALIFIED HANDICAPPED INDIVIDUAL SHALL, SOLELY BY REASON OF HANDICAP, BE EXCLUDED FROM PARTICIPATION IN, BE DENIED THE BENEFITS OF, OR BE SUBJECT TO DISCRIMINATION UNDER ANY PROGRAM OR ACTIVITY RECEIVING FEDERAL FINANCIAL ASSISTANCE."

Any person having knowledge that a handicapped infant is being discriminatorily denied food or customary medical care should immediately contact:

Handicapped Infant Hotline
U.S. Department of Health and Human Services
Washington, D.C. 20201
Phone 800-368-1019 (Available 24 hours a day) · TTY Capability

In Washington, D.C. call 863-0100

OR

Your State Child Protective Agency

Federal Law prohibits retaliation or intimidation against any person who provides information about possible violations of the Rehabilitation Act of 1973.

Identity of callers will be held confidential.

Failure to feed and care for infants may also violate the criminal and civil laws of your state.

Fig. 11-1. Facsimile of "Baby Doe Regulation" Notice.

appropriate to hydrate them at least enough to prevent suffering. Enteral or parenteral supplementation may not be in the patient's best interests, however, and can only prolong the suffering of the patient's loved ones.

Accurate and timely assessment of the patient's condition, appropriate consultation, and rapid and honest review of decisions will expedite the appropriate management of the seriously ill patient. In teaching hospitals, the need to learn, combined in a particularly potent manner with the technological imperative, often urges aggressive and hasty interventions. Senior physicians have stringent obligations to supervise the practice of their junior colleagues to

Table 11-1
Treatment of Seriously Ill Newborns

- Parents should be the surrogates for a seriously ill newborn unless they are disqualified by decision-making incapacity, an unresolved disagreement between them, or their choice of a course of action that clearly is against the infant's best interests.
- Therapies expected to be futile . . . need not be provided; parents, health care professionals and institutions and reimbursement sources, however, should ensure the infant's comfort.
- Within the constraints of equity and availability, infants should receive all therapies that are clearly beneficial to them . . . The concept of benefit necessarily makes reference to the context of the infant's present and future treatment, taking into account such matters as the level of biomedical knowledge . . . and the availability of services necessary . . . [this] underlines the ethical duty of the community to ensure equitable access for all persons to an adequate level of health care.
- Decision-makers should have access to the most accurate and up-to-date information . . . Physicians should obtain appropriate consultations and referrals. The significance of the diagnoses and the prognoses under each treatment option must be conveyed to the parents (or other surrogates).
- The medical staff, administrators, and trustees of each institution . . . should take the responsibility for ensuring good decision-making practices. Accrediting bodies may want to ensure that institutions have appropriate policies in this area.
  - An institution should have clear and explicit policies that require prospective or retrospective review of decisions when life-sustaining treatment for an infant might be foregone or when parents and providers disagree about the correct decision for an infant. Certain categories of clearly futile therapies could be explicitly excluded from review.
  - The best interests of an infant should be pursued when those interests are clear.
  - The policies should allow for the exercise of parental discretion when a child's interests are ambiguous.
  - Decisions should be referred to public agencies (including courts) for review when necessary to determine whether parents should be disqualified or decision-makers . . .
- The legal system has various—though limited—roles in ensuring that seriously ill infants receive correct care.
  - Civil courts are . . . the appropriate decision-makers concerning the disqualification of parents . . . and the designation of surrogates to serve in their stead.
  - Special statutes requiring providers to bring such cases to the attention of civil authorities do not seem warranted . . . nevertheless, educating providers about their responsibilities is important.
  - Although criminal statutes should be available to punish serious errors, the ability of criminal law to ensure good decision-making . . . is limited.
  - Governmental agencies that reimburse for health care may insist that institutions have policies and procedures regarding decision-making, but using financial sanctions . . . to punish an "uncorrect" decision is likely to be ineffective and to lead to excessively detailed regulations . . .

From Deciding to Forego Life-Sustaining Treatment. Report of the President's Commission for the Study of Problems in Medicine and Biomedical and Behavioral Research. Washington, DC, U.S. Government Printing Office, March 1983, pp. 6-8.

prevent or mitigate the tragedy of overtreatment and inhumane prolongation of inevitable death. Ill-conceived attempts to shorten the life of a seriously ill newborn, though well-intentioned, demand the immediate intervention of superiors. Sensitive consultation, counsel, and supervision are as necessary for young professionals, both physicians and nurses, as they are for parents.

DOES OFFERING THE PATIENT WITH A HOPELESS PROGNOSIS FOR RECOVERY A NUTRITIONAL LIFE SUPPORT SYSTEM CONSTITUTE AN INHUMANE PROLONGATION OF INEVITABLE DEATH?

In situations in which death is inevitable and the conditions of living intolerable, highly sophisticated means of feeding are not in a patient's best interests and may be withheld or withdrawn. These situations involve extensive technological isolation from human touch, futile pain, and pointless extensions of dying.

AFTER ITS INITIATION, CAN NUTRIENT THERAPY LEGITIMATELY BE WITHDRAWN WHEN ITS REMOVAL CAUSES DEATH?

In situations when sentient life is a reasonable expectation, nutritional life support measures generally should be continued unless a rational adult patient refuses them. When permanent unconsciousness can be reliably predicted, artificial nutritional life support may be terminated. The President's Commission had the following to say:

> Most patients with permanent unconsciousness cannot be sustained for long without an array of increasingly artificial feeding interventions—nagogastric tubes, gastrostomy tubes, or intravenous nutrition. Since permanently unconscious patients will never be aware of nutrition, the only benefit to the patient of providing such burdensome interventions is sustaining the body for a remote possibility of recovery. The sensitivities of the family and of care giving professionals ought to determine whether such interventions are made . . . When all remedial attempts have failed to bring the patient out of chronic coma, but where the patient is able to spontaneously maintain respiration and circulation, it would seem to be a matter between physician and family as to whether or not other, more mundane, care would continue . . . if the family feels the emotional or financial drain too great and the physicians in attendance indicate no reasonable possibility of any recovery, then it can be anticipated that the courts, when presented with petitions for appointment of a conservator with power to refuse consent to further treatment of any kind, including I.V. drip . . . can be expected to grant such requests.[7]

DOES PARENTAL PERMISSION FOR A MINOR CONSTITUTE A SUFFICIENT AS WELL AS A NECESSARY RATIONALE FOR WITHHOLDING OR WITHDRAWING PARENTERAL AND ENTERAL FEEDING?

Parental permission is a necessary but not sufficient precondition for withholding or withdrawing nutritional life support. The President's Commission holds that parents who make decisions that are "clearly against the infant's best interests" be disqualified and that civil courts appoint surrogates.[7] Judge Gesell, in his comments on the Baby Doe regulation, noted that "the effort to preserve an unwanted child may require concurrent attention to procedures from adoption or other placement."[8] The right of parents to direct the future of their children is cherished and legally protected, but it is not absolute. Parental rights do not include a right to abandon or to endanger their children or to let their children die when readily attainable assistance is available.[10] In short, physicians, nurses, and institutions are not relieved of their moral and legal responsibilities for a seriously ill newborn when parents choose a course of action clearly contrary to an infant's best interests; rather, their responsibilities are increased and judicial intervention must be sought.

COMMENTS ON THE CASES

Given these general reflections on these important ethical and legal issues, it seems that a grave injustice was done in each of the three situations presented at the beginning of this article. Baby "Doe" in Arizona, although untreatable surgically, was subjected to an unnecessarily painful and prolonged death. It seems that Baby "Doe" in Indiana was denied his civil rights under section 504 of the Rehabilitation Act of 1973 if, indeed, he was denied lifesaving surgery solely because he had Down's syndrome. The fact that he died before his case could be appealed to the United States Supreme Court underscores provider responsibility for maintaining nutritional life support while the issue is in litigation. His death under these circumstances also produced unprecedented controversy that yielded the Baby Doe Regulation that, in turn, resulted in unwarranted intrusions in several situations. Although a case could be made for withholding intravenous hyperalimentation from Baby "Doe" in Texas, its withdrawal from a sentient and "thriving" child was not morally justifiable and may not be legally justifiable. Surely and particularly in the absence of parents or other surrogates, court intervention should have been sought.

CONCLUSIONS: THE ROLE OF ETHICS COMMITTEES

Certainly the Baby Doe situations considered in this chapter are the exception rather than the rule. Far more likely are situations such as the "Baby Boy Houle"[11] case in which vigorous, unnecessary, and even inhumane interventions were undertaken in futile attempts to preserve an irremedially damaged infant.

By and large, courts are not necessarily the best places to make care decisions. As the President's Commission pointed out: "judicial review is costly in terms of time and expense; it can disrupt the care of the patient; it can create unnecessary strain between professionals and surrogate decision-makers; and it exposes private matters to public scrutiny and to the glare of public media."[7] Occasionally, it may be wiser to request judicial review, but in most instances internal review by an appropriate committee is far more desirable. Institutions are urged to develop "clear, explicit and publicly available policies regarding how and by whom decisions are to be made for patients who lack adequate decision-making capacity."[7]

Moreover, institutions are urged to exercise their responsibility to protect patients' well-being by establishing ethics committees. The recommended role and functions of such committees include the following:

- They can review the case to confirm the responsible physician's diagnosis and prognosis of a patient's medical condition.
- They can provide a forum for discussing broader social and ethical concerns raised by a particular case; such bodies may also have an educational role, especially by teaching all professional staff how to identify, frame, and resolve ethical problems.
- They can be a means for formulating policy and guidelines regarding such decisions.
- Finally, they can review decisions made by others (such as physicians and surrogates) about the treatment of specific cases.[7]

By and large, it seems most appropriate for such committees to concentrate initially on the development of rational policies regarding withholding and withdrawing life support, surrogate decision-making, cardiopulmonary resuscitation, and the like. Such policies, once agreed on by the committee, would be recommended to administration for adoption. Once the policies are adopted, the ethics committee can serve as a valuable resource for education of staff to ensure that the policies are appropriately promulgated. Not all ethicists concur with the Commission's recommendation that the Ethics Committees should serve to review particular case situations: "When ethics committees serve as reviewers, they do not supplant the principal decision-makers . . ."[7] Presumably, they can serve in an advisory capacity, and they can ensure that appropriate cases are taken to the courtroom. Nonetheless, the problems of patient and family privacy, diffusion of personal accountability, and professional liability loom large. There is no guarantee that a committee will make a sounder or more humane decision than an individual. Whatever else the ethics committees may be, they should be primarily counselors—not deciders.

The make-up of the committee is also of concern. The President's Commission recommends diverse membership: members of the medical, nursing, pastoral, and legal profession, and at least one public member.[7] Other disciplines could be represented as members of the ad hoc committees of the committee when policy or practice touches on their areas of expertise. Long experience of committees suggests that a committee that is too large (1) will never reach a decision[12] and (2) will have a great difficulty gathering members for a meeting.

Humane and compassionate care for patients—and for families—can no more be guaranteed by a committee than by a court. The American Medical Association's 1986 statement on withdrawal of nutritional life support is the most significant private sector attempt to date to bring compassion and rationality to these decisions.[13] (See Appendix, Editor's Note #2, following Chapter 15.) Compassion resides in human beings and is demonstrated in human relationships. Courts and committees can ensure appropriate procedure—and undoubtedly will contain abuses—but, in the end, individual health professionals in their intimate interpersonal contacts with patients and their families determine the quality of the caring.

ACKNOWLEDGMENTS

This chapter is reprinted in part with permission from Curtin L: Should We Feed Baby Doe? Nursing Management 15:22–28.

REFERENCES

1. *The Arizona Republic* January 16, 1974

2. Court decisions and the Feds: Travesty of tragedy? (editorial). Nursing Management 12:7;1982

3. Bandman B, Bandman E: Bioethics and Human Rights. Boston, Little, Brown and Company, 1978, pp 322–323

4. Grassian V: Moral Reasoning: Ethical Theory and Some Contemporary Moral Problems. Englewood Cliffs, NJ, Prentice-Hall, 1981, p 285

5. Rawls J: A Theory of Justice. Cambridge, MA, Harvard University Press. 1971, p 114

6. McCormick RJ: How Brave a New World. New York, Doubleday & Company, 1981, pp 339–351

7. Deciding to Forego Life-Sustaining Treatment. Report of President's Commission for the Study of Ethical Problems in Medicine and Biomedical and Behavioral Research. Washington, DC, U.S. Government Printing Office, March, 1983

8. *American Academy of Pediatrics v. Heckler*, 83-0774 U.S. District Court (1983)

9. Annas GJ: Law and the life sciences: Disconnecting the Baby Doe hotline. The Hastings Center Report 13(3):15–16, 1983

10. Larsen G: Child neglect in the exercise of religious freedom. Kent Law Review 32:283, 1954

11. Hellegers AE: Obstet Gynecol News 1977

12. Friedman B: One philosopher's experience of an ethics committee. Hastings Center Report 11:20–21, 1981

13. American Medical Association House of Delegates' Statement on Withdrawal of Nutritional Life Support. Chicago, IL, American Medical Association, 1986

Mary Williams Cazalas

12

Nutritional Support Nursing Medico-Legal Concerns

This chapter provides nurses with basic information about the law as it pertains to the practice of nursing with particular emphasis on nutritional support nursing.

THE MEDICAL MALPRACTICE CRISIS

Definition of Medical Malpractice

Medical malpractice is defined in Black's Law Dictionary[1] as ". . . . any professional misconduct, unreasonable lack of skill or fidelity in professional or fiduciary duties, evil practice, or illegal or immoral conduct." Applied to physicians, it is defined as professional misconduct toward a patient that is considered reprehensible because it is either immoral in itself or contrary to or expressly forbidden by law. It is further defined as meaning bad, wrong, or injudicious treatment of a patient, professionally and in respect to the particular disease or injury, resulting in unnecessary suffering or death to the patient, and proceeding from ignorance, carelessness, want of proper skill, disregard of established rules, principles, neglect, malicious or criminal intent.[1]

Medical malpractice may be by breach of a contract or it may be a tort, which is a civil wrong. When the rules of contract law have appeared to lead to unreasonable and unjust results, lawyers have simply bypassed traditional contract doctrine by invoking tort, and when tort law appeared to be unsatisfactory for some reason, lawyers have developed alternative legal approaches by invoking contract. Duties of conduct that give rise to tort actions are imposed by

NUTRITIONAL SUPPORT IN NURSING
ISBN 0-8089-1889-3

319

law and based primarily on social policy and not necessarily on the will or intention of the parties as is true in contracts. In tort, duties may be owed to all individuals and classes who fall within the range of harm from which they are to be protected. Contract actions protect the interest in having promises performed. Contractural obligations are imposed because of conduct of the parties who manifest consent. Contractual obligations are owed only to the particular individuals named in the contract. Recoverable damages for breach of a contractual duty are limited to those individuals reasonably within the contemplation of the defendant when the contract was made. In a tort action, a much broader measure of damages is applied. Medical malpractice suits are usually filed as tort actions.[2-4]

Past History of Medical Malpractice

The first recorded medical negligence suit in the United States was *Cross v. Guthery*, 2 Root 90 (1794). It was not until the 1930s that filing of medical malpractice suits began to increase in number. Following World War II, the number of claims increased steadily. During the early 1970s, the growth rate became so alarming that it received national attention for the first time and was called a "crisis." The peak of the crisis was reached in 1975. The withdrawal of many insurers from the market left health care providers without insurance and a "crisis of availability" developed.[5,6]

State legislatures throughout the country reacted by passing legislation curtailing access to the courts and facilitating the means by which health care providers could obtain liability coverage unavailable to them on the commercial market. Health care and malpractice litigation costs continued to rise. However, the crisis faded from public view in the late 1970s and early 1980s. In the mid 1980s a new medical malpractice crisis arose with the advent of available but cost-prohibitive insurance. The new crisis has been called the "crisis of affordability."[5]

Causes of the Medical Malpractice Crisis

Much controversy surrounds the causes of the medical malpractice crisis. Insurance companies have been accused of manipulating the medical malpractice insurance market to eliminate competition among insurers. The insurance industry has the power to accomplish this because of its unique immunity from federal antitrust laws and the absence of any effective state regulation.[5] The insurance industry denies being a cause, however, and it places the blame on liberal doctrines adopted by the courts. Such doctrines include eliminating the locality rule in defining the standard of care required of the health care provider, adopting discovery of the injury as the beginning of the statute of limitations (the time within which a suit must be filed) tolling the statutes of limitations pending the age of majority for minors, adopting the tort of emotional distress as a cause of action, allowing recovery for pain and suffering, accepting the lack of an informed consent as an independent tort, and adopting the loss of a chance of recovery due to the defendant's negligence as a basis for recovery.[5,7]

Blame has also been placed on advances in technology that began in the 1960s. This has caused the role of many physicians to change from that of family friend and confidant to that of an anonymous technician who treats the ailment that falls within the physician's particular specialty. Physicians who engage in general or family practice may have a closer and more traditional relationship with their patients.[5]

Advanced technology has improved treatment modalities, but it has also increased the opportunities for errors to occur and caused patients and their families to have greater expectations than may be obtainable from treatment.

The political climate of the 1960s and 1970s set the stage for reform, agitation, broader entitlement to social welfare, and stricter regulation of industry, including the health industry. The general public came to regard medical care as a right and not just a privilege.[5]

Another cause is physicians themselves. Malpractice is widespread, but there has been an insufficient disciplinary process.[5] A report of the Federation of State Medical Boards published the Health Lawyers News Reports dated December, 1986, revealed that a record number of physicians had their licenses revoked for incompetence in 1985, and the number of lesser disciplinary actions increased. About 20 states have revised their laws between 1984 and 1986, and these revisions removed impediments that have blocked disciplining physicians.[8]

Hospitals and professional associations may be reluctant to invoke disciplinary actions when professionals fail to comply with proper standards because they may find themselves sued for defamation of character. Failure to exercise care in granting staff privileges and in reviewing and supervising the treatment given by staff members may result in liability of the hospital. In *Darling v. Charleston Community Memorial Hospital*, 38 Ill.2d 211, 211 N.E. 2d 253, cert. den. 383 U.S. 946 (1965), the hospital was held liable for failure to review and supervise treatment given to a patient by a staff physician.

The medical profession has been accused of forming a conspiracy of silence to protect its members. In the case of *Hart v. Browne*, 103 Cal. App.3d 947, 163 Cal. Rptr. 356 (1st Dist., 1980), a physician wrongfully stated that Dr. Nark was not negligent. When the patient learned of the incorrect statement, the time for filing suit against Dr. Nark had passed. The physician who had been consulted was sued for damages and a judgment was rendered against him.

Incompetence of members of the nursing profession may be a contributing cause of the crisis. It has been estimated that 40,000 nurses in the United States are alcoholics. According to the National Council of State Boards of Nursing, more than 1 out of 3 disciplinary cases are drug-related. In the case of *United States v. Doremus*, 249 U.S. 86 (1919), the Supreme Court of the United States stated that drug addiction is not a crime. It is an illness for which competent and compassionate nursing care is needed.[9] Hospitals and the nursing profession owe a duty to patients and their families to police the nursing profession so that only competent nurses will be permitted to render care. The low costs of malpractice for nurses reflects that nurses have not been a high risk insured. As nurses assume duties that have been traditionally performed by physicians, however, their risk of being sued increases.

Attorneys must also share the blame for the crisis. They have been characterized as greedy, exploitive, and wholly unethical in seeking large damage awards. The contingency fee has been criticized as creating a personal interest in the attorney which gives incentive for the attorney to encourage the public to litigate for excessive damages. To counteract this, states have passed statutes authorizing courts to approve reasonable fees and set limits on the maximum fee attorneys may collect. Traditionally, attorneys have charged one-half to one-third of the amounts recovered. Justification for the contingency fee is that without it persons who are unable to pay legal costs might be denied their day in court. It is pointed out by the legal profession that a large fee received in one case is balanced by the loss sustained in other cases that are lost and no payment for services is received.[5]

Health care providers may bring countersuits against attorneys and plaintiffs to combat frivolous and nonmeritorious medical malpractice claims. A malicious prosecution claim may be filed when there is no probable cause for initiating the underlying medical malpractice action. Abuse of process claims can be pursued when the underlying action has been initiated for an invalid reason such as the desire to institute a nuisance suit to obtain a settlement. The health care provider may be able to restore a damaged reputation and receive compensation for having to endure a frivolous malpractice suit.[10]

Reform Legislation—An Attempted Solution

Modifying Access to the Courts

Statute of limitations. A statute of limitations is a statute that prescribes limitations to the right of action on certain described causes of action; that is, declaring that no suit shall be maintained on such causes of action unless brought within a specified period after the right accrued.[1] State legislatures have shortened the statutes of limitation for medical malpractice causes of action. The majority of statutes provide that the period of limitations begins to run and the cause of action accrues when the negligence occurs. Some have adopted the discovery rule that provides that the period begins to run when the plaintiff discovers or should have discovered the injury through the use of reasonable diligence. Over half of the states have provided a maximum time within which a claim may be brought.[5]

Arbitration. Some states have enacted statutes permitting arbitration in medical malpractice cases. Arbitration is usually a voluntary alternative to litigation. The patient and health care provider enter into an agreement for arbitration as a substitute for a jury trial. Usually the decision of the expert fact-finder is subject to only limited judicial review by a court on appeal.[5]

Pretrial screening. Pretrial screening panels designed to screen out nonmeritorious claims prior to trial have been established by many states. The panel is usually composed of physicians and attorneys. A hearing is generally conducted before the panel, and this hearing is mandatory prior to filing suit. The panel's decision is not binding on the parties, and the plaintiff is not precluded from bringing a lawsuit.[5]

Shifting Costs and Burdens

Awarding costs. Some states have enacted statutes that provide that courts may award payment of attorney's fees and expert witness fees against the unsuccessful party when the action brought is frivolous. Costs of the litigation may be awarded to the prevailing party.[5]

Limiting attorney's fees. Several states have statutes that limit the maximum fee attorneys can charge, and they provide for court approval of reasonable fees.[5]

Altering the collateral source rule. The collateral source rule prevents the value of any benefits received by the injured party from sources other than the defendant to offset the damage recovery. Under this rule, the plaintiff may receive double recovery for the same injury. Insurance benefits and an award of damages may be paid for the same injury.[5]

Limiting damages. Several states have enacted legislation that restricts the amount of the recovery for particular types of damages. These are implemented by statutes that place caps on the amount of damages a plaintiff may recover or by statutes that limit liability of health care providers who participate in state patient compensation funds. Damage caps will have an adverse effect only on severely injured persons, since damage awarded to those with lesser injuries will not reach the ceiling amounts.[5]

In *Fein v. Permanente Medical Group*, 38 Cal.3d 137, 695 P.2d 665, 211 Cal. Rptr.368 (1985), the court modified the award of damages and entered a judgment pursuant to the California Civil Code Section 3333.2, which places a $250,000 limit on noneconomic damages. The California Supreme Court affirmed the finding of the lower court that the statute did not violate either the due process or the equal protection clauses of the 14th amendment to the Constitution of the United States. The Supreme Court of the United States dismissed the appeal for want of a substantial federal question.[11]

Creating a patient compensation fund. Some states have established a fund with which to pay the portion of a judgment or settlement that is in excess of the statutory amount the health care provider must carry to participate in the patient compensation fund. Funds are usually financed through annual surcharges assessed against the health care providers.[5]

Mandating periodic payments. Damages may be awarded for future anticipated medical care, loss of future earning capacity, and future pain and suffering. If a lump sum is paid, the plaintiff who recovers or dies sooner may be overcompensated. An award paid by the insurance company over a period of time is favorable for the company because funds can be used to earn income over that payment period. Some states have enacted legislation that permits or requires medical liability judgments to be paid on installments.[5]

Modifying Evidentiary and Procedural Requirements

The expert witness standard. Expert witnesses play an important role in establishing liability in a medical malpractice case. State legislatures have attempted to curtail malpractice claims by restricting the qualifications of expert witnesses. The witness may be required to practice in the state in which the claim is brought. It may be required that the witness has practiced a certain percentage of time in the specialty of the defendant.[5]

Limiting the standard of care of the health care provider. To prevail in a medical malpractice action, the plaintiff has the burden of proving that the health care provider departed from accepted standards of medical practice. Each state has its own standard with which the defendant must comply. Some states have limited or modified the standard of care, and most of these statutes have codified the "locality rule."[5]

Ad damnum clause. The ad damnum clause is the part of the plaintiff's complaint that states the recovery being sought. States have enacted statutes that exclude or limit the monetary amount claimed in an ad damnum clause. The purpose is to reduce publicity of medical malpractice suits in order to discourage the public from seeking large recoveries.[5]

Legal Challenges

Alleged constitutional violations. The constitutionality of reform legislation discussed above has been challenged. It has been argued that such legislation is in violation of the due process and equal protection clauses of the 14th amendment to the Constitution of the United States.[5]

CAUSES OF ACTION AND THE NUTRITIONAL SUPPORT TEAM

Contracts and Nursing

Elements of a Contract

A *contract* has been defined as a promise or a set of promises, the performance of which the law recognized as a duty. When that duty is not performed, it is called a breach of contract and this gives rise to a cause of action in contract. Every enforceable contract must contain the following elements: (1) an agreement between the parties; (2) based on the assent of the parties; (3) supported by valid consideration (something of value); (4) made for a lawful object; (5) the parties to the contract must be competent (persons with a legal capacity to make a contract); and (6) the contract must be in the form required by law. The party who makes the contract is called the *promisor*. If the contract is binding, it imposes on this individual duty or obligation and he or she is called an *obligor*. The person to whom the promise is made and who can claim the benefit of the obligation is called a *promisee* or *obligee*. A party to a contract may be an individual, a partnership, a corporation, or a government. A person may act for himself or herself or another may act on his or her behalf.[12,13]

In any contract, there must be an offer and an acceptance. An acceptance is good only if it comes from the party to whom the offer is made. The acceptance must be unconditional and in accordance with the terms of the offer as to price, amount, time of delivery, and so on. The person who makes the offer can terminate it at any time prior to acceptance unless a payment has been made to the offeror in return for the offeror's agreement not to revoke the offer for a specified period of time. Termination of the offer is effective when it is communicated by the person who made the offer.[12,13]

Kinds of Contracts

Contracts are classified as *formal* and *simple* or *parol* (verbal), *implied*, and *express*. A formal contract is one that is required by law to be in writing. Each state has a Statute of Frauds that requires written contracts in certain cases in order to prevent fraudulent practices. Other contracts are simple or parol contracts, whether written or oral. An express contract is one in which the terms and conditions of the contract are given orally or in writing by the parties. An implied contract is one in which evidence of the agreement is not shown by words, written or spoken, but by acts and conduct of the parties. Such a contract arises when one person, without being requested to do so, renders services under circumstances indicating that he or she expects to be paid for them, and the other person, knowing such circumstances, avails himself or herself of those services. Under certain circumstances the law creates and enforces legal rights and obligations when no real contract, express or implied, exists. These obligations are known as *quasi-contracts*, and they rest on the equitable principle that a person shall not be allowed to enrich himself or herself at the expense of another.[12-14]

Nurses' Contracts

A nurse may enter a professional employment agreement verbally or in writing. A written contract is desirable, particularly if the employment is to last for one year or longer. A verbal contract is enforceable; however, the terms of a verbal agreement are more difficult to prove than are terms enumerated in a written document. The employment agreement is a binding contract for personal services of the nurse. The nurse has a duty to perform her nursing assignment in accordance with the standards of professional nursing practice as defined by the profession and in the nursing practice act of the state. The employer has the duty to provide a safe place to work and safe equipment with which to work. The employer also has a duty to provide properly trained and qualified co-workers.[13]

Termination of Contracts

A contract will be terminated when each person has duly carried out all obligations in accordance with the terms of the contract. It terminates on the expiration of a fixed period or on the occurrence of a particular event as specified by the terms of the contract. The parties to the contract may agree to substitute a new obligation or a new person. A party to a contract can generally assign or transfer the right to receive money without the agreement of other parties; however, assignment of duties of a personal nature cannot be assigned unless this is acceptable to the other parties to the contract.[12-14]

Breach of Contract

If a party to a contract does not perform his or her obligations as required under the terms of the contract, that party commits a breach of the contract unless the performance has been excused. There are three remedies for breach of contract, and one or more is available to the injured party. The injured party may bring an action for damages; in some instances, the contract may be rescinded, and in some instances a suit may be brought to obtain specific performance. Damages refers to a sum of money awarded to a person because another has disregarded the rights as established by law. Damages are given if it is shown that the breach caused a money loss. When a breach occurs and the injured party has completed a portion of the obligation, a claim can be made for the value of what has been done. Under certain circumstances, an injured party may obtain a judgment ordering specific performance of the contract or an injunction to prevent a breach of the contract. This remedy is not usually applied to contracts for nursing service.[12-14]

Most malpractice suits against health care providers are brought on tort law, not on contract law. If there is no specific promise to cure, the law does not consider the physician to be an insurer of a particular outcome. However, in

Guilmet v. Campbell, 385 Mich. 57, 188 N.W.2d 601 (1971), the physician did promise to cure a bleeding ulcer. Although he was not negligent, he did not cure the ulcer. The court found him liable for his breach of promise to cure.

Tort—A Civil Wrong

Definition

A *tort* has been defined as a private or civil wrong or injury, which is independent of contract, and it is a violation of a duty imposed by general law or otherwise on all persons occupying the relation to each other that is involved in a given transaction. There must always be a violation of some duty owing to the plaintiff. Generally, the duty must arise by operation of law and not by a mere agreement between the parties.[1]

Tort liability is usually based on fault. The act giving rise to the suit is something that was done wrong, or the omission that gives rise to the suit was something that should have been done but was not. Strict liability may be imposed for all consequences of certain activities regardless of fault. The intentional torts include assault, battery, false imprisonment, invasion of privacy, defamation, intentional infliction of emotional distress, malicious prosecution, and abuse of process.[15,16]

Intentional Torts

Assault and battery. Assault is an intentional act designed to place another in apprehension of a battery. A battery is an unwanted, not consented to, intentional touching of another. Liability for these acts is based on one's right to be free from invasion of one's person. A patient may sue for lack of informed consent or for assault and/or battery when medical and/or surgical treatment has been rendered without informed consent.[15,16]

False imprisonment. False imprisonment is the unlawful restriction of a person's freedom. Holding a person against his or her will by physical restraint, barriers, or threats of harm can be false imprisonment if the holding is not legally justified. There is a common law authority to hold persons who are disoriented. All states have a procedure for the commitment and holding of persons who are mentally ill, infected with a contagious disease, or abusers of drugs.[15,16]

Invasion of the right of privacy. The right of privacy is the right to be left alone and free from unwarranted publicity and exposure to public view. Hospitals, nurses, and physicians may be liable for divulging information about a patient to an improper source or for committing unwarranted intrusions into the patient's personal affairs. Truth is not a defense.[15,16]

Defamation. Defamation is a written or oral communication to someone other than the person who is defamed, concerning a living person, which tends to injure that person's reputation. Libel is written and slander is oral. A report that a nurse is abusing drugs or that a nurse or a physician is incompetent may result in an action for defamation.[15,16]

Usually limited immunity is available when a report is made in good faith to an authority such as a state licensing board. Most courts apply a qualified immunity privilege to statements made during medical staff peer review activities and during due process procedures for medical staff actions.[15,16] In *Spencer v. Community Hospital of Evanston,* 87 Ill.App.3d 214, 408 N.E.2d 981 (1980), the court found a qualified privilege and dismissed an action alleging defamation where no malice was proved. This same reasoning is applicable to nurses.

Intentional infliction of emotional distress. Intentional infliction of emotional distress can result in liability. Such an action can be prevented by treating patients and their families with understanding and kindness.[16]

Malicious prosecution and abuse of process. The plaintiff who sues for malicious prosecution or abuse of process must prove perversion of legal process for improper ends. It must be proved that the defendant brought an action against the plaintiff; the proceeding was terminated in favor of the party who was sued; probable cause for the proceeding was lacking; and the defendant brought the action because of malice. Health care providers who have received favorable judgments in malpractice suits against them have brought countersuits against the attorneys and plaintiffs based on malicious prosecution and abuse of process.[15,16]

Negligence

Elements. Negligence has been defined as the omission to do something that a reasonable person, guided by those ordinary considerations that ordinarily regulate human affairs, would do, or the doing of something that a reasonable and prudent person would not do.[1,3] It has also been defined as conduct that falls below the standard established by law for protection of others against unreasonable risk of harm. For liability to be found from a cause of action based on negligence, the following elements must be proved by the plaintiff, who is the party suing and filing suit:

1. The defendant must have had a duty or obligation recognized by law to conform to a certain standard of conduct for the protection of others against unreasonable risk of harm.
2. The defendant must have failed to conform to the standards required by either an act of omission or an act of commission.

3. A causal connection between the conduct of the defendant and the injury that results, which is referred to as "legal cause" or "proximate cause."
4. Actual loss or damage resulting to the interest of another.[3,13,15]

A nurse who causes injury to a patient may be liable for damages regardless of who employed the nurse and who pays for services rendered. Liability for negligence is not dependent on a legal or contractual relationship between the nurse and the patient. A nurse may be liable for services rendered gratuitously. Most states have enacted good samaritan laws that relieve physicians, nurses, and in some instances lay persons from liability in emergency situations. Some states have enacted statutes that apply to medical care providers such as emergency medical technicians, medics, and ambulance attendants. The purpose of such legislation is to encourage persons who are trained in the health care field to render service to victims of accidents and catastrophies. Few suits have been filed against health care professionals who have rendered emergency care; however, there is always the possibility that a suit may be filed.[17]

Proof of negligence. The plaintiff who files a suit alleging negligence as the basis for the claim for damages must prove that the defendant owed a duty to the plaintiff, that the duty was breached, and that the breach of that duty was the proximate cause of the injury for which damages are sought. Common law does not impose a duty on individuals to come to the rescue of persons for whom they have no responsibility such as accident victims. If one does undertake to render care, it must be done in accordance with the accepted standard of care. Existence of a duty of a hospital and employees of a hospital may be established by proof of admission of the patient to the hospital. Proof of an agreement between a nurse and a patient for the nurse to render services to that patient will prove existence of a duty owed by the nurse to that patient. Once a duty is established, the plaintiff must prove the scope of the duty, which is the obligation to conform to the standard of care. The standard of care varies in each state to some extent.[18]

The Standard of Care

Nurses. The general duty required of a nurse is to exercise ordinary or reasonable care to see that no unnecessary harm comes to the patient. Usually, the standard of care required is that of other nurses practicing their profession in the same or a similar locality.[18] In the case of *Norton v. Argonaut Insurance Company*, 144 So.2d 249 (La. App. 1st Cir. 1962), the court recognized the duty of the nurse to be the exercise of the degree of skill ordinarily employed, under similar circumstances, by members of the nursing profession in good standing in the same community or locality, or those similar to it, and to use reasonable care and diligence, along with his or her best judgment, in the application of that skill.

Hospitals. The standard of care for hospitals is usually the degree of reasonable care the patient's known or apparent condition requires.[18,19] In *Hunt v. Bogalusa Community Medical Center,* 303 So.2d 745 (La. 1974), the court found the standard of the hospital to be that it must exercise the requisite amount of care toward a patient that the particular patient's condition may require, and it must protect the patient from dangers that may result from the patient's physical and mental incapacities as well as from external circumstances peculiarly within the hospital's control. A determination of whether a hospital has breached the duty of care it owes to a particular patient depends on the circumstances and facts of that case. A hospital is not an insurer of a patient's safety.[19]

Vicarious liability—Respondeat superior. A hospital may be sued for the negligent acts of its employees. *Respondeat superior* is the term for this form of vicarious liability wherein the employer is held liable for the wrongful acts of an employee although the employer was without fault. Liability based on respondeat superior will be imposed only if there was a master-servant relationship between the employer and employee and the wrongful act of the employee occured within the course and scope of the employment. A master-servant relationship exists when the employer has control of the physical conduct of the employee in the performance of duties. The act is within the course and scope of employment when it is so clearly related to what the employee was hired to do that it may be regarded as carrying out the orders of the employer.[15]

Who can diagnose and treat. The general rule of law is that only a physician can diagnose the cause of an abnormal condition and prescribe treatment for it. Those functions of a physician cannot be delegated. Once treatment is prescribed, however, a registered professional nurse can carry them out. A licensed practical nurse may be authorized to perform certain tasks in the treatment of a patient, usually under the direction or supervision of a physician or a registered nurse. The role of a student nurse usually is limited by the degree of experience and education at the time. All nurses are required to have the same basic concepts of patient care and manual skills incidental to the practice of nursing. The registered nurse has a much greater responsibility for assessing the nursing needs of the patient.[18,19]

Breach of Duty

After proof of a duty owed, the plaintiff must prove a breach of that duty by the defendant. A breach of duty is a deviation from the standard of care. A breach of an act of omission is failure to do something that should have been done. Failure of a nurse to raise a bed rail after caring for a comatose patient is negligence by an act of omission. A breach by an act of commission is doing something that should not have been done. The administration of a wrong medication or the wrong dose of a medication are examples of a breach of duty by an act of commission.[15,16]

Injury

The plaintiff must prove physical, financial, or emotional injury. Generally, negligently inflicted emotional injuries are compensated only if there are also physical injuries. Intentionally inflicted emotional injury is compensated without proof of any physical injury. It is necessary that the plaintiff prove the amount of the injuries.[15,16]

Cause of the Injury   The plaintiff must prove that the breach of duty by the defendant was the legal or proximate cause of the injury suffered.[15,16] In the case of *Lenger v. Physician's General Hospital*, 455 S.W.2d 703 (Tex.1970), a nurse gave a patient solid food immediately after colon surgery. This was a breach of duty. Eight days later, the ends of the sutured colon came apart. This is an injury. The court did not find that the injury was caused by the breach of duty because of the length of time between the breach of duty and the injury.[16]

Res Ipsa Loquitur

Res ipsa loquitur literally means that the thing speaks for itself. The usual criteria for application of this doctrine are:

1. The accident or injury must be one that usually does not occur in the absence of negligence.
2. The accident or injury must have occurred through an instrumentality or agency within the exclusive possession or control of the defendant.
3. The accident or injury must not have been the result of the plaintiff's contributory negligence or assumption of risk.
4. Sometimes it is required that the evidence explaining the accident should be more accessible to the defendant than to the plaintiff.

If these are met, a rebuttable presumption of negligence is created.[18]

Defenses to Allegations of Negligence

Contributory Negligence

Contributory negligence of the plaintiff can be raised by the defendant. The elements of contributory negligence include the following: (1) the plaintiff's conduct is below the required standard of care, and (2) there is a connection between the plaintiff's careless conduct and the injury suffered by the plaintiff. In some states, contributory negligence is a bar to recovery.[15,16]

Comparative Negligence

Comparative negligence is recognized in some states. Where both parties are found to be negligent or careless, the degree of negligence or carelessness of each party must be determined by the trier of fact. Each party is held to be responsible for an appropriate proportion of the injuries.[15,16]

Assumption of the Risk

Assumption of the risk means that the defendant took the chance of injury from a known risk arising from the defendant's conduct.

Unavoidable Accident

Unavoidable accident may be raised when an injury occurs, but the elements of negligence are not present. If a patient falls only because an ankle turned, an unavoidable accident has occurred. There is no liability.

Legal Aspects of Nutritional Support Services

Total Parenteral Nutrition

Total parenteral nutrition (TPN) was introduced in 1968 by Dudrick, who described the techique of intravenous feedings via a central venous catheter. In slightly more than a decade, virtually every area of medical and surgical practice utilized enteral and parenteral nutrition. Pharmacy departments in hospitals have been affected greatly by the increase in nutritional therapy prescribed in hospitals. Medical literature has advocated use of aggressive nutritional support for critically ill patients with many types of problems. Patients receiving TPN often have highly complex medical problems and a variety of health care professionals are involved in their care. The nutritional team is composed of physicians, surgeons, nurses, dietitians, social workers, psychiatrists, and pharmacists.[20]

Research has progressed so that nutritional needs of the acutely and chronically malnourished patient can be provided. The nutrition team must know the avenues of nutrient administration in order to tailor the best approach to each individual patient. Failure to remain current in medical and nutritional advances may result in failure to properly prescribe and administer the nutritional support needed by patients. If this breach of duty occurs and is the proximate cause of injury, liability may be incurred.[21]

Improvement of the quality of care reduces the probability of injury to patients and also reduces the chance of liability for damages imposed on the nutritional support team. Education of the team members and the hospital and medical staff is most important. Careful monitoring of patients is essential for timely discovery and remedy of problems. Use of proper procedures and careful monitoring can minimize complications and avoid a basis of liability. Caution must be used in selecting patients to receive particular treatment modalities. In addition to patient eligibility, other factors requiring knowledge and skill are selection of the most suitable equipment (catheters needles, tubing, filters, and solutions); the best site of injection; proper preparation of the intravenous site; and assessment and care of infusion sites. The team has a duty to observe local inflammation at intravenous sites so that needles and catheters can be removed to prevent thrombosis and/or sepsis. Injury may occur from negligent administration of drugs and solutions. Intravenous administration of fluids may cause harm as the result of infiltration of solutions, infection, and broken needles. Pumps may fail to function properly and filters may clog. Establishment of protocols for monitoring of administered fluids and proper maintenance of equipment are duties of the nutritional support team.

The Food and Drug Administration has established rules and regulations for reporting defective medical devices in 21 Code of Federal Regulations Sections 803.1 through 803.36. These rules provide that a manufacturer or importer must file a report with the Food and Drug Administration whenever it learns that, in the opinion of a nurse, its product is or might be hazardous. If a nurse reports to a manufacturer that its device might cause death or serious injury, the manufacturer must file a written report with the Food and Drug Administration within 15 working days. If a manufacturer fails to notify the Food and Drug Administration, it can be penalized, even though the manufacturer believes that the device is not faulty.

Home Care With TPN

Some patients may be treated with TPN in the home. Physicians and nurses who care for these patients have a duty to know and understand the techniques their patients use and the complications that may arise. They must maintain a close liaison with the patients and those aiding the patients in the home. Early detection and treatment of complications is the duty of the members of the health care team.[22,23] Physicians who refer patients to home nutritional support services have a duty to refer them to only those that will render care in accordance with the standard of care that meets proper quality control.

Informed Consent and Refusal of Treatment

Consent for Treatment

Consent may be either oral or written, unless a statutory provision of a particular state requires that the consent be written. A written consent for medical treatment is preferable as it is more difficult to deny.

The foundation for the consent to medical treatment requirement is the torts of assault and battery, which are based on the legal right of each individual to be touched only when and in the manner authorized by that individual. In recent years, courts have ruled that the patient's consent to treatment must be an informed consent if it is to be legally valid. The old rule was the "professional community" standard that required the physician to disclose only those disclosures that a reasonable medical practitioner would make under the same or similar circumstances. The new rule is the "reasonable patient" standard, which places emphasis on the informational needs of an average, reasonable patient rather than on professionally established standards of disclosure. Under the new rule, a physician can be held liable if the court finds that the patient did not receive information material to the decision to accept the proposed treatment.[24] The landmark case upholding the new rule is *Canterberry v. Spence*, 464 F.2d 772 (D.C. Cir.1972).[25,26] Physicians who fail to obtain an informed consent before performing any medical or surgical procedure such as TPN expose themselves to claims of battery, medical malpractice, and civil rights violations. It is the physician who knows best what he or she intends to do in treating the patient. It is the physician, therefore, who should obtain the consent. Discussing the patient's condition and proposed treatment with the patient and providing an opportunity for the patient to ask questions assist in maintaining a good personal relationship between the patient and the physician. People are less likely to sue people they like, and this may reduce the likelihood of a suit.[24]

Refusal of Treatment

Treatment may be refused as well as consented to. Such cases fall into four general categories: (1) the competent adult who refuses treatment; (2) the incompetent adult whose own wishes were never expressed but whose family or guardian refuses treatment; (3) the incompetent adult who expressed the desire, before becoming incompetent, not to be treated; and (4) the minor child patient who refuses treatment. Courts have recognized the right of competent adults to refuse treatment, but the patient's wishes are not always granted. Court decisions are divided as to the right of families to refuse treatment of incompetent patients. If parents refuse treatment for their minor children, child neglect statutes may be invoked.[26]

Patients refuse treatment for many reasons such as religious beliefs, fears of disfigurement or discomfort, and the desire not to have life prolonged artificially when there is no hope of recovery. The distinction between "extraordinary" treatment like respirators and ordinary treatment like nutrition is beginning to blur.[27]

In the case of *In re Conroy*, 98 N.J. 321, 486 A.2d 1209 (1985), the New Jersey Supreme Court decided that life-sustaining treatment, including artificial feeding, may be withdrawn from incompetent, institutionalized, elderly patients with severe and permanent mental and physical impairments and a limited life expectancy under detailed guidelines. The subjective standard is first used, under which the court reviews the evidence presented to it and determines that life-sustaining treatment may be withheld or withdrawn from an incompetent patient when it is clear that the patient would have refused treatment under the circumstances. Living wills provide evidence of the patient's desires. The limited objective test can be invoked to withhold or withdraw life-sustaining treatment when there is some trustworthy evidence that the patient would have refused treatment and the burdens of the patient's continued life with the treatment outweigh the benefits of that life. Under the pure objective test, where there is no reliable or trustworthy evidence of the patient's wishes, life-sustaining treatment may still be withheld or withdrawn when the net burden of the patient's life with the treatment clearly and markedly outweighs the benefits that the patient derives from life. The recurring, unavoidable, and severe pain suffered by the patient with the treatment should be such that the effect of administering the life-sustaining treatment would be inhumane.[27]

On March 22, 1983, Paul E. Brophy became unconcious after the rupture of an aneurysm. On February 6, 1985, his wife, after consulting with her children and a priest, requested a court in Massachusetts to authorize discontinuance of all life-sustaining treatment including nutrition and hydration. On October 21, 1985, the court denied her petition in the case entitled *Patricia Brophy v. New England Sinai Hospital, Inc.*, No. 85 E0009-Gl slip. op. (Mass. Probate Ct. Norfolk Div.). On September 11, 1986, the Supreme Court of Massachusetts reversed the trial court and authorized the termination of nutrition and hydration; the United States Supreme Court denied the appeal to that court.[28]

On October 23, 1986, Paul E. Brophy, who was 49 years of age, became the first American to die after the highest court in the land permitted removal of hydration and nutrition from this comatose patient. It is estimated that there are 10,000 cases in the United States of persons who are permanently comatose. Ethical dilemmas about the care given to permanently comatose patients are not yet resolved. On October 16, 1986, the New Jersey Catholic Conference expressed opposition to the removal of feeding tubes in cases involving comatose patients. It stated that the Supreme Court of New Jersey should not sanction starvation of persons who are not on the verge of dying.[28] This position has been described as wholly contrary to the centuries long tradition of the church on the duty to preserve life. It is contrary to the Vatican's recent "Declaration on Euthanasia" and the recent policy on "The Rights of the Terminally Ill" issued by the Pro-Life Committee of the United States Catholic Conference, which stated that: "Laws dealing with medical treatment may have to take account of exceptional circumstances where even means of providing nourishment may be too ineffective or burdensome to be obligatory."[29] The nutritional support team is directly affected by these court decisions authorizing or denying removal of life-sustaining treatment that includes nutrition and hydration.

Medical Records

Purpose and Content of Medical Records

The primary purpose of medical records is for diagnosis, treatment, and care of the patient. Records document what was found and what was done. They are of use in hospital educational and research programs. Accurate and complete medical records and a medical records library are required and regulated by both governmental and nongovernmental agencies. The Joint Commission on Accreditation of Hospitals has established high standards for maintenance of medical records.[16]

The medical record consists of personal, financial, and medical data pertaining to the patient. Entries should usually be made when treatment is given or when observations are made. Entries made during or immediately after a patient's hospitalization have greater credibility than those made several days, weeks, or months later.[16] The medical record should be a complete, accurate, up-to-date report of the medical history, condition, and treatment of the patient. Medical records are important evidence in legal proceedings. They are used to determine the cause of death, the time of death, the extent of the patient's injuries, the degree of pain and suffering endured by the patient, and the mental competency of the patient. Witnesses are permitted to refresh their recollection of facts and circumstances by reviewing medical records. Medical records may be introduced into evidence in legal proceedings. Whether medical records are admitted or excluded is governed by the rules of evidence that have been established to ensure that introduced information is trustworthy.[15]

The original record should be introduced in legal proceedings under the best evidence rule. If only a copy is available, however, a copy may be introduced if proof is presented that the original is not available and that the copy is a true copy of the original. If the original is introduced, a party may make a motion to substitute it with a copy.

Owner of the Record and Right of Access

The medical record is owned by the health care provider; however, the patient has a property right to the information contained therein and must be given access to that information. The procedure for obtaining medical records is controlled by state and federal statutes and rules of procedure in state and federal courts.[16]

It was held in *Rabens v. Jackson Park Hospital Foundation*, 40 Ill. App.3d 113, 351 N.E.2d 276 (1976), that a hospital may charge a reasonable amount for a copy of the record. Competent persons can generally give authority for themselves and others to have access to medical records concerning their own care and treatment. An exception to this has been recognized when release of the information would be detrimental to the patient's health.[16]

If a patient is not competent to authorize access to the medical record, someone else may be able to authorize access. It is necessary that the health care provider be certain that the one authorizing access has legal authority to do so. State statutes may set forth who has such authority. Guardians of minors and mentally ill persons and executors of estates of deceased persons usually have such authority. Parents of minors may have authority. Some statutes prohibit disclosure of medical information such as venereal disease, drug abuse, and pregnancy, and abortion pertaining to minors.[16]

There was no physician-patient privilege in the English common law, and this has been followed by most courts in the United States. Approximately two-thirds of the states have enacted a statutory physician-patient privilege, however, and some of these extend to nurses. The physician-patient privilege is the rule that a physician is not permitted to testify as a witness concerning certain information gained in the physician-patient relationship. Privilege statutes address only situations in which the physician is being compelled to testify as in a deposition, administrative hearing, or trial.[16]

Patients can waive the physician-patient privilege. Some statutes that establish the privilege may also enumerate exceptions thereto and may specify the way in which the privilege is waived. Some statutes require that certain reports such as information pertaining to abused children and communicable diseases must be made. Information that would be an invasion of a patient's privacy, even if true, cannot be disclosed under tort law.[16]

Subpoena for Persons and Records

A subpoena may be issued ordering that medical records be provided to the court or to a party to a suit. A subpoena may also be issued to a person to submit to questioning under oath prior to trial. This is called a *deposition*, and it is recorded by a court reporter. The deposition can be introduced at trial under certain circumstances as provided in the rules of procedure for the state and federal courts. If a witness cannot be present at the time of trial, the deposition testimony may be introduced. It can be used to attack the credibility of a witness when inconsistent statements are made. Depositions are excellent tools for discovering the facts and circumstances prior to trial. A request for admission of facts may be made by one party to a suit to another party in the suit. Interrogatories are questions that are served on parties to a suit and must be answered. If a party does not wish to answer questions or produce documents, a protective order must be obtained from the court. Evidence must be presented to the court, and the court must be convinced that the request for a protective order is justified under the circumstances. Otherwise, the party must answer the questions asked. The rules of procedure provide the basis for granting protective orders.

In *Marchand v. Henry Ford Hospital*, 398 Mich. 163, 247 N.W.2d 280 (1976), the defendant hospital in a medical malpractice action was ordered to answer interrogatories requesting information about how many patients the procedure of hyperalimentation had been used on before it was used on the deceased and of those patients how many died. The court determined that the information sought by the interrogatories was not protected from disclosure by Section 12(2) of the act regulating licenses of hospitals, 1968 P.A. 17, M.C.L.A. Section 331.411 et seq.; M.S.A. Section 14.1179(1) et seq., because the information sought was not collected pursuant to a directive from a hospital committee assigned the function of reviewing professional practices of the hospital for the purposes of reducing morbidity and mortality. The fact that the physician who had voluntarily collected the information sought had presented it at a general staff meeting did not satisfy the "collection" criteria of the Hospital Licensing Act and it was not brought within the ambit of the evidentiary privileges of the Act. The party was required to answer the question asked.

CONCLUSION

There can be no doubt that a medical malpractice crisis exists. The excessive costs of medical malpractice litigation and the practice of defensive medicine are passed on to the consumer by increasing the costs of medical care and treatment. Insurance premiums have increased so that the "crisis in availability" has become a "crisis in affordability."

The costs of medical litigation are emotional as well as monetary. No one can predict how a court will rule. Even if a judgment is favorable to the health care provider, the mere filing of the malpractice litigation and the publicity incident thereto can damage the reputation of the health care provider.

Tort reform legislation has not eradicated the crisis. The common goal of health care providers, the legal profession, state and local government, the insurance companies, and the general public should be a reduction in the occurrence of medical malpractice, a high quality of health care, adequate compensation to victims of medical malpractice and a decrease in the costs of health care. Health care providers should make every effort to maintain a high quality of care through education, licensing requirements, and adequate disciplinary measures. Health care professionals should be aware of and participate in passage of proposed reform legislation.

REFERENCES

1. Black: Law Dictionary (ed 4). St. Paul, MN, West Publishing, 1951
2. Atiyah P: Medical malpractice and the contract/tort boundary. Law and Contemp Prob 49:287–303, 1986
3. Prosser W: Law of Torts (ed 4). St. Paul, MN, West Publishing, 1979, pp 139–290, 416–496, 613–640
4. Danzon P: The frequency and severity of medical malpractice claims: New evidence. Law and Contemp Prob 49:57–60, 1986
5. Qual S: A survey of medical malpractice tort reform. William Mitchell Law Review 12:418–457, 1986
6. Robinson G: The medical malpractice crisis of the 1970's: A retrospective. Law and Contemp Probs 49:5–35, 1986
7. Posner J: Trends in medical malpractice insurance. Law and Contemp Probs 49(2):37–56, 1986
8. Health lawyers news report 14(12):7–8, 1986
9. Lachman V: Why we must take care of our own. Nursing 86 16(4):41, 1986

10. Sokol D: The current status of medical malpractice countersuits. Am J Law Med 10(4):339–457, 1985
11. Jones D: *Fein v. Permanente Medical Group*: The Supreme Court uncaps the constitutionality of statutory limitations on medical malpractice recoveries. University of Miami Law Review 40:1075–1099, 1986
12. Corbin A: Corbin on Contracts. St. Paul, MN, West Publishing, 1952, pp 37–358, 923–939
13. Creighton H: Law Every Nurse Should Know (ed 3). Philadelphia, WB Saunders, 1975, pp 29–57
14. Anderson R, Pomeroy D, Kumf W: Business Law (ed 4). Cincinnati, South-Western Publishing, 1952, pp 33–151
15. Cazalas M: Private practice and the law, in Koltz C: Private Practice in Nursing. Germantown, MD, Aspen Systems, 1979, pp 165–196
16. Miller R: Problems in Hospital Law (ed 4). Rockville, MD, Aspen Systems, 1983, pp 177–200, 271–299
17. Rosoff A: Informed Consent. Rockville, MD, Aspen Systems, 1981, pp 1, 33–38
18. Averbach A: Handling Accident Cases. Revised. Vol 3A. Rochester, MN, The Lawyer's Co-operative Publishing Co., 1970, pp 15–16, 133–135
19. Pegalis S, Wachsman H: American Law of Medical Malpractice. Vol 1. Rochester, MN, The Lawyer's Co-operative Publishing Co., 1980, pp 45–303
20. Levenson J: Psychiatric aspects of total patenteral nutrition. Nutr Supp Serv 2(7):38–40, 1982
21. Rodgers L, Moss J, Wright R: New developements in enteral feeding techniques. Nutr Supp Serv 2(10):17–20, 1982
22. Ament M: Home TPN. Nutr Supp Serv 2(10):47–48, 1982
23. Masser E: Nursing management of peripheral parenteral nutrition patients. Nutr Supp Serv 2(8):43–44, 1982
24. Meyers D: Medico-Legal Implications of Death and Dying. Rochester, MN, The Lawyers Co-operative Publishing Co., 1981, pp 59–98
25. Rothman D, Rothman N: The Professional Nurse and the Law. Boston, Little, Brown and Company, 1977
26. Swartz M: The patient who refuses medical treatment: A dilemma for hospitals and physicians. Am J Law Med 11(2):147–194, 1986
27. Siegal H: *In re Conroy:* A limited right to withhold or withdraw artificial nourishment. Notes and comments. Pace Law Review 6:219–265, 1986
28. Drinan R: Should Paul Brophy have been allowed to die? America 155:324–325, 332, 1986
29. Paris J, McCormick R: The Catholic tradition on the use of nutrition and fluids. America 156:356–362, 1987

Bonnie L. Metzger
Barbara C. Hansen

13

Research Opportunities: Dimensions in Nutritional Support Nursing

Research is the process by which facts and laws are established. The purpose of nursing research is to generate those facts and laws that serve as the basis for efficient and effective nursing practice.

As integral parts of a nutritional support team, nurses assume both dependent and independent roles in delivering a unique service to the individual in need of nutritional support. In addition, nurse scientists are actively applying the scientific method to those phenomena that underly nursing practice in the nutritional support area.

In a presidential address of the American Society of Parenteral and Enteral Nutrition (ASPEN), it was stated that ". . . the scientific disciplines with which we in ASPEN are primarily concerned are nutrition and medicine."[1] We look forward to the day when nursing, too, will be listed as such a scientific discipline contributing to the improvement of enteral and parenteral nutrition.

Nursing is a developing science. It is only within the past several decades that nurses have begun to critically examine the basis of nursing practice. A first step in this critique was the acknowledgement that little systematically-derived nursing science existed and our practice was based instead on traditional trial and error, individual problem solving, and a borrowed assortment of eclectic facts. The next logical step in the development of a firm foundation of scientific nursing knowledge was the education of nurse scientists trained in the systematic precise process of scientific inquiry. With a significant increase in the number of nurses educated to carry out research, nursing has moved to the threshold of discipline development and recognition. The actual building blocks of a discipline, however, consist of contributions to scientific knowledge and recognition

NUTRITIONAL SUPPORT IN NURSING
ISBN 0-8089-1889-3

of the discipline by others. These are dependent on the successful communication of new facts and laws throughout the larger scientific community. Finally, research in nursing, unlike that of nonapplied sciences, is not focused on the development of knowledge for the sake of only knowing. The overall test of nursing as a discipline and a science will be successful demonstrating of that knowledge by the professional practitioner of nursing.

TARGETED ISSUES OF NURSING RESEARCH

Examination of the scientific literature dedicated to nursing research and to research focused on parenteral or enteral nutrition suggests that nurse scientists have, since the early 1970s, been actively engaged in examining those phenomena related to efficient and effective nursing care of individuals receiving enteral or parenteral nutritional support.[2]

Nutritional and Therapy Assessment

One of the primary responsibilities of all nurses involved in the daily care of *any* patient is assessment of that person's overall nutritional status. Furthermore, it is the nurse who performs the day-to-day overall assessment of the patient receiving either enteral or parenteral nutrition (TPN) and who continuously analyzes the success or failure of the medical and nutritional therapies. Further research aimed at the development of noninvasive, eclectic nutritional assessment tools is clearly needed. Some beginning work on nutritional assessment has been reported by Jones et al.,[3] Johnson et al.,[4] and Courtney et al.[5] Another related area of nursing research includes the development and testing of methods of instructing all nurses, especially those not specifically oriented to nutritional support, in the art of nutritional assessment.

Containment of Cost

All nurses on the nutritional support team are acutely aware of the high cost of this service, especially TPN. The reduction of patient care costs through the prevention of waste of equipment and time, as well as the promotion of safe, effective home care for patients in need of long-term nutritional support, will be enhanced by additional nursing research. Specific research questions to be addressed include (1) methods to enhance catheter life, including specific questions of heparinization, techniques, volume, type, and frequency of solution administration, (2) catheter types, and (3) sepsis prevention. Psychosocial research also has its place in nursing research to improve nutritional support. Identification of family support systems, the most effective use of support systems in home care, adaptation of the home environment for chronic nutritional supprt,[6,7] and the emotional needs of persons receiving long-term nutritional support are a few examples.[8–11]

Prevention of Sepsis

The day-to-day safety and well-being of the individual receiving TPN is the responsibility of the nurse and is highly dependent on the prevention of sepsis. The nurse caring for that patient needs the knowledge derived from research directed toward identifying sepsis in patients on immunosuppressants; differentiating the source of infection—the catheter, solution, tubing, or a secondary site; and identifying insertion-site care that is associated with the lowest occurrence of insertion site infection.[12-16]

Promotion of Comfort

One of nursing's historical challenges is to promote comfort and well-being in situations characterized by discomfort, pain, and fear. The administration of nutritional support, parenteral or enteral, is no exception. It is the responsibility of nursing research to identify methods of administration that will induce the minimal amount of intolerance symptoms. Significant work has been done in this area by a consortium of nurse researchers and others interested in enteral feeding.[17-26] Another area of research focus deals with the exploration of refeeding and appetite alteration as a function of nutritional support.[27-30]

IMPEDIMENTS TO NURSING RESEARCH

Although there are some reports of nursing research focused on the needs of the patient receiving nutritional support, in many cases the reported investigations are beginning exploratory studies, and although important contributions have been made by nurse researchers to the general knowledge base, these efforts have usually been isolated from the research efforts of other scientists. Few attempts have been made by nurse researchers to draw together their research findings or consolidate their efforts. A fact here and an observation there do little to influence nursing practice or impact on the scientific community.

Many factors interfere with the scientific investigation itself. One factor is the high cost of research in a time of fiscal constraints. Another is the fact that the nursing scientific community is still in its infancy. Other impediments to nursing research are the inadequate sample sizes frequently associated with clinical research and the nonsupportive attitudes of other disciplines and other nurses themselves toward nursing research in general. These attitudes, combined with the general shortage of research funding and proven nurse scientists, compound the problem of inadequate funding for independent nursing research projects.

All nurses can be actively involved in nursing research, but not all nurses possess the skills essential to planning and directing a scientific investigation. In addition, although all nurses involved in the direct delivery of care should be able to systematically observe and intuitively examine identified relationships as a basis for a research project, the pool of nurses trained to design the study, manage the data, and obtain the financial support necessary to the actual research is still very small.

One solution to many of the identified problems is the development of a consortium research effort among nurses interested in common phenomena. A consortium needs nurses who deliver care and value research to identify the problems of nutritional support delivery, the complications of parenteral supplementation, the possible emotional needs and adjustments of the patients, potential ways to cut costs, and methods to adequately assess care and nutritional status. A consortium effort would also require research-prepared nurses with the knowledge and self-discipline essential to systematic collection and meticulous handling of data. The final ingredients for a successful research consortium are nurse scientists who can design an effective study, manage data, obtain necessary funds, and effectively communicate the results of the study.

The Tube Feeding Consortium established by a grant awarded to the Western Interstate Council for Higher Education in Nursing serves as a model for collaborative nursing research. Reports of this consortium's achievements present both the advantages and disadvantages of this type of group approach to scientific inquiry.[31] One distinct advantage of bringing together scientists interested in the same research problems, but from different areas of the country and representing multiple agencies, is the significant increase in the size of the potential subject pool. A second plus reported by the consortium is the research cost advantage of using one subject for more than one study. For example, questions related to emotional adjustment to long-term TPN could be addressed in subjects who are on an experimental protocol designed to examine the effect of a unique sepsis prevention routine. Obviously, the pool of research-prepared nurses is expanding with an associated increase in creative suggestions for study focus, in available resources for grant writing and development of measurement tools, and in the understanding of research design and methodology, data management and analysis, and the use of the computer. In addition, there is a significant increase in the number of persons committed to research and available to assist in data collection. Maybe the most important advantage of collaborative research is that it provides an ongoing communication link essential to drawing together the generated facts and extending the research in multiple directions. Collaborative research provides the framework essential to more rapid expansion of the existing knowledge base through systematic replication of ongoing studies.

The disadvantages of collaborative research are those inherent in any group effort. It is often difficult and expensive to communicate when great distances are involved. In most instances, the work of the consortium is not the primary professional concern of its members and scheduling of meetings or conference calls will be difficult because of distance and many different schedules. Plans must be made in establishing a collaborative research effort to overcome these communication difficulties. Money for phone calls, computer communication conference calls, and travel to meetings are essential budget items. The size of the group and selection of membership are clearly important. Complementary skills and knowledge may be highly cost effective.

Another problem associated with data collection in multiple agencies by many different persons is a legitimate concern about the consistency of data collection, the reliability of the data, and of the data-collector. This problem can be addressed by clear, detailed preparation of research protocols prior to data collection and systematic training programs for each person hired to collect data.

As with any group project, individual ambitions and egos are a factor. Issues of responsibility and credit, including publications, must be acknowledged by the group, and guidelines must be established to deal with the identified problem areas, as well as for handling unanticipated group or personal crises.

One alternative to the nursing consortium is the involvement of nurses in interdisciplinary research. Nutritional support of individuals is a multidisciplinary effort and naturally lends itself to interdisciplinary research. It is important that nurses be involved not only in the collection of data directed toward specific problems, but also in the initial design and planning of such studies. Only in this way will nursing involvement in interdisciplinary research on nutritional support lead to advances in nursing's understanding of those phenomena underlying its own independent practice.

RESEARCH PROCESS AND FUNDING

The research process has many steps. To begin the process of inquiry, the researcher should develop a well-reasoned and convincing rationale for the importance of the study to the expansion of the knowledge essential to safe, effective, efficient delivery of nursing care to the enteral or parenteral nutritional support patient. This rationale is essential to all aspects of the study, but it is imperative to the development of a proposal for research support. The first step toward obtaining this essential support is identifying what data concerning the problem area already exist. It is highly unlikely that funding will be made available to researchers who have not done their homework or have underestimated the knowledge of the grant reviewers.

The next step in applying for research support is the identification of the appropriate funding source. Many health-care agencies have in-house or institutional sources of funds. From what sources are the physicians, pharmacists, and nutritionists on the support team receiving research funds? Are these funds set aside for multidisciplinary research? It is often useful to get to know the in-house grantors and processes for competing for local funds.

Specific private and federal agencies are established to support nursing research. The American Nurse's Foundation (ANF), a nonprofit organization, was founded to support research aimed at the improvement of patient care. Sigma Theta Tau, the nursing honor society, provides small money grants to members engaged in nursing research.

The National Center for Nursing Research (NCNR) at NIH (formerly the Division of Nursing) is well established as the major source of federal funding for nursing research. A committee made up of both nurse and non-nurse researchers carefully reviews every proposal submitted, recommends approval or disapproval, and indicates the degree of priority a proposal should receive for funding. A council then reviews those recommendations from the peer review group and provides guidance to the staff of the NCNR, where final decisions are made about funding.

Several foundations have been historically generous to nursing or health care research projects: Russell Sage Foundation, Rockefeller Foundation, W.K. Kellogg Foundation, PEW Foundation, and the Robert Wood Johnson Foundation. Other nongovernmental research grant fellowship organizations providing opportunities for scientists interested in the phenomena related to total nutritional support are the American Cancer Society and the P.D.A. Foundation of Pharmaceutical Sciences, Inc. Other potential sources of research funding seldom used by nurse researchers are private corporations. Those private industries most likely to support TPN and enteral nutrition research are those companies involved in the production of TPN and enteral solutions and equipment.

The next step in applying for funding is to contact the potential funding source. Share your goals and resource needs with them, and let them help you decide if they are the appropriate funding source for your research. Once the potential funding source is identified, develop the proposal. The process and product are oriented to selling the need for research on a particular topic to the reviewers, then providing sufficient documentation to support the need for the studies as specified, and finally demonstrating the competence to design the study and analyze the data effectively. To do these, one must be thoroughly familiar with the research process and the science of proposal development. The remainder of this chapter provides a primer to those who would actively pursue nursing research related to nutritional support.

Once the research problems have been delineated and the aims, rationale, and significance of the study have been spelled out, the next step in the process of scientific inquiry and the preparation of the proposal for funding is the development of the research blueprint. Integral pieces of the study model include the following:

- What does the study population look like?
- What kinds of persons should be selected to make up the sample?
- How will the sample be selected?
- What are the controls that will be built into the systematic design and colleciton of data, so that both scientist and consumer of the research will have confidence in the fact and/or laws generated?
- What is the information essential to answering the research question?
- How will that information be obtained and measured?

- Are the methods of data collection valid (do they measure what they were designed to measure) and reliable (do they consistently measure what they were designed to measure)?
- How will the reliability and validity of the collection tools be demonstrated so that others will have confidence in the findings?
- Finally, how will the collected data be condensed, described, and analyzed?

Answers to all of these questions prior to the actual colleciton of data are important to the formal, systematic process of scientific inquiry, to communication of the final research findings, and to successful research funding.

Study Design and Sampling

Experimental research design provides the most powerful scientific method for answering many biomedical and health questions. The optimal research design is the one that controls or eliminates bias. Eliminating bias does not imply reducing the researcher's prejudices; it means instead that the researcher has chosen a sample that truly represents the population to be studied and has chosen measurement devices of criteria that are likely to objectively measure the phenomenon of concern. The most effective way to eliminate bias is to use an experimental research design and randomly selected sample.

Although experimental research (hypothesis testing) is the most powerful research design, it is not always possible to conduct experimental research in nursing. Further, it is not always the appropriate research design based on the research questions being asked or the current status of the discipline's knowledge base. In nursing there are many research areas where it would be more appropriate for the nurse scientist to design a study specifically to describe a phenomenon and its relationships with other phenomena. These studies of nonbiased observations of ongoing phenomena are essential to the generation of hypotheses for future testing and are appropriate to new, developing disciplines.

Despite the need for descriptive, exploratory research in nursing, there are still many instances where the nurse researcher avoids clinical experimentation because it is just too difficult to accomplish. For example, to truly eliminate bias a sample must not only be random but sufficiently large to compensate for the expected differences, not experimentally-induced differences, within any group of individuals. Sample size inadequacy is not the only problem of small clinical subject pools. Many times clinical subjects are not available as research subjects.

Among nurses themselves there must be support and encouragement for those already engaged in research activities. Workshops for nurses should be based on current research. It is important for clinical nurse practitioners and nursing staff to get to know nurse researchers interested in the problems related to enteral and parenteral nutrition. The support and advice of active clinicians are crucial to researchers. As mentioned before, the legitimacy of nursing research can be enhanced by participation in interdisciplinary research and the involvement of nurses in the planning and conduct of research. The development of nursing research activity must be encouraged in every care setting. The support and encouragement of nursing administration is also crucial to the facilitation of nursing research in the agency. Such support requires active efforts through budget, released time and support staff.

Measurement and Data Collection

Research is a tool for describing relationships between things and the things themselves. Things are not beliefs about what is real; things can be seen, felt, heard; they can be quantified. There is a prescribed range within which anything may vary. If some things exhibit differences beyond the parameters set to describe that specific thing, the guidelines set for describing it may be inadequate or it may be a different thing altogether. The important points here are that things are expected to differ from similar things within a certain range, and this variance can be measured. Research provides us with the formal process by which we can determine if changes in one thing (independent variable) influence or affect another (dependent variable) as well as a systematic basis for describing the parameters of a phenomenon, the thing itself.

A research proposal must precisely define what is to be measured and how the subtle changes in the variable will be identified. In general, a number represents the degree to which a specific thing may vary from another. These numbers are synonymous with quantification of the thing and allow the scientist to communicate the findings of the research to others who use similar numerical systems and to mathematically manipulate these numbers for the purpsoe of describing the phenomenon and the effect of one variable on another. Statistics are a set of mathematical theories that guide the researcher in understanding the relationships and differences implied by the numbers derived from the measurement (data).

Statistics are a tool. As researchers we must not stand in awe of the tool. Just as experimental design may not be appropriate to the type of research questions being asked, so, too, may classic statistics be inappropriate to the description of the data collected. Each craftsman should have a sound understanding of and the ability to use and manipulate the tools of the trade. The tools of measurement, data management, and data analysis are some of the basic tools of the scientist.

Not all nurses have the ability to develop measurement tools and to skillfully manage and analyze data. As mentioned before, collaborative research provides one framework for dealing with the small pool of research-prepared nurses. An important guideline to use in seeking collaborative or consultive assistance with these problems is to value the uniqueness of nursing phenomena. Classic statistical measurement techniques may not be appropriate to what is to be measured. Nursing is a relatively new scientific discipline and may need to develop novel techniques and tools. Research-prepared nurses are available to consult with clinicians, are able to understand nursing research goals, and may not require significant amounts of explanation or time before they can help identify or develop the tools needed to measure and discriminate the similarities and differences within the phenomena of interest.

Data collection is not a simple process. Quality research requires a systematic, consistent approach to measurement not necessarily similar to observations performed by clinical nurses. Nurses are skilled in systematic observation and are often good collectors of research data. They are trained to see changes in the whole person, as well as specific small alterations. Restlessness, a behavioral change, combined with subtle physical changes in the patient's skin color or color and amount of drainage will alert a nurse to a patient's status long before that change could be quantified by a single change in urine volume or hematocrit. Clinically, therefore, it is an advantage for a nurse to synthesize many things into a conceptual whole. Detailed protocols assist an excellent clinical nurse to become an excellent collector of research data.

Research Proposal Preparation

The review panel that determines the scientific merit of proposed research has as its primary source of information the written blueprint of that research. The preparation of a concise, adequate request for funding thus requires considerable care and time. After identifying the appropriate funding agencies, the grant application and instructions for preparing the application should be obtained. In-house or institutional sources of "grantsmanship," both experienced researchers or grants reviewers, should be recruited to assist in the preparation and review of the grant application. Obviously, ready assistance in preparation and review of research protocols is a distinct advantage of optimal collaborative research since honest critique of the proposal prior to submission is imperative to the development of a clear, adequate request for research funding.

One component of a research grant application is a current literature review. This review includes an adequate coverage of the current work in the area and it strengthened by describing the relevant research of the investigative team. Any grant proposal is strengthened by the presence of pilot study data. Pilot studies demonstrate that the persons requesting funds are not novice investigators in the area and have some inquiry currently underway. It is imperative that this part of the proposal is current, complete, detailed, and logical. Again, an honest critique will help ensure that this introduction to the research, which provides the rationale and framework of the study, possesses all of the above qualities.

The second step in preparing a grant proposal is the preparation of a concise statement of research aims—the specific research questions to be answered, outcomes to be expected, or hypotheses to be tested by this scientific inquiry. These concise statements of research goals should flow logically from the study rationale. Again, an honest critique is imperative to the presentation of sufficiently clear, concise, and logical aims. An honest appraisal of available resources is essential to the preparation of specific aims that are not overly ambitious. Reviewers of grant applications are very aware of the resources essential to achievement of research goals. Common bases for disapproval of grant applications are insufficient understanding of the problem on the part of the investigator, insufficient available resources and unrealistic research aims.

The next step essential to the development of a fundable grant proposal is a clear presentation of the study plan, including scientific rationale for the strategies of measurement, data collection, and analysis.

A clear statement of the significance of the proposed research is a requirement of most grant proposals. In this section, the individual seeking funding must demonstrate that the study logically extends and builds other research in the area. At the same time, it is imperative that the unique aspects of the proposed study be clearly presented, with a heavy emphasis on how the collected data will make a *unique* contribution to the knowledge basis and/or clinical practice. It is important to establish a strong match between the proposed contributions of the scientific inquiry and the goals of the granting agency. To achieve this match, the goals of the granting agency must be understood by the investigator. What information do they want and are they ready to pay for? This section and the granting agencies goals should also be shared with an appropriate colleague for critique before revision and submission.

The final step in the preparation of a grant proposal is the preparation of the budget request. Using the research plan, a flow chart that includes time and personnel should be developed. Budget planning includes an estimate of time needed to complete the project and its different phases. Do the different phases of the inquiry require different amounts and types of personnel? What and who are the personnel needed to accomplish the study? Could some of the personnel effort be better accomplished through consultation or collaboration? What equipment and supplies are essential to the achievement of the research goals? A strength of any grant proposal is the identification of institutional resources, including equipment, supplies, available research laboratories or clinical research units, consultants, and/or computer use and accessibility that are to contribute to the study. The availability of resources and facilities to the investigator suggests to the review panel that this scientific inquiry may be conducted more efficiently in this setting by this researcher, than in another setting.

A rationale for each budget item is required. Part of this item justification is a description of the personnel and their research experience. Most beginning investigators need experienced professional assistance in the preparation of the budget request.

In summary, the preparation of a grant proposal requires significant planning and lead time. Presubmission communication with funding agencies is essential to assist in the identification of the appropriate agency and clarification of their funding goals. A systematic review of the current state of the research in the area is the framework on which the proposed scientific merit of the study is built—the introduction, the specific aims, and the significance of the study. The methods and procedures of the study must be appropriate, and scientific rationale to support the use of each must be clearly stated. The budget request must be realistic, and available resources should be emphasized. Possibly the most important step in the preparation of the grant application is the identification and use of research-experienced colleagues who will give an honest critique of the request at every stage of the grant proposal development process. Finally, the final package, the proposal itself, should be concise, free of error, neat, and attractive.

Research Ethics

Nursing is a humanistic science and service. By its very nature, nursing mandates that the ethical and moral concerns associated with experimental manipulation and data-gathering must be systematically raised and examined by its scientists. Although ethical guidelines exist that clearly delineate certain limitations for human and animal research, many ethical and moral questions are still unclear. For example, are we as morally responsible to maintain an individual's right to privacy as we are to protect that individual from psychological stress or physical harm? In health-related research, it is sometimes suggested that the value of a scientific fact that could improve the public well-being justifies the possible invasion of privacy associated with gathering data about personal habits, illness and loss. Other issues that scientists should examine include the following:

- Who is responsible for the overgeneralization of research findings that results in inappropriate changes in clinical practice?
- How do we safeguard the generated scientific facts from premature or inappropriate application by the research consumer?
- How do scientists balance the amount of information essential to informed consent and the amount that will bias the subject's response?
- In addition, how do we quantify the things from which we are required to protect subjects—physical or emotional stress and invasion of privacy?

The development of a new discipline demands that its scientists struggle with the moral questions and ethical concerns unique to that discipline. At some point, quality humanistic research requires the use of human subjects and the protection of those subjects. Nursing's unique commitment to the well-being and comfort of their clients has implications for the moral and ethical guidelines of their research.

SUMMARY

The purpose of nursing research is to generate knowledge that serves as the basis for effective clinical practice. Within the past decade nurse scientists have been actively engaged in research focused on the nursing care of the individual receiving enteral or total parenteral nutritional support: nutritional and therapy assessment, containment of cost, prevention of sepsis, and promotion of comfort.[2]

One impediment to nursing's development as a science is that few systematic attempts are being made to draw together or build on the isolated facts generated by nursing's small pool of scientists. A research consortium was one solution proposed to resolve both the problems of isolated research and the inadequate supply of nurses educated to design studies, manage data, and obtain financial support essential to research. This type of collaborative research effort has several distinct advantages. It increases the sizes of both the potential subject and research-prepared nurse pools and, probably most importantly, the consortium has a built-in mechanism for pulling together isolated facts and expanding and extending the subsequent consolidated knowledge base. An alternative solution to the proposed consortium research effort is the active involvement of nurses in interdisciplinary research efforts.

Finally, research is a conscious, systematic process of inquiry. The confidence others have in the validity of the generated knowledge is directly related to the rigor applied to each of the steps of the scientific process. Indeed, research support, whether collegial or financial, is highly dependent on a demonstrated ability to systematically identify relevant problem areas and current knowledge about the problems, to develop significant research aims form the existing data base, and to design research protocols and manage resultant data. In conclusion, the generation of nursing knowledge must be conducted within the moral and ethical boundaries dictated by nursing's unique commitment to the well-being and comfort of their clients.

REFERENCES

1. Blackburn GL: Presidential address. Interaction of the science of nutrition and the science of medicine. *JPEN* 3(3):131–136, 1979
2. Moore MC, Guenter PA, Bender JH: Nutrition-related nursing research. *Image* 18(1):18–21, 1986
3. Jones TN, Moore EE, Van Way CW III: Factors influencing nutritional assessment in abdominal trauma patients. *JPEN* 7(2): 115–116, 1983
4. Johnston CA, Keane TJ, Prudo SM: Weight loss in patients receiving radical radiation therapy for head and neck cancer: A prospective study. *JPEN* 6(5):399–402, 1982

5. Courtney ME, Green HL, Folk CC, et al: Rapidly declining serum albumin values in newly hospitalized patients: prevalence, severity and contributing factors. *JPEN* 6(2):143–145, 1982

6. Montague N, Srp F, Steigner E: Emergency catheter repairs in the home parenteral nutrition (HPN) patient. *JPEN* 4(6) (abstr 86): 1980

7. Newmark SR, Simpson MS, Beskitt MP, et al: Home tube feeding for long-term nutritional support. *JPEN* 5(1):76–79, 1981

8. Hughes BA, Fleming CR, Berxner S, et al: Patient compliance with a home parenteral nutrition program. *JPEN* 4(1):12–14, 1980

9. Lyons JM, Falkenbach LA, Cerra FB: Home parenteral nutrition with full-time home care nurses. *JPEN* 5(6):528–530, 1981

10. Perl M, Hall RCW, Dudrick SJ, et al: Psychological aspects of long-term home hyperalimentation. *JPEN* 4(6):554–560, 1980

11. Price BS, Levine EL: Permanent total parenteral nutrition: Psychological and social responses of the early stages. *JPEN* 3(2):48–52, 1979

12. Jarrard MM, Olson CM, Freeman JB: Daily dressing change effects on skin flora beneath subclavian catheter dressings during total parenteral nutrition. *JPEN* 4(4):391–392, 1980

13. Jarrard MM, Freeman JB: The effects of antibiotic ointments and antiseptics on the skin flora beneath subclavian catheter dressings during intravenous hyperalimentation. *J Surg Res* 22:521–526, 1977

14. Palidar PJ, Simonowitz DA, Dreskovich MR, et al: Use of op-site as an occlusive dressing for total parenteral nutrition catheters. *JPEN* 6(2):150–151, 1982

15. Powell C, Regan C, Fahri PJ, et al: Evaluation of op-site catheter dressings for parenteral nutrition: A prospective, randomized study. *JPEN* 6(1):43–46, 1982

16. Crocker KS, Noga R, Filibeck DJ, et al: Microbial growth comparisons of five commercial parenteral lipid emulsions. *JPEN* 8:391–395, 1984

17. Crocker KS, Krey SH, Steffer WP: Performance evaluation of a new nasogastric feeding tube. *JPEN* 5(1):80–85, 1981

18. Hanson BC, Martyn PA, Jen K-LC: Sequential change in hunger and gastric motility patterns during periods of initiation and termination of parenteral nutrition. *JPEN* 5(6)(abstr 14):560, 1981

19. Hansen BW, DeSomery CH, Hagedorn PK, et al: Effects of enteral and parenteral nutrition on appetite in monkeys. *JPEN* 1(2):82–88, 1977

20. Hanson RL: Predictive criteria for length of nasogastric tube insertion for tube feeding. *JPEN* 3(3):160–163, 1979

21. Heitkemper ME, Martin DL, Hansen BC, et al: Rate and volume of intermittent enteral feeding. *JPEN* 5(2):125–129, 1981

22. Kagawa-Busby K, Heitkemper MM, Hansen BC, et al: Effects of diet temperature on tolerance of enteral feedings. *Nurs Res* 29(5):276–280, 1980

23. Padilla GV, Grant M, Rains B, et al: Distress reduction and the effects of preparatory teaching films and patient control. *Res Nurs Health* 4(4):375–387, 1981

24. Padilla GV, Grant M, Wong H, et al: Subjective distresses of nasogastric tube feeding. *JPEN* 3(2):53–57, 1979

25. Walike BC, Padilla GV, Bergstrom N, et al: Patient problems related to tube feeding. *Communicating Nursing Research* 7:89–112, 1975

26. Dixon J: Effect of nursing interventions on nutritional and performance status in cancer patients. *Nurs Res* 33:330–334, 1984

27. DeSomery C, Hansen BW: Regulation of appetite during total parenteral nutrition. *Nurs Res* 27:19–24, 1978
28. Martyn PA, Hansen BC, Jen KC: The effects of parenteral nutrition on food intake and gastric motility. *Nurs Res* 33:336–342, 1984
29. Metzger BL, Bodkin N, Jen K-LC, et al: Effect of varying nutrient compositions on food intake. *JPEN* 8:1, 1984
30. Metzger BL, Bodkin N, Jen K-LC, et al: Effects of high protein enteral formulas on appetite. *JPEN* 9:113, 1985
31. Bergstrom N, Hansen BC, Grant M, et al: Collaborative nursing research. Anatomy of a successful consortium. *Nurs Res* 33:20–25, 1984

Linda Carrick Torosian
Margaret Cunliffe

14

Nutritional Support Nursing in a Changing Health Care Environment: Administrative Issues

The American health care industry is experiencing a revolution that is dramatically changing the delivery of health care. It is a time when nurses in specialty fields must assume leadership roles in protecting and advancing quality health care. This is particularly true for the field of nutritional support.

Accompanying this movement is an attitudinal change on the part of the public. Individuals accept and are expected to play an active role in retaining and regaining their health. This active role in health care requires that patients and their families be well-educated and supported, particularly when they are involved in decision-making. This change in patient involvement is manifested in the successful treatment of home parenteral nutritional patients. The first home parenteral nutritional patient was treated in 1970; currently, several hundred patients are maintained on home parenteral nutrition.[1] Nutritional support nurses are needed to coordinate and direct the education, monitoring, and support of these patients.

There is an increasing demand by the public for delivery of quality health care. Many patients are no longer willing to accept the complications of medical treatment without questioning health care professionals. The media abounds with news of medical litigations, and the fear of a lawsuit strikes every health care professional practicing medical and nursing science. Nutritional support nurses must demonstrate a prospective strategy for ensuring quality and safety in this new, rapidly expanding, technology-dependent field.

In addition, society has recognized that health care can no longer be considered a bountiful service to be enacted for everyone at any price. Health care is a limited and costly product that needs to be carefully monitored and appropriately delivered. The current source of the economic revolution is the initiation of diagnosis-related groups (DRGs), one form of a prospective payment system that attempts to quantify health care costs. The DRG system, however, represents only a *tool* that is being used to implement changes in society's philosophy of health care delivery.

Over future years the tools will change, but the philosophic impetus will remain. Prospective payment systems (PPSs) are having a great impact on health care providers in both hospitals and community agencies. All professional disciplines are critically reviewing their practices searching for more economical and effective methods of providing patient care. Survival of efficiency has become a key concept in professional practice. To thrive in a contained environment requires an understanding of the current health care climate, a willingness to evaluate our method of health care delivery (type of structure, kinds of resources, standards of practice), and a creative fervor to develop proactive strategies to meet current and future challenges.

NUTRITIONAL SUPPORT TEAM IN A CHANGING ENVIRONMENT

The prevailing focus in health care has shifted from "more of everything," including costs, to "less of most things," especially costs. In 1983 Congress changed the Medicare reimbursement system from a retrospective per diem charge system to a prospective cost per discharge system. Under this system, hospitals no longer get reimbursed for charges the patient incurred for treatments, length of stay, diagnostic tests, and soon; instead, hospitals receive a predetermined amount of money based on the discharge diagnosis of the patient. Since 1983, other types of insurers have joined the PPS of reimbursement. Some economists believe that by 1995 all insurers will be functioning under a PPS, although perhaps not DRGs.

All these changes were precipitated by the tremendous increases in the cost of providing health care. In 1950, health care expenditures totaled $10.8 billion; in 1982, that figure rose to $322 billion, which equals 10.5 percent of the Gross National Product (GNP).[2] Since the enactment of PPSs, health care expenditures in 1984 reached $387 billion, 10.6 percent of the GNP. Although this is still a significant percentage of the GNP, the growth rate for health care expenditure has declined slightly.

Under the PPS, hospital administrators, nurses, physicians, and all other care providers are working together to achieve the following four goals to remain solvent:

1. Decrease the length of stay for all patients since a longer stay only adds to the overall costs.
2. Increase the hospital's mix of patients for whom reimbursement is profitable.

3. Increase turnover of patients so that bed occupancy and admissions are increased resulting in increased revenue.
4. Decrease costs of providing care.

Many hospitals that have not been able to achieve these goals have been forced to close.

The role of the primary physician and primary nurse have become increasingly important in achieving the aforementioned objectives. The role of consultative services, however, are being carefully scrutinized by hospital administrators and insurance providers. The nutrition support service represents an important interdisciplinary consultative team whose role is currently being examined for efficacy in numerous hospitals throughout the country.

Studies have documented the prevalence of malnutrition as ranging from 30 to 50 percent in hospitalized patients.[3,4] Based on the widespread incidence and clinical impact of malnutrition, it is imperative that there be experts in the field of nutrition to meet these patient care needs. The complexity and high technological skills required for optimal nutritional support makes a multidisciplinary team approach necessary. Studies by Dalton and Jacobs demonstrate improved clinical monitoring and treatment through the use of a structured nutritional support team.[5,6] The team typically consists of nurses, dieticians, pharmacists, and physicians. The clinical objectives of a nutritional support team include the following:

1. Identification of patients who are nutritionally impaired.
2. Performance of a nutritional assessment that can adequately monitor nutritional therapy.
3. Provision of nutritional support in a safe and effective manner.
4. Monitoring and evaluation of treatments related to the nutritional care of the patient.

Improving clinical standards and establishing goals is an important function of the nutritional support team. It remains controversial, however, whether the nutrition support team assists the hospital in providing cost-effective care by achieving the four goals previously mentioned. A superficial review of nutritional support teams indicates that they are associated with high cost. It must be realized that nutritional support services are extended to patients with increased complexity and severity of illness and length of hospital stay. On a typical nutritional support team, 20–30 percent of the patients are critically ill, and the administration of forced feeding adds to their daily cost of care. For a patient receiving parenteral nutrition, this additional cost may amount to hundreds of dollars per day. Under a PPS hospitals can suffer a dramatic financial loss on these patients; consequently, expert judgment is required in the selection and administration of parenteral and enteral nutrition.

Hospitals are currently expanding revenue-generating programs and are scrutinizing nonrevenue-generating programs and positions. There is uncertainty regarding whether nutritional support teams ultimately generate revenue through the use of solutions and equipment, decreased complication rates, and decreased length of stay. Most health care providers admit that nutritional support is a very expensive treatment modality. Focusing only on total cost for providing this service is an inadequate means for assessing efficacy.

Decisions regarding allocation of resources are difficult but are essential to financial survival in the health care industry. Clinical effectiveness is an important but difficult component to evaluate. The need for improved methods of determining resources based on efficacy has led to the use of three methods of analysis: cost benefit, cost-effectiveness, and risk-benefit analysis.

Cost-benefit analysis relates the cost of a therapy or strategy to the benefits produced. Cost-effectiveness analysis identifies the goal to be achieved and then reviews the cost of various strategies to achieve it. Risk-benefit analysis compares the morbidity and mortality of the proposed treatment to actual reductions in these parameters and the improved quality of life that results.[8] Studies in the field of nutritional support using these methods are currently being initiated. Determining costs for nutritional support services are difficult because they are not adequately measured under DRGs. In addition, although nutritional support teams are labor-intense, the majority of the costs are for solutions and materials rather than services. As outlined by Twomey and Patching in a preliminary study, cost-benefit analysis showed a net savings of $1720/patient by using parenteral nutrition in patients with gastrointestinal (GI) cancer.[8] These savings occurred as a result of decreased complications observed in patients receiving parenteral nutrition.

The future existence of interdisciplinary nutritional support teams will be determined based on data supporting their clinical effectiveness and cost-effectiveness. The organizational structure of the nutritional support team should facilitate maximum resource utilization. All disciplines must work both individually and collectively to provide data determining their impact on patient outcomes. Quality control and nutritional surveillance are the responsibility of the nutritional support team. Data must be collected, analyzed, and reported in the literature to document the overall effect of these teams on clinical care and prevention of nutrition-related complications. Although the health care environment is focusing on cost containment, it is the responsibility of all health care providers to discourage the assessment of clinical practice in terms of cost only. We must remain cognizant of legal responsibilities, quality care, ethical practice, and standards of practice. Each member of the team must consider his or her role in today's health care environment and identify strategies for role justification and promotion.

NURSING STRATEGIES IN TODAY'S HEALTH CARE INDUSTRY

The reimbursement changes are primarily affecting direct patient care activities. Hospital administrators encourage nurses to take leadership in developing new strategies to deliver quality patient care at reduced costs. In response to this challenge, several innovative methods for quantifying and controlling nursing costs have been developed. Organizational restructuring, patient classification systems, concurrent quality monitoring, and cost accounting for nursing services are several responses to the changing health care system. In the forefront of these innovations are nursing specialists, many of whom are academically prepared as clinical nurse specialists and whose positions are on the frontiers of nursing science. Nutritional support nurses constitute an important contingency of this group. Nutritional support nurses seek to provide patients with safe and effective parenteral and enteral nutritional care while aiding these individuals and their families in coping with illness in collaboration with other health care professionals.

Organizational Structure

Nutritional support nurses typically function as one component of a multidisciplinary nutritional support service. Their scope of practice incorporates all nursing activities that facilitate and optimize nutritional status in accordance with the patient's life goals. The practice areas of nutritional support nursing include direct and indirect patient care, consultation, education, research, and administration. The functions of this role differ according to the philosophy and objectives of the agency in which the nurse practices. Employers, health legislation, professional organizations, and payment systems provide structural determinants for the level of care that is delivered.

The impact that the PPS is having on the practice of nutritional support nursing is dependent on several factors:

1. The financial status of the institution.
2. The clinical activity of the nutritional support team.
3. The organizational structure and effectiveness of this service.
4. The perceived value of the team to the institution based on clinical effectiveness data and marketing.
5. The strength of the nursing care delivery system.
6. Justification based on research, quality control, and cost-effectiveness.

The organizational structures in which nutritional support nurses practice differ greatly among institutions. Many nutritional support nurses report to the nursing department; however, others report to medical departments, pharmacy, or hospital administration. The structural organization of an institution determines to a great extent the role and power of the nutritional support nurse.

Employers determine the type of authority and possible sphere of influence an individual practitioner may command within the position description. Nutritional support nurses need to scrutinize these position descriptions to ensure that they include the following:

1. Define responsibilities as an individual nurse and as a nutritional support team member.
2. Provide access to patients.
3. Establish communication channels to hospital committees where practice issues such as infection control and product review committees are decided.
4. Provide for an evaluation system that will reflect the necessity of the position.

In general, the position description must be sufficiently defined so that common goals can be achieved and must be sufficiently vague to allow for growth and change. Finally, the strength of one's role may depend on the department to which one reports. Nutritional support nurses who report to nursing service acquire strength for identification of the expansion and limitations of their professional practices. Because the majority of nutritional support nurses report either jointly or exclusively to nursing service, comments regarding organizational structure will focus on this group.

Depending on the volume of nutritional support patients, there may be one or more nutritional support nurses. In centralized nursing services, the reporting structure may be to staff development or directly to nursing administration. The advantage of this relationship is that other nurse clinicians or clinical specialists may be reporting in this manner, so there is a high potential for a peer support group. One disadvantage for this centralized approach is that these nurses are seen as "additional or supportive" nursing resources. During times of budget cuts, such a position in the organization is more vulnerable. Another disadvantage is that this resource group may be neglected when tools are being developed in the clinical departments to quantify nursing care costs.

Over the past decade, many nursing services have decentralized in an attempt to increase accountability and allow for more participation in decision-making. In a decentralized nursing service, the nutritional support nurse will most likely report to a clinical nursing department. The advantage of this reporting relationship rests with the direct clinical line to patient care units. Clinical practice input and decision-making are strengthened. Another advantage is that when nursing costs are being analyzed, the department will vigorously attempt to quantify the impact of the nurse consultant on staff-nurse productivity and patient outcomes. The major disadvantage of this structure is that the span of practice of nutritional support nurses often extends beyond one clinical nursing department; therefore, when reporting departmentally, communication with the other clinical nursing departments might become more difficult.

A matrix organization represents another possible design that provides for simultaneous coordination in two directions. Specialized groups such as nutritional support nurses may be organized in this manner. The advantage of this design is that it allows nutritional support nurses to have a direct reporting relationship. This also demonstrates their expanded scope of practice, which interfaces with all patient care units. The potential disadvantage is possible conflict between the two sides of the matrix, which could result in the nutritional support nurse feeling pulled in different directions.

The optimal organizational placement for nutritional support nurses remains dependent on the structure, philosophy, and operations of each individual organization. When determining organizational placement and design, the following are important considerations:

1. A mechanism for efficient and effective communication within the division of nursing, nutritional support team, and hospital.
2. An opportunity for professional and clinical practice growth.
3. A clear mechanism for input into direct care and clinical decision-making.
4. The department director should be an advocate for the role (market to administration, nurses, and other health care providers).

Structures will continue to change over the years to meet current and future challenges. Organizations that survive and function efficiently are those that consistently adapt to their external environments.[9]

Justification for Nutritional Support Nursing Roles

The impact of the PPS has been felt by many nurses in specialized roles. The effects on nutritional support nurses range from elimination of positions to frequent justifications for existing positions. In these times of careful financial scrutiny, the employer and nutritional support nurse must be able to justify positions that influence overall quality of patient care. It must be remembered that strategies for justification are only effective when based on data and information. Many strategies can be used to justify nutritional support nursing resources. The initial strategies should be focused on measuring the efficacy of the nutritional support team. Second, a major effort must be placed on strategies that emphasize the contribution of nutritional support nurses to affect nursing care delivery and patient outcomes. Finally, it is essential to select strategies that incorporate the agency's financial resource allocation.

Strategy 1: Efficacy of the Nutritional Support Team

Studies that evaluate the impact of the nutritional support team on length of stay, readmission rates, and complication rates are extremely important. If the use of nutritional support ultimately decreases the patient's length of stay, it may be very cost-effective. Studies by Ryan et al.[10] and Dalton et al.[11] are examples of demonstrated cost-effectiveness through reduction of catheter complications. The study by Robinson et al.[12] of the impact of nutritional status on DRG allowances and the study by Neill et al.[13] on the effect of parenteral nutrition on hospital costs and length of stay also provide important data that establish the need for nutritional services. Several other studies attempting to document cost effectiveness are currently in progress. Nutritional support nurses are working with the team to justify the effectiveness and economy of their service.

Strategy 2: Nursing Activity and Patient Care Impact

Utilizing the second strategy, nurses must examine their expert contribution as it relates to nursing practice standards and patient outcomes. The Standards of Practice for Nutrition Support Nursing developed by the American Society for Parenteral and Enteral Nutrition (ASPEN) establishes a framework for evaluating practice and outcome standards. The following outcomes have been developed for patients who require nutritional support nursing care:[14]

1. The individual and/or significant other demonstrate a knowledge of nutritional requirements and measures to meet these requirements.
2. The individual and/or significant other utilize nutritional support methods that maintain or improve status.
3. The individual demonstrates the desired response(s) to nutritional support intervention.
4. The individual suffers no preventable complications from nutritional support interventions or related nursing care.

Nutritional support nurses working with the division of nursing should conduct audits using process and outcome standards to evaluate their impact on patient outcomes. The clinical role of the nutritional support nurse should support and complement the nursing care delivery system in the institution. All clinical specialists and nurse clinicians should have input into the patient classification and/or task quantification systems used by the nursing division. We believe that the quality and quantity of direct nursing care delivered by the staff is influenced by using clinical specialists.

Several studies currently underway are attempting to relate clinical acuity and classification systems to DRG case groupings. The clinical specialist role, however, is not currently captured by these tools. Data must be collected to support the resource utilization of nutritional support nursing using patient classification and DRG classifications.

A daily activity log is currently being used by several nutritional support nurses and clinical specialists to categorize and quantify workload. The computer has made this approach more feasible and less time-consuming. This system is based on the major role components of the clinical nurse specialist: patient care, education, consultation, administration, and professional activities (Fig. 14-1). It is possible to produce activity summaries as well as trends. This tool can be very useful in justifying existing resources or the need for additional resources. In addition, by reviewing trends, correlations between changes in practice, patient population, and nursing activity can be examined. For example, with earlier discharges the shift to greater outpatient activity and follow-up should become

MONTH:		1	2	3	4	5	→ 31 days
EDUCATION	Program Preparation						
	Hospital-Wide						
	Department						
	Division						
	University-Formal						
	Precepting						
	Community						
	Education Total						
CONSULTATION	Nursing Staff						
	Physician						
	Other						
	University						
	Community						
	Consultation Total						
INPATIENT	Direct Care						
	Teaching						
	Coordinating						
OUTPATIENT	Direct Care						
	Teaching						
	Coordinating						
	Practice Total						
RESEARCH							
QA	Prod. Eval.						
	General						
RESEARCH &	QA TOTAL						
ADMINISTRATIVE	Meetings						
	Projects						
	Paperwork						
	Policy Development						
	Admin Total						
PROF. DEVEL.	Organizations						
	Projects						
	Publication						
	Prof Dev. Total						
TIME	Hours Worked						
	Holiday—Earned						
	—Taken						
	Sick Time Taken						
	Vac Time Taken						
	Conference Time						

Fig. 14-1. Daily Activity Log.

apparent from the activity log. This log is also helpful for individuals with joint appointments. Percentages of time spent in various components can be easily determined and should be billed appropriately. Further studies in these areas are essential for justification of the nurse specialist role.

Strategy 3: Financial Resource Allocations

The third justification strategy focuses on financial resource allocation formulas. Determination of resources for the nutritional support nursing staff requires that several basic decisions be made about the caregivers and the environment in which they operate. The first major concern is the time framework in which the care will be given, including the numbers of days per week and number of hours per day for care to be delivered. The number of patients to be seen by each nurse daily must be determined. The level of activity and workload must be determined for both inpatient and outpatient care.

Whereas the above questions quantify the operating time framework, the next questions are concerned with the caregivers. Most important is the question of the productivity rate. *Productivity rate* is the number of hours paid and worked divided by the number of hours paid. A standard full-time employee is paid for 8 hours a day, 5 days a week, and 52 weeks a year, for a total of 2080 hours. This total of hours is the definition of a Full Time Equivalent (FTE). Most, if not all employers, however, pay employees for various categories of nonproductive time, usually vacation, sick, holiday, and continuing education. This nonproductive time is important to know because staff coverage must be provided during these expected absences.

The number of hours paid and worked can be simply calculated by subtracting the hours paid and not worked from the total hours paid. The productivity rate generated from this calculation is then divided into the total number of hours of service to be provided. The result is the total number of hours required to be paid in order to produce the desired number of productive hours. The total hours required to be paid is divided by the number of paid hours per employee to determine the number of paid FTEs required.

For example, given the following data: (1) 7 day a week operation, (2) 8 hours a day on-site coverage, (3) nurse to patient ratio of .05 (i.e., 1 RN to 20 patients), (4) predicted nonproductive hours of 354/year, and (5) average daily census of 45 patients, the FTE can be calculated as follows:

$$\text{Productive hours} = \text{Total paid hours} - \text{Nonproductive hours}$$
$$= \quad 2080 \quad - \quad 354$$
$$= 1726 \text{ Productive hours}$$

$$\text{Productive rate} = \frac{\text{Productive hours}}{\text{Total paid hours}}$$

$$= \frac{1726}{2080}$$

$$= 83\% \text{ Productivity rate}$$

Paid hours required $= \#$ Days operating $\times$ Average daily census $\times$

$$\frac{\text{RN: patient ratio} \times \text{Hours care day}}{\text{Productivity rate}}$$

$$= \frac{365 \times 45 \times .05 \times 8}{83\%}$$

$$= 7916 \text{ Paid hours required}$$

FTEs required $\quad = \dfrac{\text{Paid hours required}}{\text{Total paid hours per FTE}}$

$$= \frac{7916}{2080}$$

$$= 3.81 \text{ FTEs required}$$

Four full time employees or three full time and one part-time employee working four days a week should be hired to provide the staffing resources required to support operations and practice requirements.

Financial resource allocation strategies address the amount of staff needed to provide care. It must be realized, however, these formulas are based on predetermined clinical practice assumptions regarding the nurse:patient ratio. In justifying resource allocations for nutritional support nurses, one must consider the following: the activity and functions of the nutritional support team nursing practice and standards and daily operations including productivity and nurse:patient ratios.

PROFESSIONAL ORGANIZATIONS

Professional organizations provide a vehicle for development, communication, and recognition of the standard of care and quality care. For many nutritional support nurses this is accomplished through ASPEN. ASPEN maintains several nursing committees, and nurses also participate in organizational committees. Acknowledging its obligation as a professional barometer for quality care, ASPEN has published standards of care as they apply to specific patient populations such as the home parenteral patient. Communication of new clinical and research developments have a forum in the Association's journal and its annual clinical congress. ASPEN's obligation to define quality practice has led to the development of the Nutrition Support Nursing Certification Program. As nursing leaders, nutritional support nurses must take an active role in professional organizations that seek to improve the field of one's clinical expertise.

In addition, the State Boards of Nursing are particularly significant for nurses in specialty roles who expand the common practice of nursing. These groups are responsible for defining the scope of nursing practice. It is imperative that nurses practicing on the frontier of health care communicate with these groups on practice issues.

NURSING PRACTICE

Nutritional support nursing practice is the care of individuals with potential or known nutritional problems. Nutritional support nurses utilize specific expertise to enhance the restoration and maintenance of an individual's nutritional status.[14] A detailed discussion of the many facets of the nutritional support nurse's role have been outlined in various chapters of this book. The emphasis of this section will therefore, be the interface of the nutritional support nursing role and the staff nurse role.

Actualizing the nutritional support nurse role is partially dependent on the nursing care delivery system in any particular institution. Traditionally, nutritional support nurses have been responsible for all catheter care including teaching and dressing changes. With the expansion of primary nursing care delivery systems, the functions of nutritional support nurses have changed. In several institutions, it is the primary nurse who assumes responsibility for the majority of the direct patient care. The nurse specialist serves as a resource to the staff and assists in monitoring the quality of care being delivered.

The role of the nutritional support nurse is significantly influenced by the clinical activity of the nutritional support team. If a nutritional support nurse is responsible for more than 20 inpatients receiving parenteral nutrition, it becomes difficult to administer direct care and continue to participate in education, research, and consultation activities. During times of cost containment and limited resources, it is our belief that the nutritional support nurse will administer less direct patient care and more indirect care by providing specialized teaching for both the staff and patients. A certain level of direct care, however, must be provided by the nutritional support nurse.

Another current trend is the increasing number of nutritional support outpatients. Incentives under the PPS have encouraged shortened hospitalizations resulting in increased outpatient activity. Nutritional support nurses have taken leadership in coordinating much of the outpatient activity. Because nursing is frequently the vital link between inpatient and outpatient care, nutritional support nurses play a key role in discharge planning and outpatient evaluation. In the near future we are hopeful that more nurses will get directly reimbursed for their outpatient activities.

Nutritional support nurses are expanding and constantly modifying their role depending on patient and particular institution needs. In addition, some nurses have combined specialty positions such as critical care/nutrition or nutrition/oncology. These specialists are nutritional support nurses who specialize in the needs of patient subpopulations. Depending on the nutritional support service activity and the needs of the institution, nutritional support nurses are creating innovative roles to meet patient care needs in an efficient and effective manner. Today's specialists must plan for the future and adapt their roles to meet current and future health care demands.

NURSING PRACTICE STANDARDS

Based on the assumption that nursing contributes positively to health, accountability for the nutritional support nurse is the promise of delivering direct and indirect quality nursing care to the patient receiving specialized nutritional support. Indirect care is achieved through standard-setting. It includes practice guidelines, standards of care, standard care plans, patient education material, form development, and product selection. Nursing practices of importance to the nutritional support nurse include administration of parenteral and enteral nutrition, assessment of nutritional status, insertion and maintenance of intravenous catheters and feeding tubes, use of intravenous and enteral pumps, product selection, referrals, and consultations. The nursing practice reflects the identified values of the agency as well as those found in published professional organization standards. Nursing practice standards are defined by their purpose and should flow from one to the other.

Below is an example of standard setting:

Issue: Patient Education
Source Documents:
   Nursing Service Philosophy: Nurses have an obligation to teach patients.
   ASPEN Standard: The individual and/or significant other demonstrates a knowledge of nutritional requirement. [15]
   A.N.A. Code: Assist patients and their families to assume responsibility for their own health and illness care. [16]
Standards:
   Standards of care (published statements of minimally accepted level of nursing care; they highlight the critical behaviors and are often considered process and/or outcome standards): Patient will demonstrate correct technique of capping and flushing the right atrial catheter.

Practice Guidelines:

(Also termed policy or procedure, these are step-by-step explanations of the practice, detailing assessments, actions, and resolving problems): Instruct patient to cap and flush a Hickman catheter.

Standard Care Plans:

(These plans are patient-directed statements that actualize the practice guidelines and standards of care): Each morning the patient will cap and flush their Hickman catheter. Try to decrease verbal cuing each day.

Patient Education:

(These materials reflect the rationale for the practice and translate from the nursing standard care plan to a patient, self-directed plan of action): Follow these steps in capping and flushing your right atrial catheter. . . . .

Closely related to standards is the evaluation of equipment. The selection of equipment should be dictated by set standards. Proper choice of equipment is especially important in nutritional support because of the rapidly expanding market and the fact that malfunctioning equipment is a growing cause for litigation against nurses. The equipment must be critically evaluated for accuracy, patient safety, and cost.

An example of equipment assessment was performed by Powell et al. in examining transparent dressings and the incidence of catheter infection.[17] Kellem and Fraze (1986) similarly studied central-line dressing material in the neonate.[18] These studies may have a direct impact on practice; however, assessment typically occurs when a product is being introduced into an agency during a cost and safety analysis.

QUALITY ASSURANCE

The companion to standard-setting is evaluation, which frequently is the thrust behind change and quality assurance activities. Evaluation of nursing care ranges from simple data collection to complex statistical and measurement techniques used to isolate quality identifiers. In the mid 1970s the focus of quality assurance was very structured and outcome-oriented. The technique employed at that time was multidisciplinary, retrospective chart review. For example, Srp et al. examined the cause for rehospitalization of home parenteral nutritional patients and Burchett et al. documented complications following gastric bypass surgery.[19,20] These studies provide practitioners with a more descriptive picture of the patient, but they do not answer the questions why and how. Prospective evaluation tools are more frequently used today. Prospective evaluation offers two distinct advantages over retrospective audit: (1) review is concurrent with practice, and (2) chart review is combined with observation of patient and/or nurse. The use of these instruments requires more time and labor but provides greater accuracy and timeliness of information. Two areas of concern are associated with these systems: (1) criteria selection for patient acuity, and (2) validation of the instrument items in predicting desired quality. Of importance to nutritional support nurses would be the verification that these instruments accurately evaluate the quality of nursing care for the patient with nutritional deficits. Specific quality questions such as: "Is the level of nursing care at or above the standards for patients receiving parenteral nutrition?" must be answered with other evaluation techniques.

The evaluation process is guided by the severity and frequency of the problem and be the ability to control the practice. To highlight possible strategies, the above question will be outlined below.

Step 1.   *Examine local standards for consistency among themselves.*

Step 2.   *Compare local standards to current literature and published standards*: The quantity of heparin flush varies among institutions. To provide a rationale for practice change Cariello et al. studied the complication rate of right atrial catheters after changing the heparin flush quantity to determine the efficacy of the new practice. Comparison of patients before and after the practice change showed no difference in infection or occlusion rates.[21] Therefore, the new flush quantity was accepted.

Step 3.   *Examine the details of the practice by identifying critical elements*: Several studies have been done utilizing this principle in areas other than nutritional support nursing. This process is useful in determining safety and efficiency of a practice as well as providing an evaluation tool for practitioners.

Step 4.   *Determine if practice problems are occurring by a review of incident reports*: This evaluation will detect evidence of noncompliance with critical elements or inadequacy of essential processes in meeting safe practice requirements. If a problem is identified, this problem becomes a priority for further evaluation and action. One such problem is disconnection or intravenous tubing. A problem was detected, solutions were sought, and luer-locked tubing is now used in most agencies for attachment of central intravenous catheters and tubing.

Step 5.   *Select strategy for identified problem*: Compliance with dressing standard lends itself to an observational audit performed periodically. Specific observations to be made are outlined and standardized. Precise details of how the observations are to be carried out is essential for consistency. Subsequent quality assurance activity may be generated by the results of this review.

Compliance with standards regarding the insertion and maintenance of central intravenous lines requires routine daily monitoring and alternate strategies. The availability and cost of resources to monitor this problem must be compared to the usefulness and significance of the information gained. The monitoring system must be designed to allow for rapid, easy retrieval and recording of critical elements. A system of this design leads to identification of unexpected problems such as an unannounced change in catheter manufacturing and to rapid resolution.

Other issues may focus on documentation of intravenous catheter sites and dressings. Corrective action may consist of the design of a flow sheet. Critical elements from the standard need to be scrutinized a format identified. A subsequent audit would be required to verify if the change in practice corrected the identified deficiency.

Quality assurance activities should be generated and directed by the standards set and identification of real and/or potential problems. The techniques used to evaluate the practices vary according to the problem and its complexity. To be effective a quality assurance program must design flexible strategies capable of evaluating general as well as specific practices. All nurses should participate in the identification and correction of problems as an ongoing component of nursing practice. The result of all quality assurance activities should be a higher level of nursing practice. A systematic review of our practice using relevant outcomes provides a data base to support our impact on the patient and the institution.

MARKETING AND NETWORKING

Health care providers continue to react to the effects of the new payment policies and resultant changes within the system. The climate in the health care industry is one of competition. Institutions are competing for clients/patients. New and innovative marketing strategies are being used to sell available services and increase the provider's visibility.

Marketing is the successful selling of a product or service. It has been difficult for nurses to accept the idea of "selling their services." To some, this idea conflicts with the traditional image of nurses as self-denying care givers. Fortunately, these traditional views are changing. As institutions plan to market their services, nursing must be an integral part of the strategic planning.

Marketing is a process that considers product, promotion, price, and place. Nurses are still attempting to define the product, quality care, and are just beginning to promote the services delivered. Marketing nursing can result in internal and external benefits. Internal benefits include a greater appreciation of nurses, a sense of pride among nurses, and increasing institutional awareness of nursing's role in the organization. External benefits include recruitment and retention of high quality nurses, initiation of joint ventures with other organizations, and generation of revenue by attracting additional patients.

Nurses are capable of marketing themselves everyday to a consumer—the patient. Nurses should capitalize on their ability to impact the consumer. Physicians may be primarily responsible for bringing patients into a particular hospital, but it is the nursing care that most influences a patient's perception of that hospital's quality.

Publicity and advertising are two marketing methods. Publicity is differentiated from advertising in that the former is achieved without direct costs. Health care professionals have a tremendous opportunity to use publicity in marketing through public speaking, publishing, and organizational activities including professional, interdisciplinary, and community organizations.

Networking is another vehicle for marketing. Networking has been used for years in corporations and is tremendously underutilized in health care, especially in nursing. According to Mary Scott Welch, "networking is the process of developing and using your contacts for information, advice and moral support as you pursue your career."[22] Networks include groups such as business, professional, sports, politics, and support groups. Women seem to have more difficulty in networking than men for two reasons. First, networking often takes place after normal working hours. Women frequently have time constraints because of responsibilities at home, including a husband and children. Second, the perception that networkers manipulate people makes some women uncomfortable.[23] Finally, networking is seldom taught but is learned by experience or from a mentor. Nurses may have difficulty identifying an appropriate mentor. This problem is resolving as the nursing profession grows and develops.

Nutritional support nurses are in the unique position of being part of a specialized interdisciplinary team. They may choose several individuals with different strengths as mentors. Individual growth is also facilitated as the team grows and advances. In addition, nutritional support teams began marketing their services several years ago. For consultative services to be effective, marketing was essential from the onset. Present strategies for marketing the nutritional support team, however, are quite different than those of the past. Marketing in the past focused on improved care for the malnourished patient. Today's marketing focus also addresses cost-benefit analysis.

Nutritional support nurses must publicize their contribution to the team and to the consumer. The consumers are both the patient and the institution. Through the use of quality assurance data, research data, and patient audits, nutritional support nurses have the ability to market their role internally in the institution. Their impact on patient care and overall nursing practice must be emphasized. Their consultative support for the staff nurses should be evidenced because internal nursing support is an important component.

Through publications, public speaking, and organization activities, nutritional support nurses become visible to the public. If nutritional support nurses are providing services that potentially generate revenue such as outpatient care these should be marketed. If their teaching protocols decrease the length of hospital stay for patients, this aspect should be marketed. ASPEN provides an excellent vehicle for marketing and networking for nutritional support nurses. This organization provides a forum for experts to address issues related to clinical practice, reimbursement, marketing, and the future direction of the Nutrition Support Team.

SUMMARY

Rapid and continual changes exist in the health care industry. Given the nature of the challenges that face nutritional support nurses, the strategies devised must incorporate input from clinicians, educators, researchers, and administrators. The nutritional support team must collaborate to define innovative and efficient methods of delivering nutritional care. Nutritional support nurses must take leadership in the designing of the future. We must act rather than react.

REFERENCES

1. Jeejeehboy K, Zohrab W, Longer B, et al: Total parenteral nutrition at home for 23 months without complication and with good rehabilitation. Gastroenterology 65: 811–820, 1973
2. Califano J Jr: American Health Care Revolution. New York, Random House, 1986
3. Bistrian BR, Blackburn GL, Vitale J, et al: Prevalence of malnutrition in general medical patients. JAMA 235:1567–1570, 1976
4. Mullen JL, Gertner MH, Buzby GB, et al: Implications of malnutrition in the surgical patient. Arch Surg 114:121–125, 1979
5. Dalton MJ, Schepers G, Gee JP, et al: Consultative total parenteral nutrition teams. The effect on the incidence of TPN related complications. JPEN 8:146–152, 1984
6. Jacobs DO, Melnik G, Forlaw L, et al: Impact of a nutritional support service on VA surgical patients. J A Col Nutr 3:311–315, 1984
7. Hamaoui E, Rombeau J: The nutrition support team, in Rombeau J, Caldwell M (eds): Total Parenteral Nutrition. Philadelphia, WB Saunders, 1985, p 237
8. Twomey PL, Patching SC: Cost-effectiveness of nutrition support. JPEN 9(1):3–10, 1985
9. Charns MP, Schaefer MJ: Health care organizations—a model for management. Englewood Cliffs, NJ, Prentice-Hall, 1983, p 77
10. Ryan JA, Abel RA, Abbott WM, et al: Catheter complications in total parenteral nutrition. A prospective study of 20 consecutive patients. N Engl J Med 290:757–761, 1974
11. Dalton MJ, Schepers G, Gee JP: Consultative total parenteral nutrition teams. The effect on the incidence of TPN related complications. JPEN 8:146–152, 1984
12. Robinson G, Goldstein M, Levine G: Impact of nutritional status on DRG allowances. JPEN 10(1):22, 1986
13. O'Neil M, Marein C, Steigar C, et al: Effect of total parenteral nutrition on hospital costs and length of stay. JPEN 10(1):22, 1986
14. Standards of Practice—Nutrition Support Nursing. Committee for Nursing Standards. ASPEN, January, 1985
15. American Society for Parenteral and Enteral Nutrition Standards for Nutrition Support: Home patients. Silver Springs, MD, ASPEN, 1985
16. American Nurses Association. A statement on the scope of medical-surgical nursing practice. Kansas City. American Nurses' Association, 1980
17. Powell C, Tractow M, Fabri P, et al: Op-site dressing study: A prospective

randomized study evaluating providine iodine ointment and extension set changes with 7 day op-site dressings applied to total parenteral nutrition subclavian sites. JPEN (9)3:443–446, 1985

18. Kellem B, Fraze D: A neonatal central line dressing material: Preliminary study. Nutr Supp Serv 6(2):66–71, 1986
19. Srp F, Steiger E, Montague N, et al: Causes for rehospitalization of home parenteral nutrition patients. 6th Clinical Congress Abstracts. JPEN 5(6):574, 1981
20. Burchett H, Freeman J; Gastric partitioning for morbid obesity. 6th Clinical Congress Abstracts. JPEN 5(6):562, 1981
21. Cariello F, Cunliffe P, et al: Standard of care for right atrial catheters. Unpublished paper. Philadelphia, Hospital of the University of Pennsylvania
22. Welsh MS: Networking. Orlando, FL, Harcourt Brace Jovanovich, 1980, p 15
23. Puetz B: Networking for Nurses. Rockville, MD, Aspen Publications, 1983, p 4

Marsha Evans Orr

15

Future Directions

We should all be concerned about the future because we will have to spend the rest of our lives there.

CHARLES FRANKLIN KETTERING

What will the world be like in the next fifteen years? Who will be the major consumers of health care? What will be the nature of the health care delivery system? Where will nurses be employed? What will happen to nursing specialty groups such as nutritional support nurses? Attempting to predict the future of nutritional support nursing may seem somewhat akin to consulting a crystal ball, but to be only concerned with the here and now would result in reactive instead of proactive planning. The nutritional support nurses who are practicing now are helping to create the future of nutritional support nursing.

THE ENVIRONMENT

Trends occurring in the environment and the nursing profession are helpful predictors of factors that will also affect the future of nutritional support nursing.

The Elderly Boom Generation

During the next several decades, America will be growing slowly and graying rapidly. The increased percentage of elderly Americans will be most dramatic as the baby boom generation reaches and surpasses the age of 65. By the year 2000, the median age of the population will be thirty five.[1] Health care needs of persons in the middle and later years thus will be emphasized in the next century.

NUTRITIONAL SUPPORT IN NURSING
ISBN 0-8089-1889-3

375

The "me" generation tends to be more quality-of-life conscious, affluent, pleasure seeking, and isolated. Although the median income is projected to increase as 1990 approaches, there will still be an even more stratified poverty level that will include single heads of household (most often female) and the elderly who have no income except social security. Persons in the poverty level will continue to depend on financial support from the government to meet health care costs.

Diseases of the gastrointestinal tract or the cardiovascular, pulmonary, renal, and endocrine systems occur more frequently in the elderly, and these diseases can lead to the need for specialized nutritional support. Although advances seem likely in the treatment of cancer, cardiovascular disease, and other diseases, progress toward cures has been painfully slow. The enlarging elderly population is likely to require more nutritional services unless cures are developed.

An increased use of nutritional support services by the elderly has already become apparent in the home care arena. Data collected by the New York Academy of Medicine (currently by OASIS) indicate an 8 percent increase from 1980 to 1983 in the number of persons aged 65 and over who were receiving home parenteral nutrition. In addition, the major diagnosis associated with the need for home parenteral nutrition changed from inflammatory bowel disease which typically affects young adults, to cancer which more often occurs in the middle to later years.[2,3] Because the benefit of specialized nutritional support in cancer treatment has not been unequivocally demonstrated, there remains controversy over when, what, and how much, and how long it should be provided, especially to the terminally ill. Perhaps some of these questions will be answered in the next decade by high quality, prospective, randomized clinical research studies. In the meantime, a larger proportion of elderly people with cancer and other diseases will be receiving parenteral (PN) and enteral (EN) nutrition, and these people will need nutritional support nurses.

They're Everywhere, They're Everywhere

Dramatic changes are occurring in the settings, organizations, and patterns of health care services. Cost-containment efforts by the federal government have lead to a prospective payment system (PPS) that is based upon diagnosis-related groups (DRGs). The shorter length of stays (LOS) that many patients experience under the DRG system have caused a concomitant increase in the utilization of home care services. Patients go home "quicker and sicker" and many need substantial home health care services to achieve a safe and adequate level of care. Health care services that were once offered only to hospitalized patients are now commonly offered on an outpatient basis in clinics, free-standing surgical centers, and emergency care centers. Hospitals, long-term care facilities, and home health care agencies are being purchased by proprietary chains. Practitioners are employees or owners of an ever-increasing variety of health care organizations. These changes bring new opportunities and challengers but the effect on the quality of health care services to the consumer is not yet clear, and the changes in health care delivery systems are likely to continue into the next decade before stabilization occurs.

Bottom Line—Cost

In the future patients will need and use more specialized nutritional support services and will receive these services in a variety of settings. Scrutiny of the cost-effectiveness (cost:benefit ratio) and appropropriate use of nutritional support services by third party payers and all levels of government, however, is certain to continue. Because a greater proportion of services will be offered in the home, and nurses will continue to be the primary providers of home care, the nurses' role in nutritional support will be of great importance. Research will be needed to further substantiate the cost-effectiveness and value of nursing services.

In hospitals, a greater percentage of patients are likely to need nutritional support even though the hospital's census may be smaller than in the past. Only the frailest, most acutely ill patients will require hospitalization, and these are the patients most likely to need nutritional services. Patients will continue to come to hospitals to receive medical treatment and nursing care, and nurses will continue to need expertise in the area of specialized nutritional support. Nutritional products are becoming more specialized and disease-specific, but, at the same time, practitioners are being asked to clearly demonstrate that these more costly products are necessary (i.e., to examine the cost:benefit ratio). Products will no longer be chosen because they are theoretically sound, but rather because clinical research studies unequivocally demonstrate the efficacy of the products. Hopefully, cost constraints will not erode the quality of care too deeply before a balance is struck.

Horizontal Violence

Shrinking resources, diversification of health care settings, and changes in health manpower will contribute to an increasingly competitive environment. Marketing, a vital aspect of the business world for decades, is also a health care tool in the middle 1980s. Services, organizations, institutions, and even professionals are marketed. Competition has forced hospitals to expand into nontraditional areas of health care services and to adopt businesslike attitudes. Large corporations continue to purchase hospitals, causing experts to predict that by 1995, 53 percent of all hospitals will be owned or managed by multihospital systems.[1]

Manpower needs within health care professions are shifting. Enrollments in schools of nursing have dropped precipitously at a time when nursing shortages are already evident.[4] At the same time, there is an expanding supply of physicians. The Department of Health and Human Services estimates that by 1990, there will be a 60 percent increase in practicing physicians above the current level.[5] Distribution of physicians to areas of need may be a continuing problem, and the need for primary care physicians is likely to continue. Unfortunately, the atmosphere of competition will extend into interdisciplinary relationships as health care professionals compete with one another for patients and profit.[1]

THE NURSING PROFESSION

Where Have All The Nurses Gone?

With decreasing LOSs and hospital patient populations, the idea of a nursing shortage seems somewhat inconceivable, but a nursing shortage is occurring. Many hospitals are switching to a predominantely registered nurse staff, and there is a tremendous increase in the need for critical care nurses as the acuity level rises for hospital inpatients. In addition, enrollment in schools of nursing is down by approximately 30 percent and, as a consequence of this decreased enrollment, the shortage is likely to intensify before things get better.[6] The need for critical care nurses or specialty nurses may enhance job prospects for nutritional support nurses, especially if they are experienced in dual specialties (i.e., critical care and nutritional support) or if they are willing to diversify their specialty practice. For example, nutritional support nurses who have entered the home care arena are usually involved in other types of parenteral therapies such as chemotherapy and antibiotics.

Perhaps some of the nurses who seem to have disappeared from the hospital marketplace can be found in other health care delivery systems. In 1983, employment growth was an outstanding 129 percent in outpatient facilities compared with 39 percent in hospitals.[6] As health care settings have continued to diversify in recent years, additional employment opportunities have arisen for nurses, overshadowing the hospital as the traditional place of employment. A number of nutritional support nurses have left the hospital setting to work for home care companies.

Toward A Long-Range Plan

Following an extensive assessment of the environmental changes predicted to occur over the next decade and beyond, the American Nurses' Association (ANA) developed a 15-year plan for the nursing profession. The ANA long-range plan targeted seven goals:

1. Expand the scientific and research base for nursing practice.
2. Clarify and strengthen the educational system for nursing.
3. Develop a coordinated system of credentialing for nursing.

4. Restructure the organizational arrangements for delivery of nursing services.
5. Develop comprehensive payment systems for nursing services.
6. Achieve effective control of the environment in which nursing is practiced.
7. Enhance the organizational strength of ANA.[7]

An eighth goal was added following action by ANA's House of Delegates in 1986:

8. Maintain and strengthen nursing's role in client advocacy.[8]

The long range goals of ANA are intended to promote and strengthen the nursing profession in the primary areas of research, education, and practice but the goals also include statements about client advocacy and public policy. As the official voice of the nursing profession, ANA's goals will have a major influence on the goals and long-range plans of specialty nursing organizations.

Within the context of environmental changes and the future goals of the nursing profession, a clearer picture emerges of future directions for nutritional support nursing.

NUTRITIONAL SUPPORT NURSING

Reflections

Nurses have been concerned with the nutritional status of their patients from the inception of nursing as a profession. Florence Nightingale's *Notes on Nursing* included two chapters about the role of nutrition in nursing care.[9] Nutritional support nursing as a specialty practice arose from the development of technology enabling a person to receive nutrition by vein and by tube and from the nursing care requirements of patients who received specialized nutritional support. Nurses and other health care professionals used this technology to provide nutrients to patients who might otherwise have perished from starvation. The recognition that practitioners needed special expertise to provide quality care to patients receiving PN and EN, however, led to the formation of the American Society for Parenteral and Enteral Nutrition (ASPEN) in 1975.[10]

ASPEN's founders wisely recognized the need to establish a multidisciplinary society that could promote excellence in practice for each discipline within a cooperative and collaborative atmosphere. The structure of ASPEN today continues to recognize the unique contribution of each discipline and to foster interdisciplinary interactions. The internal structure is composed of "Discipline Committees" (i.e., Nurse's Committee, Pharmacist's Committee, Dietitian's Committee) who plan activities to promote excellence in practice within the discipline, and also "Society-wide Committees" composed of representatives from each discipline who plan activities for the society as a whole. The total number of nutritional support nurses in the United States is not known but during 1986, 492 nurses were members of ASPEN.

Directions

In 1986, ASPEN created a multidisciplinary long-range planning committee. Representatives of each discipline are examining trends within the environment, the health care delivery system, the health care professions, and ASPEN to develop the organization's future plans. Nutritional support nursings' goals will be articulated by the Nurse's Committee and by the society within the context of the long-range plan. Education, research, and practice are key areas of consideration in determining the future of nutritional support nursing.

Education

During the 1960s, nutrition ceased to be taught as a discrete course in the curricula of many schools of nursing and, instead, became integrated into content presented about diseases or conditions. Nurses began to view nutritional needs of their patients as low priority needs, and, subsequently, the role of the dietitian was strengthened.[11] Even into the 1980s, the number of questions about nutrition on the State Board Test Pool Examination has decreased by almost one-half.[11] If this current trend continues, new graduates from schools of nursing may have less knowledge about basic nutrition than in the past. Nutritional support nurses may find themselves educating their colleagues about basic nutrition as well as specialized nutritional support, and basic nutritional concepts will need to be offered in continuing education courses to nurses entering the specialty practice.

Declining enrollment in schools of nursing will exacerbate the nursing shortage in general and specialty practice in particular. Aggressive recruiting and marketing strategies will undoubtedly occur in the next decade. Efforts to recruit the best and brightest into the profession will be planned. Enterostomal therapy (ET) nurses began marketing themselves in 1985 with an advertisement in nursing journals entitled "Beat the DRG Clock with an Enterostomal Therapy Nurse." The advertisement cited the ET nurse's expertise in four specific areas of direct patient care and in staff education.[12] Other nursing specialty practice groups are sure to follow suit.

Nutritional support nurses originally became members of a specialty practice group through clinical practice in the specialty rather than through a formal educational process. Continuing education courses offered by ASPEN and other nutrition-oriented organizations have provided a major means for nurses to gain expertise and stay abreast of new developments in the field. Hospitals have cut back on the amount of funding provided to nurses who wish to attend continuing education courses, and, consequently, nurses' attendance of seminars that involve significant cost is decreasing or has leveled off. In the future, continuing education may be offered by more cost-effective methods and on a more regional or local basis. Among the methods apt to be popular in the 1990s will be interactive computer-assisted learning, teleconferences, and videoconferences.

Until 1985, there was no means of certifying to the public or to employers that a nurse possessed the knowledge needed to practice nutritional support nursing. With ASPEN's support, a Nutrition Support Nursing Core Curriculum was published and a certification examination was offered by the National Board of Certification in Nutritional Support.[13] The Core Curriculum acts as a means of identifying the body of knowledge that encompasses nutritional support nursing practice. Nurses who have successfully passed the certification examination have an objective measure of their level of expertise.

Certification is offered in a variety of specialty practices. As certification examinations proliferate, nurses may find themselves making difficult decisions about which certification is the most beneficial and appropriate for them. Nurses working in home care already find themselves choosing between certification in nutritional support or intravenous therapy.

Efforts by the ANA to develop a coordinated credentialling system may move the educational levels of all nurses in specialty practice (clinical or functional) to the master's degree level. Within nutritional support nursing, there has been no minimal educational level for nurses to enter the specialty practice, and the certification examination is offered to registered nurses of all educational levels. The nursing shortage will cause a delay in upgrading the educational levels of nurses, but eventually a higher level of education will likely be required for entry into specialty practice.

Research

Research provides the scientific basis on which a profession or specialty practice is founded. Data from research studies may be used to change clinical practice, develop new procedures or policies, change the content of curricula or teaching methods, set public policy, determine reimbursement schemes, conduct subsequent research, or any number of other significant uses. Nutritional support research may be collaborative multidisciplinary studies, collaborative single-discipline studies, or single-investigator, single-discipline studies.

The number of nutrition-related nursing research articles has increased significantly in recent years; two-thirds of the 104 articles identified in the literature were published since 1980.[14] Nevertheless, a great deal more research is needed to enrich, define, and refine the practice of nutritional support nursing. Moore, et al. identified the following areas in which research in nutritional support nursing is absent or incomplete: psychosocial responses to artificial feeding, nutrition and the very young and elderly, nutrition in specific disease states, prevention and health maintenance, nutrition education in schools of nursing, nutrition-related nursing diagnoses, cost containment and nutritional support nursing, and role development of the nutritional support nurse.[14]

Practice

In 1985, Standards of Practice for Nutritional Support Nursing were published by ASPEN.[15] This document described the scope of practice, standards of practice, rationales, and outcome criteria for nutritional support nursing. The standards are being revised and will continue to need to be revised periodically as changes in practice occur. Research findings, economic factors, changes in health care delivery, changes in the nursing profession, social factors, consumer issues, and other factors impact on and mold the practice of nutritional support nursing.

The settings in which nutritional support nurses are employed, either directly or by contract, will continue to diversify. Health maintenance organizations (HMOs), preferred provider organizations (PPOs), clinics, free-standing surgical centers, home health agencies, hospitals, and nursing homes are among the future employers of nutritional support nurses. The job market will remain competitive for as long as the shortage of nursing specialists continues, but nutritional support nurses may have to practice in dual or multi-specialties. Two opposing forces will be present. Advances in medicine and technology create pressures toward specialization, but the need for a "generalist" specialist (e.g., a specialist who can practice in more than one specialty area) will exert an opposing force. Nutritional support nurses will have to decide how far they can generalize yet still be able to identify with nutritional support specialty practice.

Advances in medicine are unlikely to make nutritional support an obsolete technology in the near future. Innovations may occur in access devices, feeding formulations, and technological equipment, but gut transplants seem decades away. Patients who cannot eat, digest, or absorb nutrients will still need to be fed. Patients who receive PN or EN and their families will continue to need nursing care. Nutritional support nurses make unique, irreplaceable contributions to patient care whether the nurses work within a team or as individual practitioners.

SUMMARY

The future of nutritional support nursing is a melding of the environment, the nursing profession, and the specialty practice. Never before has the health care system been in such a dynamic state, and health care professionals are struggling to find their niche. The future holds dilemmas, opportunities, changes, and challenges. The future directions of nutritional support nurses are to solve the dilemmas, use the opportunities, plan for the changes, and meet the challenges.

REFERENCES

1. Environmental Assessment: Factors Affecting Long Range Planning for Nursing and Health Care. American Nurses Association, 1985, p 1
2. New York Academy of Medicine; Registry of Patients on Home Total Parenteral Nutrition (TPN). Questionnaire No. 5 New York, 1982
3. New York Academy of Medicine: Registry of Patients on Home Total Parenteral Nutrition (TPN). Questionnaire No. 8 New York, 1985

4. AJN survey shows a new RN shortage sprouting: Rising acuity falling enrollments are blamed (news). Am J Nurs 86:969, 1986
5. Johnson EA, Everett A, Johnson RL: Hospitals in Transition. Rockville, MD, Aspen Systems Corporation, 1982, p 7
6. A recruiter's-eye view of the new shortage (news). AJN 86:1054, 1064, 1986
7. Selby TL: House to act in 15-year plan for nursing. The American Nurse, May, 1986, p 1
8. Report of ANA Board of Directors. Long-Range Strategic and Business Planning for the American Nurses Association. 1986, p 4
9. Nightingale F: Notes on Nursing: What It Is and What It Is Not. London, Harrison and Sons, 1859, pp 36–44
10. Seltzer MH: A.S.P.E.N.: The genesis. JPEN 10:9–16. 1986
11. Englert DM, Crocker KS, Stotts NA: Nutrition education in schools of nursing in the United States. Part 1. The evolution of nutrition education in schools of nursing. JPEN 10:522–527, 1986
12. Beat the DRG Clock with an Enterostomal Therapy Nurse. Newport Beach, CA, International Association of Enterostomal Therapy, Inc, 1985
13. Kennedy-Caldwell C (ed): Nutrition Support Nursing Core Curriculum. Silver Spring, MD, American Society for Parenteral and Enteral Nutrition, 1985
14. Moore MC, Guenter PA, Bender JH: Nutrition-related nursing research. IMAGE 18:18–21, 1986
15. Forlaw L, Crocker K, Muttart C, et al: Standards of Practice, Nutrition Support Nursing. Silver Spring MD, American Society of Parenteral and Enteral Nutrition, 1985

APPENDIX

EDITORS NOTE #1

The United States Supreme Court has upheld lower court findings that the Department of Health and Human Services does not have the right to intervene in decisions made about the medical treatment of handicapped newborn babies (Bowen v. American Hospital Association et.al.). The recent ruling adds final invalidation to the 1984 "Baby Doe" rules permitting HHS employees to investigate suspected violations of Section 504 of the Rehabilitation Act of 1973, which prohibits discrimination against handicapped persons in federally funded programs and activities.

The reader is referred to the American Nurses' Association "Code for Nurses" which dictates that respect for human dignity and support of the patient's rights to self-determination are an integral part of nursing practice (American Nurses' Association. Code for nurses with interpretive statements. Kansas City, Mo.: American Nurses' Association, 1985). In addition "Ethics Reference for Nurses" lists hundreds of reference material concerning the complex ethical dilemmas confronted in contemporary nursing (Pub. No. G-159. American Nurses Association, Kansas City, Mo., 1982).

EDITORS NOTE #2

Following are excerpts from *Current Opinions of the Council on Ethical and Judicial Affairs of the American Medical Association—1986*. Chicago: American Medical Association, 1986. Reprinted with permission.

2.18 WITHHOLDING OR WITHDRAWING LIFE-PROLONGING MEDICAL TREATMENT. The social commitment of the physician is to sustain life and relieve suffering. Where the performance of one duty conflicts with the other, the choice of the patient, or his family or legal representative if the patient is incompetent to act in his own behalf, should prevail. In the absence of the patient's choice or an authorized proxy, the physician must act in the best interest of the patient.

For humane reasons, with informed consent, a physician may do what is medically necessary to alleviate severe pain, or cease or omit treatment to permit a terminally ill patient whose death is imminent to die. However, he should not intentionally cause death. In deciding whether the administration of potentially life-prolonging medical treatment is in the best interest of the patient who is incompetent to act in his own behalf, the physician should determine what the possibility is for extending life under humane and comfortable conditions and what are the prior expressed wishes of the patient and attitudes of the family or those who have responsibility for the custody of the patient.

Even if death is not imminent but a patient's coma is beyond doubt irreversible and there are adequate safeguards to confirm the accuracy of the diagnosis and with the concurrence of those who have responsibility for the care of the patient, it is not unethical to discontinue all means of life-prolonging medical treatment.

Life-prolonging medical treatment includes medication and artificially or technologically supplied respiration, nutrition or hydration. In treating a terminally ill or irreversibly comatose patient, the physician should determine whether the benefits of treatment outweigh its burdens. At all times, the dignity of the patient should be maintained. (I, III, IV, V)

2.19 **WITHHOLDING OR WITHDRAWING LIFE-PROLONGING MEDICAL TREATMENT-PATIENTS' PREFERENCES.** A competent, adult patient may, in advance, formulate and provide a valid consent to the withholding or withdrawal of life-support systems in the event that injury or illness renders that individual incompetent to make such a decision. The preference of the individual should prevail when determining whether extraordinary life-prolonging measures should be undertaken in the event of terminal illness. Unless it is clearly established that the patient is terminally ill or irreversibly comatose, a physician should not be deterred from appropriately aggressive treatment of a patient. (I, III, IV, V)

Index

Page numbers in *italics* indicate illustrations.
Page numbers followed by *t* indicate tables.

O